RESPIRATORY SENSATION

LUNG BIOLOGY IN HEALTH AND DISEASE

Executive Editor

Claude Lenfant
Director, National Heart, Lung and Blood Institute
National Institutes of Health
Bethesda, Maryland

1. Immunologic and Infectious Reactions in the Lung, *edited by Charles H. Kirkpatrick and Herbert Y. Reynolds*
2. The Biochemical Basis of Pulmonary Function, *edited by Ronald G. Crystal*
3. Bioengineering Aspects of the Lung, *edited by John B. West*
4. Metabolic Functions of the Lung, *edited by Y. S. Bakhle and John R. Vane*
5. Respiratory Defense Mechanisms (in two parts), *edited by Joseph D. Brain, Donald F. Proctor, and Lynne M. Reid*
6. Development of the Lung, *edited by W. Alan Hodson*
7. Lung Water and Solute Exchange, *edited by Norman C. Staub*
8. Extrapulmonary Manifestations of Respiratory Disease, *edited by Eugene Debs Robin*
9. Chronic Obstructive Pulmonary Disease, *edited by Thomas L. Petty*
10. Pathogenesis and Therapy of Lung Cancer, *edited by Curtis C. Harris*
11. Genetic Determinants of Pulmonary Disease, *edited by Stephen D. Litwin*
12. The Lung in the Transition Between Health and Disease, *edited by Peter T. Macklem and Solbert Permutt*
13. Evolution of Respiratory Processes: A Comparative Approach, *edited by Stephen C. Wood and Claude Lenfant*
14. Pulmonary Vascular Diseases, *edited by Kenneth M. Moser*
15. Physiology and Pharmacology of the Airways, *edited by Jay A. Nadel*
16. Diagnostic Techniques in Pulmonary Disease (in two parts), *edited by Marvin A. Sackner*
17. Regulation of Breathing (in two parts), *edited by Thomas F. Hornbein*
18. Occupational Lung Diseases: Research Approaches and Methods, *edited by Hans Weill and Margaret Turner-Warwick*
19. Immunopharmacology of the Lung, *edited by Harold H. Newball*
20. Sarcoidosis and Other Granulomatous Diseases of the Lung, *edited by Barry L. Fanburg*
21. Sleep and Breathing, *edited by Nicholas A. Saunders and Colin E. Sullivan*
22. *Pneumocystis carinii* Pneumonia: Pathogenesis, Diagnosis, and Treatment, *edited by Lowell S. Young*

23. Pulmonary Nuclear Medicine: Techniques in Diagnosis of Lung Disease, *edited by Harold L. Atkins*
24. Acute Respiratory Failure, *edited by Warren M. Zapol and Konrad J. Falke*
25. Gas Mixing and Distribution in the Lung, *edited by Ludwig A. Engel and Manuel Paiva*
26. High-Frequency Ventilation in Intensive Care and During Surgery, *edited by Graziano Carlon and William S. Howland*
27. Pulmonary Development: Transition from Intrauterine to Extrauterine Life, *edited by George H. Nelson*
28. Chronic Obstructive Pulmonary Disease: Second Edition, Revised and Expanded, *edited by Thomas L. Petty*
29. The Thorax (in two parts), *edited by Charis Roussos and Peter T. Macklem*
30. The Pleura in Health and Disease, *edited by Jacques Chrétien, Jean Bignon, and Albert Hirsch*
31. Drug Therapy for Asthma: Research and Clinical Practice, *edited by John W. Jenne and Shirley Murphy*
32. Pulmonary Endothelium in Health and Disease, *edited by Una S. Ryan*
33. The Airways: Neural Control in Health and Disease, *edited by Michael A. Kaliner and Peter J. Barnes*
34. Pathophysiology and Treatment of Inhalation Injuries, *edited by Jacob Loke*
35. Respiratory Function of the Upper Airway, *edited by Oommen P. Mathew and Giuseppe Sant'Ambrogio*
36. Chronic Obstructive Pulmonary Disease: A Behavioral Perspective, *edited by A. John McSweeny and Igor Grant*
37. Biology of Lung Cancer: Diagnosis and Treatment, *edited by Steven T. Rosen, James L. Mulshine, Frank Cuttitta, and Paul G. Abrams*
38. Pulmonary Vascular Physiology and Pathophysiology, *edited by E. Kenneth Weir and John T. Reeves*
39. Comparative Pulmonary Physiology: Current Concepts, *edited by Stephen C. Wood*
40. Respiratory Physiology: An Analytical Approach, *edited by H. K. Chang and Manuel Paiva*
41. Lung Cell Biology, *edited by Donald Massaro*
42. Heart–Lung Interactions in Health and Disease, *edited by Steven M. Scharf and Sharon S. Cassidy*
43. Clinical Epidemiology of Chronic Obstructive Pulmonary Disease, *edited by Michael J. Hensley and Nicholas A. Saunders*
44. Surgical Pathology of Lung Neoplasms, *edited by Alberto M. Marchevsky*
45. The Lung in Rheumatic Diseases, *edited by Grant W. Cannon and Guy A. Zimmerman*
46. Diagnostic Imaging of the Lung, *edited by Charles E. Putman*
47. Models of Lung Disease: Microscopy and Structural Methods, *edited by Joan Gil*
48. Electron Microscopy of the Lung, *edited by Dean E. Schraufnagel*

49. Asthma: Its Pathology and Treatment, *edited by Michael A. Kaliner, Peter J. Barnes, and Carl G. A. Persson*
50. Acute Respiratory Failure: Second Edition, *edited by Warren M. Zapol and Francois Lemaire*
51. Lung Disease in the Tropics, *edited by Om P. Sharma*
52. Exercise: Pulmonary Physiology and Pathophysiology, *edited by Brian J. Whipp and Karlman Wasserman*
53. Developmental Neurobiology of Breathing, *edited by Gabriel G. Haddad and Jay P. Farber*
54. Mediators of Pulmonary Inflammation, *edited by Michael A. Bray and Wayne H. Anderson*
55. The Airway Epithelium, *edited by Stephen G. Farmer and Douglas Hay*
56. Physiological Adaptations in Vertebrates: Respiration, Circulation, and Metabolism, *edited by Stephen C. Wood, Roy E. Weber, Alan R. Hargens, and Ronald W. Millard*
57. The Bronchial Circulation, *edited by John Butler*
58. Lung Cancer Differentiation: Implications for Diagnosis and Treatment, *edited by Samuel D. Bernal and Paul J. Hesketh*
59. Pulmonary Complications of Systemic Disease, *edited by John F. Murray*
60. Lung Vascular Injury: Molecular and Cellular Response, *edited by Arnold Johnson and Thomas J. Ferro*
61. Cytokines of the Lung, *edited by Jason Kelley*
62. The Mast Cell in Health and Disease, *edited by Michael A. Kaliner and Dean D. Metcalfe*
63. Pulmonary Disease in the Elderly Patient, *edited by Donald A. Mahler*
64. Cystic Fibrosis, *edited by Pamela B. Davis*
65. Signal Transduction in Lung Cells, *edited by Jerome S. Brody, David M. Center, and Vsevolod A. Tkachuk*
66. Tuberculosis: A Comprehensive International Approach, *edited by Lee B. Reichman and Earl S. Hershfield*
67. Pharmacology of the Respiratory Tract: Experimental and Clinical Research, *edited by K. Fan Chung and Peter J. Barnes*
68. Prevention of Respiratory Diseases, *edited by Albert Hirsch, Marcel Goldberg, Jean-Pierre Martin, and Roland Masse*
69. *Pneumocystis carinii* Pneumonia: Second Edition, Revised and Expanded, *edited by Peter D. Walzer*
70. Fluid and Solute Transport in the Airspaces of the Lungs, *edited by Richard M. Effros and H. K. Chang*
71. Sleep and Breathing: Second Edition, Revised and Expanded, *edited by Nicholas A. Saunders and Colin E. Sullivan*
72. Airway Secretion: Physiological Bases for the Control of Mucous Hypersecretion, *edited by Tamotsu Takishima and Sanae Shimura*
73. Sarcoidosis and Other Granulomatous Disorders, *edited by D. Geraint James*
74. Epidemiology of Lung Cancer, *edited by Jonathan M. Samet*
75. Pulmonary Embolism, *edited by Mario Morpurgo*

76. Sports and Exercise Medicine, *edited by Stephen C. Wood and Robert C. Roach*
77. Endotoxin and the Lungs, *edited by Kenneth L. Brigham*
78. The Mesothelial Cell and Mesothelioma, *edited by Marie-Claude Jaurand and Jean Bignon*
79. Regulation of Breathing: Second Edition, Revised and Expanded, *edited by Jerome A. Dempsey and Allan I. Pack*
80. Pulmonary Fibrosis, *edited by Sem Hin Phan and Roger S. Thrall*
81. Long-Term Oxygen Therapy: Scientific Basis and Clinical Application, *edited by Walter J. O'Donohue, Jr.*
82. Ventral Brainstem Mechanisms and Control of Respiration and Blood Pressure, *edited by C. Ovid Trouth, Richard M. Millis, Heidrun F. Kiwull-Schöne, and Marianne E. Schläfke*
83. A History of Breathing Physiology, *edited by Donald F. Proctor*
84. Surfactant Therapy for Lung Disease, *edited by Bengt Robertson and H. William Taeusch*
85. The Thorax: Second Edition, Revised and Expanded (in three parts), *edited by Charis Roussos*
86. Severe Asthma: Pathogenesis and Clinical Management, *edited by Stanley J. Szefler and Donald Y. M. Leung*
87. *Mycobacterium avium*–Complex Infection: Progress in Research and Treatment, *edited by Joyce A. Korvick and Constance A. Benson*
88. Alpha 1–Antitrypsin Deficiency: Biology • Pathogenesis • Clinical Manifestations • Therapy, *edited by Ronald G. Crystal*
89. Adhesion Molecules and the Lung, *edited by Peter A. Ward and Joseph C. Fantone*
90. Respiratory Sensation, *edited by Lewis Adams and Abraham Guz*

ADDITIONAL VOLUMES IN PREPARATION

Pulmonary Rehabilitation, *edited by Alfred P. Fishman*

Primary Pulmonary Hypertension, *edited by Lewis J. Rubin and Stuart Rich*

Environmental Impact on the Airways: From Injury to Repair, *edited by Jacques Chrétien and Daniel Dusser*

Inhalation Aerosols: Physical and Biological Basis for Therapy, *edited by Anthony J. Hickey*

Acute Respiratory Failure in Chronic Obstructive Pulmonary Disease, *edited by Jean-Philippe Derenne, W. A. Whitelaw, and Thomas Similowski*

Tissue Oxygen Deprivation: From Molecular to Integrated Function, *edited by Gabriel G. Haddad and George Lister*

Parasitic Lung Diseases, *edited by Adel A. F. Mahmoud*

Nitric Oxide and the Lung, *edited by Warren Zapol and Kenneth D. Bloch*

The Genetics of Asthma, *edited by Stephen B. Liggett and Deborah A. Meyers*

Topical Glucocorticoids in Asthma: Mechanisms and Clinical Actions, *edited by Robert P. Schleimer, William W. Busse, and Paul M. O'Byrne*

RESPIRATORY SENSATION

Edited by

Lewis Adams
Abraham Guz
Charing Cross and Westminster Medical School
University of London
London, England

Marcel Dekker, Inc. **New York • Basel • Hong Kong**

Library of Congress Cataloging-in-Publication Data

Respiratory sensation/edited by Lewis Adams, Abraham Guz.
p. cm.—(Lung biology in health and disease; 90)
Includes bibliographical references and indexes.
ISBN: 0-8247-8846-X (hardcover; alk. paper)
1. Dyspnea 2. Respiration. 3. Senses and sensation. I. Adams, Lewis. II. Guz, Abraham. III. Series.
[DNLM: 1. Respiration—physiology—congresses. 2. Sensation—physiology—congresses. 3. Dyspnea—physiopathology—congresses. 4. Respiration Disorders—therapy—congresses. W1 LU62 v.90 1996/ WF 102 R4365 1996]
RC776.D9R47 1996
616.2—dc20
DNLM/DLC
for Library of Congress 95-46370
CIP

The publisher offers discounts on this book when ordered in bulk quantities. For more information, write to Special Sales/Professional Marketing at the address below.

This book is printed on acid-free paper.

Marcel Dekker, Inc.
270 Madison Avenue, New York, New York 10016

Current printing (last digit):
10 9 8 7 6 5 4 3 2 1

PRINTED IN THE UNITED STATES OF AMERICA

INTRODUCTION

Respiratory sensation!

The quote from D. W. Richard cited by K. J. Killian and E. J. M. Campbell in the first chapter of this volume underscores that breathing can be conscious or unconscious. For most of us, most of the time, it is an unconscious phenomenon; sometimes, however, it becomes a conscious action that can cause discomfort, if not pain.

Ondine (or *Undine*, in the German form) was a water nymph of old German folklore. In a nineteenth-century tale written by Baron Friedrich Heinrich Karl de la Motte-Fouque, she falls in love with a mortal man whose predictable human weaknesses ultimately doom him to die. In his 1939 play, Jean Giraudoux resurrected Ondine as a fisherman's daughter who marries a knight named Hans. In the last act, Hans declares to Ondine: "Since you left me, Ondine, all the things my body once did by itself, it does now only by special order … I have to supervise five senses, two hundred bones, a thousand muscles. A single moment of inattention, and I forget to breathe. He died, they will say, because it was a nuisance to breathe."

Today, Ondine remains with us only as "Ondine's curse," a rare neurological disorder leading to chronic hypoventilation or apnea when asleep; the patient must consciously remember to breathe to stay alive.

Of course, there cannot be life without breathing. N. P. Adleon described extensively what he called *Sensation du besoin de respirer* (*Physiologie de l'homme*, 1831) and compared the need to breathe with hunger. Hunger, he said, can be fought and eating can be delayed; in contrast, one cannot resist the need to breathe. Moreover, he pointed out that the need to breathe is "pleasurable" when spontaneously met, but that it can be painful if it is opposed.

Respiratory sensation has been the object of considerable philosophical and physiological explanations. This book is about the nature and mechanisms of respiratory sensation in health and disease. That there are many views on this subject is underscored in the Preface by the editors, Lewis Adams and Abraham Guz. The viewpoints presented by the authors are many and rich in ideas. They will be both an inspiration and a challenge to researchers to come.

The Lung Biology in Health and Disease series is enriched by the inclusion of this volume. As the editor of the series, I am indebted to its editors and authors for their contributions.

Claude Lenfant, M.D.
Bethesda, Maryland

FOREWORD

Breathing is like walking; you are usually unaware of it. A quiet stroll, perhaps in deep thought, is largely automatic and unnoticed unless you stumble or come to a steep hill or merely decide to think about it. Similarly, if breathing is increased or obstructed it becomes apparent and may be unpleasant. But breathing is also unlike walking; a walk comes to an end; you reach your destination or decide to rest. You cannot stop breathing for more than a few seconds, no matter how difficult it is, or how tired you have become. Even when you are asleep, breathing must continue. To stop would remove one of the most fundamental homeostatic mechanisms maintaining the near constancy of the *milieu interieur* at optimal level.

Communication by voice and speech is another function vital to human social existence, which uses the same neuromuscular mechanisms as breathing. Control of these mechanisms requires highly complex neural programs of great sophistication and involves the highest psychological functions down to the most basic neuromuscular event. For the computer-minded, Windows 3.1 running on DOS 5.0 must be child's play by comparison, but, unlike computing, the penalties of a "bug" may be far more serious.

Apart from speech, it would seem that these neuromuscular mechanisms would be able to function insentiently—at least to the extent, for example, that digestion is insentient. So why do we become aware of breathing? Does awareness of one's breathing have purpose, or is it purely an epiphenomenon of the neuromuscular process? Is it a fortuitous result of using the mechanisms involved, or does it have a role, perhaps in optimizing the control of breathing? Why should we need to be aware of our breathing? My old teacher, Professor Samson Wright, used to caution that only the Almighty can answer "why" and only science can answer "how."

This monograph, conceived and edited by Lewis Adams and Abraham Guz, who have been in the forefront of these issues, contains accounts by those who have contributed most to current thinking about how sensations associated with breathing are generated, and, in the absence of divine guidance, occasionally about why.

Understanding in this field has advanced considerably since measurement of sensation was included in the assessment of the many physical variables of gas exchange, pulmonary mechanisms, etc., involving breathing at rest, under physical and psychological stress, and in health and disease.

In the foreword to an earlier monograph based on a symposium on breathlessness, Julius Comroe predicted that no one would talk about the only aspects that had been studied; the circumstances in which breathlessness may occur. This monograph is an authoritative compendium of the current state of objective knowledge of the mechanisms, circumstances, and consequences of the sensation of breathing and breathlessness, as well as a valuable database of facts and ideas for those who wish to research and add to knowledge. For those merely interested, it provides stimulating and thought-provoking insight into the nature of one of the most complex and challenging sensory experiences of the human condition.

J. B. L. Howell
Professor of Medicine (Emeritus)
University of Southampton Medical School
Southampton, United Kingdom

PREFACE

Over the last two millennia, respiratory sensations, particularly breathlessness, have been of interest to practicing clinicians. As well as being the principal problem for the many patients who have had a wide variety of diseases, particularly those impairing the function of the cardiovascular and pulmonary systems, breathlessness and related symptoms have clearly been of diagnostic importance. In the last half of this century, a scientific interest in this subject has evolved that attempts to characterize the nature of respiratory sensations, the mechanisms that may underlie their genesis, the parts of the brain concerned with "feeling" the sensations, and the relation of the sensations to the act of breathing. Parallel with the increase in understanding that resulted from such scientific studies, done primarily in conscious man in health and disease, there developed an interest in the therapeutics of unpleasant respiratory sensations very much along the lines of the therapeutic advances that had been made in the treatment of pain. Since the diseases that cause unpleasant respiratory sensations are often chronic and untreatable, the need to alleviate such sensations has become paramount.

In editing this volume, we were fortunate to be able to assemble a group of scientists and clinicians who have distinguished themselves in areas relevant to this subject. We did not try to present a monolithic viewpoint, and indeed our contributors would not have allowed it! The reader is therefore faced with differing viewpoints and must determine what areas of this topic to research further. We asked the authors to write in an analytical manner, and they have achieved this with considerable skill.

Our volume starts with the history of the subject and proceeds through a neurophysiological perspective toward a description of the psychophysical methods developed for the study of respiratory sensation and the perception of respiratory mechanical events, with their neurophysiological correlates. This is followed by an analysis of the qualities of respiratory sensation and the language of breathlessness. Two chapters then examine the nature and mechanisms underlying respiratory sensations generated by the activation of respiratory reflexes, while, by contrast, one chapter deals with the "sense of effort" in breathing and its relevance to breathlessness. Evidence for respiratory sensation as an optimizer of respiratory control is discussed. The final seven chapters deal with breathlessness in common clinical conditions, and the last three of these introduce therapeutics directed at unpleasant respiratory sensation.

We are especially fortunate in having an imaginative Foreword written by Jack Howell, a pioneer in this field. We are deeply indebted to Liz Murray, who administrated this project. Dr. Claude Lenfant, the series' editor, is thanked for both his patience and firm prompting.

Lewis Adams
Abraham Guz

CONTRIBUTORS

Lewis Adams, Ph.D. Reader in Respiratory Physiology, Charing Cross and Westminster Medical School, University of London, London, England

Robert B. Banzett, Ph.D. Associate Professor, Departments of Physiology and Medicine, Harvard School of Public Health and Harvard Medical School, Boston, Massachusetts

E. J. Moran Campbell, M.D., Ph.D., F.R.C.P. Professor Emeritus, Department of Medicine, McMaster University, Hamilton, Ontario, Canada

Zibin Chen, M.D., Ph.D. Associate Research Professor, Department of Physiology, University of North Carolina, Chapel Hill, North Carolina

Neil S. Cherniack, M.D. Professor of Medicine, Physiology, and Biophysics, and Dean, School of Medicine, Case Western Reserve University, Cleveland, Ohio

Andrew Clark, M.A., M.D., M.R.C.P. Robert Loff Fellow in Cardiology, Department of Cardiac Medicine, National Heart and Lung Institute, London, England

Anne Cockcroft, M.D., F.R.C.P., D.I.H., F.F.O.M. Consultant, Department of Occupational Medicine, Royal Free Hampstead NHS Trust and Royal Free Hospital School of Medicine, London, England

Lynda M. Cristiano, M.D. Instructor in Medicine, Harvard Medical School, and Division of Pulmonary and Critical Care Medicine, Department of Internal Medicine, Brigham and Women's Hospital, Boston, Massachusetts

Paul W. Davenport, Ph.D. Professor, Department of Physiological Sciences, University of Florida, Gainesville, Florida

Frederic L. Eldridge, M.D. Professor, Departments of Medicine and Physiology, University of North Carolina, Chapel Hill, North Carolina

Simon C. Gandevia, B.Sc.(Med), Ph.D., M.D., F.R.A.C.P. Principal Research Fellow, Prince of Wales Medical Research Institute, Randwick, Sydney, Australia

Abraham Guz, M.D., F.R.C.P. Professor Emeritus, Department of Medicine, Charing Cross and Westminster Medical School, University of London, London, England

Angela Heslop, M.Sc., R.G.N., R.C.N.T. Respiratory Health Worker, Respiratory Nursing Service, Charing Cross Hospital, London, England

Christopher M. B. Higgs, M.D., M.R.C.P. Medical Director, Dorothy House Foundation, Bath, England

Paul W. Jones, Ph.D., F.R.C.P. Reader in Medicine, Division of Physiological Medicine, St. George's Hospital Medical School, London, England

Kieran J. Killian, M.D., F.R.C.P.(I), F.R.C.P.(C) Professor of Medicine, Respirology Division, Department of Medicine, McMaster University, Hamilton, Ontario, Canada

Robert W. Lansing Professor Emeritus, Department of Psychology, University of Arizona, Tucson, Arizona

Gabriel Laszlo, M.D., F.R.C.P.(London) Consultant Physician, Respiratory Department, Bristol Royal Infirmary, and Senior Clinical Lecturer in Medicine, University of Bristol, Bristol, England

Donald A. Mahler, M.D. Associate Professor, Department of Medicine, Dartmouth Medical School, Lebanon, New Hampshire

Philip Poole-Wilson, M.D., M.R.C.P., F.E.S.C. Professor of Cardiology, Department of Cardiac Medicine, National Heart and Lung Institute, London, England

W. Robert Revelette, M.D., Ph.D. Resident in Pediatrics and Adjunct Associate Professor of Physiology, Department of Physiology, University of Kentucky, Lexington, Kentucky

Norman J. W. Russell, Ph.D. Manager, Biotechnology, Zeneca Pharmaceuticals, Macclesfield, Cheshire, England

Richard M. Schwartzstein, M.D. Assistant Professor of Medicine, Harvard Medical School, and Divisions of Pulmonary and Critical Care Medicine and Emergency Medicine, Beth Israel Hospital, Boston, Massachusetts

Alison Clova Stark, M.B.Ch.B., M.R.C.P. General Infirmary at Leeds, Leeds, England

Ronald D. Stark, M.D., Ph.D., F.R.C.P., F.F.P.M. Chief Physician, Department of Medical Research, Zeneca Pharmaceuticals, Macclesfield, Cheshire, England

Rachel C. Wilson, Ph.D. Research Assistant, Division of Physiological Medicine, St. George's Hospital Medical School, London, England

CONTENTS

1

Historical Aspects of Dyspnea

KIERAN J. KILLIAN and E. J. MORAN CAMPBELL

McMaster University
Hamilton, Ontario, Canada

> Breathing is truly a strange phenomenon of life, caught midway between the conscious and the unconscious, and peculiarly sensitive to both.
>
> D. W. Richards, 1953

I. Introduction

Throughout history, those of a curious mind have sought explanations for dyspnea. To early peoples, dyspnea was seen as inflicted by the gods because obvious explanations, such as structural abnormalities of the thorax, were present in only a small number of afflicted individuals. The afflicted individual was managed based on communication with the gods through the medium of dreams in sacred places. These dreams required interpretation by ministers of the gods.

These supernatural explanations persisted until the introduction of a coherent physiology by Hippocrates (460–377 B.C.) (Singer, 1957, 1959). Food, absorbed as chyle, was conveyed to the liver, where blood was formed. The blood contained natural spirit, was conveyed to the right heart, and by means of the pulmonary artery to nourish the lung and by the veins to nourish the body. Natural spirit permeated the septum to the left side of the heart, and pneuma was conveyed from the air via the pulmonary veins. The left heart was thus charged with vital spirit, generated the heat essential for life, and was transferred by bloodless arteries to the body. The brain, nourished by both vital and natural spirit, generated the animal spirit, which flowed through the nerves, driving the action of the muscles. In this system, breathing was dependent on animal spirit flowing through the nerves activating the respiratory muscles. The reality of these relationships was supported by phrenic nerve injury in gladiators and by experimental phrenic nerve section in animals. Thus, the lungs provided pneuma, a route of elimination of waste product and cooling of the heart. Within this system the body organs produced humors—blood (liver), yellow bile (liver), black bile (spleen), and phlegm (neural in origin)—and balance became a basis of various disorders and their treatment. These structural and functional properties evolved over hundreds of years and emerged as the Galenic view (Galen, 130–200 C.E.). Although in their surviving writings neither Hippocrates nor Galen explicitly examined the mechanism of dyspnea, one has little difficulty in conceiving how disturbance of several parts of this systems could be invoked.

Because prolonging life was of minor importance compared with the importance of eternal life, Galenic views continued to dominate thinking. Answers were sought in the Bible, creating an antisecular and antiscientific environment that left the work of the ancients as the only reference sources in the years between 200 and 1400 C.E. In fact, little changed until the seventeenth and eighteenth centuries, when the discovery of the circulation, the chemistry of the gases, the recognition by Lavoisier (1862) that respiration and combustion were similar, the demonstration of gas transport in the blood by Pflüger (1868), and the parallel understanding of the nervous system in movement required different conceptual models with which to make sense of the phenomenon of dyspnea.

With the Renaissance, the structural changes underlying various disorders were elucidated as anatomical dissection reappeared. "The seats and causes of disease investigated by anatomy" by Morgagni (1682–1771) proved to be a major publication, but something akin to modern views had to await Laennec (1781–1826). The presence of dyspnea in life was now characterized by its morbid anatomical appearances following death, yielding the concepts of "cardiac dyspnea," "respiratory dyspnea," and "renal dyspnea." By careful and methodical physical examination, these structural changes could be anticipated during life. The disorder was considered nervous in origin if none of these abnormalities was detected. At the same time, such expressions as exertional dyspnea, orthopnea, and paroxysmal nocturnal dyspnea and their relationship with the underlying anatomical disorder emerged. Virchow (1821–1902) voiced a cautionary note, pointing out that these morbid anatomical appearances were of limited value without knowledge of their functional effects. These advances had little immediate effect on therapeutics. Balance of the humors with bloodletting, emetics, purgatives, heating, cooling, and so on remained the cornerstone of therapy.

As these ideas evolved, various therapies for dyspnea also appeared based on collective experience. These therapies were promoted by the pragmatists who existed from the earliest times and who did not require a conceptual basis. Increasing dissatisfaction with the Galenic approach to treatment led to the emergence of Paracelsus (1493–1541) (Dawson, 1928). He popularized various agents based on folklore and ridiculed Galen. These pragmatists introduced various agents, some of which have stood the test of time: anticholinergic agents, ephedrine, and digitalis. While relieving the edema of cardiac failure, it is difficult to imagine that Withering failed to appreciate the effects of digoxin on dyspnea.

II. Nature and Mechanisms of Dyspnea

Understanding of the mechanical act of breathing begun by Erasistratus (310–250 B.C.E.) (Otis, 1986) matured with the work of Borelli (1680, 1681). The mystery of respiration unfolded with the work of Hooke (1667), Lower (1669), Boyle (1772), and Mayow (1668) and ultimately resulted in the recognition by Lavoisier (1777) that combustion and respiration were the same. The nature of respiration, the roles of oxygen and carbon dioxide, and the control of breathing provided a logical framework for thinking about the mechanism of dyspnea.

A. Neural Contribution

By the early nineteenth century, LeGallois (1813) established that breathing was dependent on neural activity in the medulla oblongata. The idea that this neural activity was sentient, giving rise to dyspnea, was implicit but this was never explicitly stated. This activity was modulated by afferent neural inputs.

> LeGallois, M. Flourens, Sir Charles Bell have erroneously considered the acts of respiration as spontaneous, and the medulla oblongata as their source and the primum mobile. I think I have, on the contrary, proved by experiments that this important function consists of excited acts, excited through a peculiar system of excitor nerves, and principally filaments of the fifth, the pneumogastric, and spinal nerves (Hall, 1836).

The activity in the medullary centers and the factors controlling this activity assumed a similar implicit importance to the mechanism of dyspnea:

> The central nervous organ for breathing movements is in a condition of continuous dependence on the prevailing state of lung distension, through the agency of vagal fibers which terminate in the lung. In other words, the prevailing degree of distension of the lung contributes a modifying influence on the movements of breathing. The lung, when it becomes more expanded by inspiration, or by inflation, exerts an inhibitory effect on inspiration and promotes expiration, and this effect is the greater the stronger the expansion. Every inspiration, therefore, in that it distends the lung

> brings about its own end by means of this distention, and thus initiates expiration. Breuer and Hering (1868)

If central respiratory neuronal activity were not inhibited, as would occur if inspiration was hindered by stiff lungs or obstructed airways, the medullary neurons would result in a prolonged forceful inspiration and would exhaust themselves, generating dyspnea. This idea was now explicit, but it was moot whether the vagus or the medullary neuronal activity was sentient and the source of dyspnea. Hering and Breuer clearly thought that hypoxia and hypercapnia gave rise to dyspnea:

> It has long been known to the physician—that the manifestations of dyspnoea are very diverse, depending on whether the respiratory surface area, e.g., in pneumonia, or by some mechanical hindrance, like stenosis of the larynx. Since it is usually considered that in both instances the cause of dyspnea lies in the defective gas exchange, it remains to be elucidated how the same cause can have such different effects. (Breuer, Hering, 1868)

These ideas persisted into the present century. Gad (1911) suggested that the vagus modified the action of the respiratory muscles to minimize dyspnea. Wright and Branscomb (1954) saw prolonged and intense activity of the inspiratory center neurons uninterrupted by appropriate vagal activity as the cause of dyspnea.

B. Respiratory Control

The respiratory physiologists of the nineteenth century were predominantly concerned with the control of breathing. Pflüger (1868) ascribed dyspnea to the accumulation of products of incomplete oxidation in the medulla oblongata, as a result of the lack of oxygen in the perfusing blood or reduction in its blood supply. The role of carbon dioxide was considered of lesser importance because under experimental conditions death from hypoxia was rapid and toleration of carbon dioxide was considerable. F. Miescher-Rüsch (1885) and Haldane and Smith (1893), realizing that CO_2 was carefully controlled, ascribed dyspnea to hypercapnia, noting "dyspneic acceleration of breathing when the CO_2 content of air in the lungs is increased." Winterstein (1921) drew attention to the central role of the hydrogen ion in the metabolic processes taking place in the medullary neurons. Medullary conditions were modulated by the hydrogen ion concentration in the perfusing blood; incomplete oxidation resulted in the generation of lactic acid under hypoxic conditions; and the acidic nature of CO_2 was also recognized. The idea that hydrogen ion concentration in the respiratory center caused dyspnea was attractive, but measurements of hydrogen ion, oxygen, and carbon dioxide were confined to blood (Winterstein, 1911; Winterstein, 1921). This idea was to emerge again and again: "The activity of the respiratory centre is fundamentally a function of its own acidity as opposed to the acidity of the arterial blood, the specificity of carbon dioxide and the direct stimulating effects of lack of oxygen" (Gesell, 1923). The assumption was that medullary neurons were directly responsible for control, with the implicit assumption that these neurons were sentient, giving rise to the sensation of dyspnea. With this background, Meakins (1923) summarized the mechanisms of dyspnea in cardiovascular disease: "How is dyspnea produced? If we confine the question to the diseases under consideration we may say that it is usually produced by two causes: (1) want of oxygen; (2) carbon dioxide retention, absolute or relative."

C. Dyspnea and Disease

Means (1924) noted that dyspnea was more intense in the presence of a reduced ventilatory capacity. The ventilatory index (minute ventilation over maximal voluntary ventilation, $\dot{V}_E$/MVV; $\dot{V}_E/\dot{V}_E$ capacity) evolved from the measurement of encroachment on capacity, and an increased ventilatory index came to be regarded as the cause of dyspnea. Cournand and his colleagues (Cournand and Richards, 1941a, b; Cournand et al., 1941) went on to quantify and classify disorders of ventilatory capacity into obstructive and restrictive based on measurements of lung volumes and their subdivisions.

D. Dyspnea and Respiratory Mechanics

As the forces generated by the respiratory muscles and the displacement achieved in the lungs and chest wall were measured (Donders, 1853; Rohrer, 1916; Wirz, 1923; Von Neergaard and Wirz, 1927; Otis et al., 1950), the work of breathing, elastance, resistance, transpulmonary pressure, the forces generated by the respiratory muscles, and the displacement achieved by the chest wall and/or lungs provided an increasing number of plausible stimuli. In addition, muscular sensations were now known to be sentient (see Chap. 7).

E. Respiratory Muscle Metabolism and Dyspnea

The oxygen cost of breathing was a special case. The oxygen cost of breathing increases in a positively accelerating manner as ventilation increases, from 0.5 ml/L ventilation at low ventilation to >2 ml/L at high levels (Liljestrand, 1918; Cournand et al., 1954; Campbell et al., 1957; Bartlett et al., 1958). The oxygen cost of breathing was increased in patients with pulmonary and cardiac diseases (Marshall et al., 1954; Fritts et al., 1959). McIlroy (1958) suggested that dyspnea results when an oxygen debt is incurred by the respiratory muscles. Afferent neural activity from intramuscular small myelinated or unmyelinated nerve fibers arising as a consequence of tissue hypoxia at the level of the respiratory muscles was the implied mechanism. Inadequate supply of oxygenated blood to the respiratory muscles similar to claudication was forwarded by Harrison (1950).

Fatigue resulting from inadequate perfusion is a present-day extension of this hypothesis (Bellemare and Grassino, 1982).

F. Chemoreceptors and Dyspnea

Preceding the contribution of the respiratory muscles to dyspnea was the discovery of the peripheral chemoreceptors and the evolving view of chemoreceptors. The peripheral chemoreceptors in the carotid body stimulated by hypoxemia discovered by Heyman and Heyman (1927) inevitably led to an idea that the peripheral chemoreceptors caused dyspnea. Surgical excision of the carotid bodies was attempted to relieve dyspnea, a practice now abandoned. Chemoreceptor function has been studied largely under conditions of hypoxemia, hypercapnia, and acidemia and alkalemia. However, chemoreceptors operate in a homeostatic fashion that is reflected in relative constancy in Pa_{CO_2}, Pa_{O_2}, and pH in the face of increasing metabolic demands. Recognition of the constancy of hydrogen ion, oxygen, and carbon dioxide during mild to modest exercise questioned the idea that acidemia, hypercapnia, or hypoxemia mediated the dyspnea experienced during exercise. Harrison (1935) noted that breathing was stimulated by passive movement of the legs (abolished by cutting the sciatic nerve and preserved during venous occlusion). Chemoreceptors, even operating in a homeostatic fashion, were no longer seen as an absolute requirement in that respiratory centers responded to reflex activity from peripheral muscle in addition to chemical stimuli. Christie (1938) summarized: "Though the conditions under which dyspnea occurs are various and manifold, giving rise to an impression of complexity, the fundamental causes are few and relatively simple. They consist of chemical and reflex disturbances." Whether the medullary neurons themselves or the afferent factors modulating their activity were sentient remained unspecified.

G. Chemoreceptors, Medullary Neurons, Respiratory Muscles, and Dyspnea

Dyspnea has been seen to accompany and to reflect respiratory muscle activity since the earliest times, and the derivation of the Greek term "difficult or labored breathing" is not surprising. From the middle of the nineteenth century, special interest has been focused on the factors controlling the extremes of respiratory muscle activity (Donders, 1853; Pflüger, 1868; Rohrer, 1925). Apnea characterizes the absence of contractile activity; dyspnea describes intense contractile activity. The idea that chemoreceptors and/or respiratory medullary neurons are sentient was broadened to include the muscular consequences of their activity. Chemoreceptors, medullary neurons, and muscular receptors could all act as sense organs and directly contribute to dyspnea. Theories about the mechanism of dyspnea never explicitly discriminated between them. Experimental clarification was difficult because when chemoreceptors are activated, medullary neural activity and motor output to the respiratory muscles increase. Furthermore, as respiratory muscle activity increases, muscle and joint receptor activity increases and pulmonary receptor activity increases. Many sensory receptors are stimulated, and each receptor type has the potential to generate dyspnea.

Recognizing that the chemical conditions of the arterial blood are dependent on alveolar levels, Fowler (1954) reasoned that chemoreceptor stimulation must increase as the duration of breath holding increases. If chemoreceptors are indeed sentient, the discomfort appearing and increasing with the duration of the breath hold should increase further if subjects breathe from a gas mixture, which would increase rather than decrease chemoreceptor stimulation at the point of termination of the breath hold. Following a breath hold to toleration, he had subjects take repeated breaths from a hypoxic and hypercapnic gas mixture. The discomfort associated with breath holding was relieved, and the subjects resumed breath holding despite further hypoxemia and hypercapnia. These studies applied to the discomfort associated with breath holding, but they were broadly interpreted to mean that chemoreceptors themselves were insentient. There was a vague idea that the intensity of dyspnea experienced by patients was inversely related to breath-holding time. Residual concerns were considered resolved when Campbell et al. (1967, 1969) reported dramatic prolongation of breath-holding times during complete neuromuscular blockade, even during hypercapnia. Hence, by the 1960s, chemoreceptors were broadly considered insentient. Sensation was generated as a consequence of their activity.

The theory of the direct sentience of chemoreceptors recently reappeared when it was reported that experimental subjects were more dyspneic in the presence of hypoxia and hypercapnia than observed for the same respiratory muscle activity under normoxic and normocapnic conditions (Guz et al., 1981; Adams et al., 1985; Chonan et al., 1987, 1990; Freedman et al., 1987; Lane et al., 1987a, b; Schwartzstein et al., 1987, 1989; Cockroft et al., 1989). However, the motor drive (effort) required to drive respiratory muscles in the presence of intramuscular hypoxia or hypercapnia might be increased. Further studies showed, however, that experimental subjects experienced discomfort when ventilation was voluntarily increased and/or decreased from that generated by normal control mechanisms. The human is apparently aware of the appropriateness of ventilation, and discomfort is experienced with deviations in either direction. The conscious awareness of the appropriateness of ventilation may be similar to the sense of hunger or thirst. Satiety is common to all, but the mechanisms remain poorly understood. Chemoreceptors must play some role in this sensory experience. All these studies were indirect, but Banzett et al. (1990) added CO_2 to the inspired circuit of four ventilated neuromuscularly paralyzed experimental subjects. All reported air hunger, and the authors again raised the issue of the direct sentience of chemoreceptors. Because of the inconsistency between these results and those reported by Campbell et al. (1967, 1969), Gandevia et al. repeated the studies looking at both breath holding and progressive hypercapnia during complete neuromuscular paralysis. Complete paralysis was ensured by supramaximal blockade, confirmed by direct phrenic nerve stimulation. Breath holding times were unchanged, and breathing discomfort was seen during both breath holding and progressive hypercapnia (Gandevia et al., 1993).

H. Psychophysical Studies

Meanwhile, there was a quiet revolution in the broad area of sensations arising in the act of breathing. The first formal psychophysical studies were modest and defined the minimum magnitude of added resistive and elastic loads that normal subjects can reliably detect, "threshold detection." Although not specifically stated, there was the belief that these studies might shed light on the mechanism of dyspnea. Normal subjects could reliably detect 2.5 cm H_2O/L in added elastance and 0.6 cm $H_2O/L/s^{-1}$ for added resistance (Campbell et al., 1961; Bennett et al., 1962). Later studies show that the threshold of detection of elastic loads is closer to 1 cm H_2O/L (Zechman and Wiley, 1986). Campbell and Howell (1963) went on to suggest that an imbalance in the relationship between tension and displacement mediated by sensory receptors in respiratory muscle might be the neurophysiological mechanism giving rise to load detection in particular and to dyspnea in general. In accordance with this view, tension is mediated by tendon organs, and length (volume or flow) is mediated by muscle spindles and joint receptors. Normally these sensory phenomena are subconscious, but consciousness is achieved on the recognition of imbalance and increases with the magnitude of inappropriateness. "Inappropriateness" was considered the fundamental basis of the sensation of dyspnea. At that time, γ efferent motor activity to intrafusal muscle fibers (spindles) was considered important as a primary motor innervation to muscle. The increase in spindle discharge, resulting from intrafusal fiber contraction, stretched the nuclear bag, causing afferent neural stimulation, which in turn intensified α-motor neuron activity (follow-up length servosystem). An imbalance between programmed length change and achieved length change would according to this view trigger dyspnea as seen when Campbell (1958, 1966) substituted length/length for length/tension. In time, Campbell and Howell further acknowledged that appropriateness was pervasive, including breathing relative to neurochemical needs, effort required relative to ventilation, and ventilation relative to the intensity of exercise.

The receptors stimulated, the route of afferent neural traffic and the central handling of the information required for load detection became major issues. Studies were performed by an increasing number of investigators to answer questions about how loads were sensed. Detection thresholds were the same before and following the application of local anesthesia to the airway (Chaudhary and Burki, 1978, 1980); detection thresholds with loads applied to the mouth and trachea were the same (Noble et al., 1972; Gandevia et al., 1981a); although detection thresholds were higher applied at the level of the trachea, the background resistance was also higher, such that in relative terms detection thresholds and sensitivity were unchanged. The conclusion was that superficial receptors in the oropharynx and trachea are not essential for detection. Detection thresholds were unchanged with loads applied with and without spinal neuromuscular blockade (Zechman et al., 1967; Noble et al., 1970; Eisele et al., 1968). The conclusion was that specific receptors in the chest cage were not required. Detection thresholds were the same with and without vagal blockade (Guz et al., 1966). The conclusion was that receptors originating in the lung are not essential. On the other hand, detection thresholds were markedly reduced during passive or artificial ventilation compared with active breathing (Killian et al., 1980). The conclusion was that muscular receptors stimulated by active contraction were particularly sentient.

Bakers and Tenney (1970) showed that the human can directly estimate the magnitude of volume, ventilation, and respiratory pressures using direct psychophysical techniques. These were followed by studies establishing that we can consciously perceive the magnitude of external loads (Killian et al., 1981; Gottfried et al., 1978) and internal loads (Burdon et al., 1982), respiratory pressures (Stubbing et al., 1983), volume (Stubbing et al., 1981; Wolkove et al., 1981; Gliner et al., 1981) and effort (Campbell et al., 1980; Gandevia et al., 1981b; Killian et al., 1984). Although previously unknown and unsuspected, a rich sensory infrastructure in the act of breathing emerged and a whole variety of respiratory sensations emerged in the act of breathing previously considered insentient.

I. Dyspnea and Sensory Physiology

The framework within which dyspnea is studied is changing. Formal psychophysical studies are now the norm. The sensory receptors activated during breathing are inferred based on the closest possible indices. For example, pressure is taken as an index of tension as long as the lung volume remains relatively constant, flow rate is taken as an index of the velocity of contraction of the respiratory muscles, lung volume and tidal volume as an index of muscle length and the extent of contraction, and flow rate expressed as a percentage of capacity or pressure expressed as percentage of capacity is used as an index of effort. Each receptor type is known to respond to a specific stimulus, and a specific qualitative dimension to the resulting sensation can be reasonably expected. Hence, respiratory sensations in the experimental setting of loaded breathing, hyperventilation, hyperinflation, and weakness caused by partial neuromuscular blockade undoubtedly have qualitative characteristics that are readily understood in terms of the specific receptors stimulated and their interactions. Clinical situations, although more complex, can be fairly well understood in the same context.

To deal with the mechanism of dyspnea, we must grapple with language.

Breathing during respiratory loading (exogenous or endogenous elastic or resistive loads), breathing during exercise, breathing following hyperinflation, breathing when the respiratory muscles are weakened by neuromuscular blockade, and breathing following the induction of fatigue are all distressing. The quality of these sensations is different. They can be crudely dissected based on the nature of stimuli and receptor types stimulated, but no current terminology has evolved to describe these different qualities. Formal attempts are being made to isolate different sensations by matching subjective descriptions of breathing to different situations or having patients with various disorders match these descriptions to their breathing (Cockroft et al., 1989; Simon et al., 1989). Precision in the use of language has not yet arisen from these studies, but progress is expected. "Dyspnea" as currently used merely represents discomfort experienced and associated with the act of breathing. This will change in the coming years.

Dyspnea experimentally induced and as a consequence of disease has common characteristics. Its presence is confined to situations in which (1) the inspiratory muscles are weak as a consequence of disease, hyperinflation, or fatigue; (2) ventilation is increased as during exercise, voluntary hyperventilation, or reflexly driven hyperventilation, such as occurs with pulmonary vascular occlusion; and (3) the action of the inspiratory muscles is impeded by the addition of resistive or elastic loads to breathing. Central motor output yielding a sense of increased effort is increased in all these situations. It may not be the sole mechanism and cannot account for the total experience of dyspnea in all circumstances, but the awareness of effort (central command) seems to be common to all circumstances and dominant in most. It should not be inferred that the other receptors are insentient, however. In the past many studies have shown that this or that mechanism is insentient, from which it may be concluded that the mechanism in question does not subserve dyspnea. We now have a number of mechanisms that have been shown to be sentient and may subserve dyspnea. But do they, and in what circumstances? These will be increasingly insistent questions.

J. Measurement of Dyspnea

In recent years a great deal of confusion has been engendered by different measurement techniques. The adage that familiarity with making measurements is not synonymous with understanding the principles of measurement is nowhere more evident. The fundamental process involved in making any measurement is the "matching" of one continuum (number continuum being one specific example) to another while conforming to preset rules. The rules and the independent continuum define a "scale." If matching is invariant, reproducible, and responsive and obeys the preset rules, then the scale is valid. The scale may be nominal and distinguish one object or event from another; ordinal, and rank objects or events in order of magnitude; interval, and determine equality and magnitude of differences in objects or events while preserving rank order; or ratio, and determine ratio relationships (Stevens, 1975).

To the skeptic, the quantitative semantics appear bogus but they have pragmatic utility. Simple descriptors, such as slight, moderate, or severe, are used to indicate sensory magnitude everyday. Precision in the use of these descriptors is variable, but it is intuitively obvious that the further apart the descriptors, the greater is the difference in sensory magnitude in and across individuals. The probability of confusing adjacent descriptors is considerable, but as descriptors are progressively separated, the probability becomes remote. Whether or not valid ratio properties or properties of absolute intensity are preserved, the Borg scale has proved remarkably easy to use in practice and is readily understood by people from a variety of educational and language backgrounds (Borg, 1960, 1962, 1964, 1972, 1980; Borg and Hosman, 1970; Borg and Lindblad, 1976). This scale has the pragmatic advantage that "moderate" conveys a meaning that "10 cm" does not. Numbers and/or line lengths are easily assumed to imply interval and ratio properties that they do not have.

III. Summary

We must have sought explanations for dyspnea since the beginning of time. These explanations were probably supernatural until the advent of the physiologies of Hippocrates and Galen. However, it was not until the middle of the last century, when the architecture of modern physiology emerged, that testable ideas came forward. Since then, the roles of many mechanisms have been examined: the respiratory centers, the motor output, respiratory muscle, sensory receptors in the chest wall, vagal receptors, blood gases, and chemoreceptors, among others.

At present it seems that although it may not be the sole mechanism and cannot account for the total experience of dyspnea in all circumstances, the awareness of effort seems to common to all circumstances and dominant in most.

The major development of the last few decades has been the application of psychophysical techniques, which have been useful in clarifying mechanisms and in the treatment of dyspnea as a quantifiable phenomenon both in research and in practice. "No natural phenomena can be adequately studied in itself alone, but to be understood must be considered as it stands connected with all of nature": Sir Francis Bacon (1561–1626).

References

Adams, L., Lane, R. Shea, S.A., Cockcroft, A., and Guz, A. (1985). Breathlessness during different forms of ventilatory stimulation: a study of mechanisms in normal subjects and respiratory patients. Clin. Sci. 69:663–672.

Bakers, J.H.C.M., and Tenney, S.M. (1970). Perception of some sensations associated with breathing. Respir. Physiol. 10:85–92.
Banzett, R.B., Lansing, R.W., Brown, R., Topulos, D., Yager, D., Steel, S.M., Londono, B., Loring, S.H., Reid, M.B., Adams, L., and Nations, C.S. (1990). "Air hunger" from increased Pco_2 persists after complete neuromuscular block in humans. Respir. Physiol. 81:1–18.
Bartlett, R.G., Brubach, H.F., and Specht, H. (1958). Oxygen cost of breathing. J Appl. Physiol. 12:413–424.
Bellemare, F., and Grassino, A. (1982). Effect of pressure and timing of contraction on human diaphragm fatigue. J. Appl. Physiol. 53:1190–1195.
Bennett, E.D., Jayson, M.I.V., Rubenstein, D., and Campbell, E.J.M. (1962). The ability of man to detect added non-elastic loads to breathing. Clin. Sci. 23:155–162.
Borelli, G.A. (1680). De Motu Animalium, Vol. I. Bernabo, Rome.
Borelli, G.A. (1681). De Motu Animalium, Vol. II. Bernabo, Rome.
Borg, G. (1960). The perception of muscular work. Pub. Umea Res. Libr. 5:1–27.
Borg, G. (1962). Physical performance and perceived exertion. Studia Psychophysiologica et Paedagogica, Series altera. Investigations, Gleerup, Lund, No. 11, pp. 1–64.
Borg, G. (1964). On quantitative semantics in connection with psychophysics. Educational and Psychological Research Bulletin, University of Umea, No. 3.
Borg, G. (1972). A ratio scaling method for interindividual comparisons. Reports from the Institute of Applied Psychology, University of Stockholm, No. 27, pp. 1–12.
Borg, G., and Hosman, J. (1970). The metric properties of adverbs. Institute of Applied Psychology Report, University of Stockholm, No. 7, pp. 1–7.
Borg, G., and Lindblad, I. (1976). The determination of subjective intensities in verbal descriptions of symptoms. Institute of Applied Psychology Report, University of Stockholm, No. 75, pp. 1–20.
Borg, G.A. (1980). A category scale with ratio properties for intermodal and interindividual comparisons. In: Psychophysical Judgment and the Process of Perception. Proceedings of the 22nd International Congress of Psychology. Edited by H.G. Geissler and P. Petzold. North Holland, Amsterdam, pp. 25–34.
Boyle, R. (1772). A Defence of the Doctrine Touching the Spring and Weight of the Air. The Works of the Honourable Robert Boyle, Vol. I. London, pp. 156–160.
Breuer, J., and Hering, E. (1868). Self-steering of respiration through the nervous vagus. Originally published in Sitzber. Math. Naturw. Cl., Vienna, 1868; 57(2):672–677. In: Pulmonary and Respiratory Physiology, Part II. Edited by J.H. Comroe, Jr., Dowden, Hutchinson & Ross, Stroudsburg, PA, 1976, pp. 108–113.
Burdon, J.G.W., Juniper, E.F., Killian, K.J., Hargreave, F.E., and Campbell, E.J.M. (1982). Perception of breathlessness in asthma. Am. Rev. Respir. Dis. 126:825–828.
Campbell, E.J.M. (1958). The Respiratory Muscles and the Mechanics of Breathing. Lloyd-Luke (Year Book Medical), London.
Campbell, E.J.M. (1966). The relationship of the sensation of breathlessness to the act of breathing. In Breathlessness. Edited by J.B.L. Howell and E.J.M. Campbell. Blackwell Scientific, Oxford, pp. 55–64.
Campbell, E.J.M., and Howell, J.B.L. (1963). The sensation of breathlessness. Br. Med. Bull. 19:36–40.
Campbell, E.J.M., Westlake, E.K., and Cherniack, R.M. (1957). Simple methods of estimat-

ing oxygen consumption and efficiency of the muscles of breathing. J. Appl. Physiol. 11:303–308.

Campbell, E.J.M., Freedman, S., Smith, P.S., and Taylor, M.E. (1961). The ability of man to detect added elastic loads to breathing. Clin. Sci. 20:223–231.

Campbell, E.J.M., Freedman, S., Clark, T.J.H., Robson, J.G., and Norman, J. (1967). The effect of muscular paralysis induced by tubocurarine on the duration and sensation of breathholding. Clin. Sci. 32:425–432.

Campbell, E.J.M., Godfrey, S., Clark, T.J.H., Freedman, S., and Jones, N.L. (1969). The effect of muscular paralysis induced by tubocurarine on the duration and sensation of breath-holding during hypocapnia. Clin. Sci. 36:323–328.

Campbell, E.J.M., Gandevia, S.C., Killian, K.J., Mahutte, C.K., and Rigg, J.R.A. (1980). Changes in the perception of inspiratory resistive loads during partial curarization. J. Physiol. 309:93–100.

Chaudhary, B.A., and Burki, N.K. (1978). Effects of airway anaesthesia on the ability to detect added inspiratory resistive loads. Clin. Sci. 54:621–626.

Chaudhary, B.A., and Burki, N.K. (1980). The effects of airway anesthesia on detection of added inspiratory elastic loads. Am. Rev. Respir. Dis. 122:635–639.

Chonan, T., Mulholland, M.B., Cherniack, N.S., and Altose, M.D. (1987). Effects of voluntary constraining of thoracic displacement during hypercapnia. J. Appl. Physiol. 63:1822–1828.

Chonan, T., Mulholland, M.B., Leitner, J., Altose, M.D., and Cherniack, N.S. (1990). Sensation of dyspnea during hypercapnia, exercise, and voluntary hyperventilation. J. Appl. Physiol. 68:2100–2106.

Christie, R. (1938). Dyspnea. Q. J. Med. 7:421–454.

Cockroft, A., Adams, L., and Guz, A. (1989). Assessment of breathlessness. Q. J. Med. 72:669–676.

Cournand, A., and Richards, D.W. (1941a). Pulmonary insufficiency. I. Discussion of a physiological classification and presentation of clinical test. Am. Rev. Tuberc. 44:26–41.

Cournand, A., and Richards, D.W. (1941b). Pulmonary insufficiency. II. The effects of various types of collapse therapy upon cardiopulmonary function. Am. Rev. Tuberc. 44:123–172.

Cournand, A., Richards, D.W., and Maier, H.C. (1941). Pulmonary insufficiency. III. Cases demonstrating advanced cardiopulmonary insufficiency following artificial pneumothorax and thoracoplasty. Am. Rev. Tuberc. 44:272–287.

Cournand, A., Richards, D.W., Bader, R.E., Bader, M.E., and Fishman, A.P. (1954). The oxygen cost of breathing. Trans. Assoc. Am. Physiol. 67:162–173.

Dawson, P.M. (1928). The heritage of Paracelsus. Ann. Med. Hist. 10:258–269.

Donders, F.C. (1853). Contribution to the mechanism of respiration and circulation in health and disease. Beitrage zum Mechanismus der Respiration und Circulation im gesunden und kranken Zustande. Z. Rationelle Med. 3:287–319; Heidelberg, 1853. Reprinted in West, J.B. (Editor). Translations in Respiratory Physiology. Dowden, Hutchinson & Ross, Stroudsburg, PA, 1975, pp. 298–318.

Eisele, J., Trenchard, D., Burki, N., and Guz, A. (1968). The effect of chest wall block on respiratory sensation and control in man. Clin. Sci. 35:23–33.

Fowler, W.S. (1954). Breaking point of breath-holding. J. Appl. Physiol. 6:539–545.

Freedman, S., Lane, R., and Guz, A. (1987). Breathlessness and respiratory mechanics during reflex or voluntary hyperventilation in patients with chronic airflow limitation. Clin. Sci. 73:311–318.

Fritts, H.W., Filler, J., Fishman, A.P., and Cournand, A. (1959). The efficiency of ventilation during voluntary hyperpnea: studies in normal subjects and in dyspneic patients with either chronic pulmonary emphysema or obesity. J. Clin. Invest. 38:1339–1348.

Gad, J. (1911). Die Regulierung der normalen Athmung. In: Human Physiology, Vol. 1, Edited by Luciani. McMillan, London, pp. 458–459.

Galen (1821). On the value of respiration; on the causes of respiration; whether blood is contained in the arteries; and on the function of the pulse. Translated into Latin by C.G. Kuhn, Leipzig, 1821–1833. Claudii Galeni Opera Omnia, Leipzig.

Gandevia, S.C., Killian, K.J., and Campbell, E.J.M. (1981a). The contribution of upper airway and inspiratory muscle mechanisms to the detection of pressure changes at the mouth in normal subjects. Clin. Sci. 60:513–518.

Gandevia, S.C., Killian, K.J., and Campbell, E.J.M. (1981b). The effect of respiratory muscle fatigue on respiratory sensations. Clin. Sci. 60:463–466.

Gandevia, S.C., Killian, K.J., McKenzie, D.K., Crawford, M., Allen, G.M., Gorman, R.B., and Hales, J.P. (1993). Respiratory sensations, cardiovascular control, kinaesthesia and transcranial stimulation during paralysis in humans. J. Physiol. (Lond.) 470: 85–107.

Gesell, R. (1923). On the chemical regulation of respiration. I. The regulation of respiration with special reference to the metabolism of the respiratory centre and the coordination of the dual function of hemoglobin. Am. J. Physiol. 66:5–49.

Gliner, J.A., Folinsbee, L.J., and Horvath, S.M. (1981). Accuracy and precision of matching inspired lung volume. Percept. Psychophys. 29:511–515.

Gottfried, S.B., Altose, M.D., Kelsen, S.G., Fogarty, C.M., and Cherniack, N.S. (1978). The perception of changes in airflow resistance in normal subjects and patients with chronic airways obstruction. Chest 73:286–288.

Guz, A., Noble, N.I.M., Widdicombe, J.G., Trenchard, D., Mushin, W.W., and Makey, A.R. (1966). The role of vagal and glossopharyngeal afferent nerves in respiratory sensation, control of breathing and arterial pressure regulation in conscious man. Clin. Sci. 30:161–170.

Guz, A., Adams, L., Minty, K., and Murphy, K. (1981). Breathlessness and ventilatory drives of exercise, hypercapnoea and hypoxia (abstract). Clin. Sci. 61:429–439.

Haldane, J.S., and Smith, J.L. (1893). Carbon dioxide and regulation of breathing. J. Pathol. Bacteriol. 1:168, 318; 1893a, b. In: Respiration. Edited by J.S. Haldane and J.G. Priestly. Clarendon Press, Oxford, 1935, pp. 16–42.

Hall, M. (1836). Lectures on the Nervous System and Its Diseases. Philadelphia, E.L. Carey and A. Hart. 1836. In: Pulmonary and Respiratory Physiology, Part II. Edited by J.H. Comroe, Jr., Dowden, Hutchinson & Ross, Stroudsburg, PA, 1976, pp. 104–107.

Harrison, T.R. (1935). Failure of Circulation. Williams & Wilkins, Baltimore.

Harrison, T.R. (1950). Shortness of breath. In: Principles of Internal Medicine. Edited by P.B. Beeson, G.W. Thorn, W.H. Resnik, and M.M. Wintrobe. Blakiston, Philadelphia, pp. 111–119.

Heyman, J.F., and Heyman, C. (1927). Sur les modifications directes et sur la regulation reflexe de l'activite du centre respiratoire de la tete isolee du chien. Arch. Int. Pharmacodyn. Ther. 33:273–372.

Hooke, R. (1667). An account of an experiment made by M. Hook, of preserving animals alive by blowing through their lungs with bellows. Philos. Trans. R. Soc. Lond. (Biol.) 2:539–540.

Killian, K.J., Mahutte, C.K., and Campbell, E.J.M. (1980). Resistive load detection during passive ventilation. Clin. Sci. 59:493–495.

Killian, K.J., Mahutte, C.K., and Campbell, E.J.M. (1981). Magnitude scaling of externally added loads to breathing. Am. Rev. Respir. Dis. 123:12–15.

Killian, K.J., Gandevia, S.C., Summers, E., and Campbell, E.J.M. (1984). Effect of increased lung volume on perception of breathlessness, effort, and tension. J. Appl. Physiol. 57:686–691.

Laennec, R. (1827). A Treatise on the Diseases of the Chest (1781–1826). Hafner Publishing, London, 1962, pp. 284–286.

Lane, R., Cockcroft, A., Adams, L., and Guz, A. (1987a). Arterial oxygen saturation and breathlessness in patients with chronic obstructive airways disease. Clin. Sci. 72:693–698.

Lane, R., Cockcroft, A., and Guz, A. (1987b). Voluntary isocapnic ventilation and breathlessness during exercise in normal subjects. Clin. Sci. 73:519–523.

Lavoisier, A.L. (1777). Reflexions sur le phlogistique, pour servir de suite a la theorie de la combustion et de la calcination. Issued with Hist. Acad. R. Sci., Paris, 1777. In: Oeuvres de Lavoisier, Vol. 2, Imprimerie Imperiale, Paris, 1862–1893, pp. 623–655.

LeGallois, C.J.J. (1813). Experiments on the principle of life, and particularly on the principle of the notions of the heart, and on the seat of this principle. Translated by N.C. Nancrede and J.G. Nancrede, Philadelphia, M. Thomas, 1913. In: Pulmonary and Respiratory Physiology, Part 2, Edited by J.H. Comroe, Jr., Dowden, Hutchinson & Ross, Stroudsburg, PA, 1976, pp. 12–16.

Liljestrand, G. (1918). Studies of the work of breathing. Untersuchungen uber die Atmungsarbiet. Scand. Arch. Physiol. 35:199–293, 1918. Reprinted in West, J.B. (Editor). Translations in Respiratory Physiology. Dowden, Hutchinson & Ross, Stroudsburg, PA, 1975, pp. 438–513.

Lower, R. (1669). Tractatus de Corde: Item De Motu & Colore Sanguinis et Chyli in cum Transitu. On the color of blood. K.J. Franklin translation, Early Science in Oxford, Vol. 9, Clarendon Press, 1932, Elsevier.

Marshall, R., Stone, R.W., and Christie, R.V. (1954). Relationship of dyspnea to respiratory effort in normal subjects, mitral stenosis and emphysema. Clin. Sci. 13:625–631.

Mayow, J. (1668). Tractatus Quinque medico-physici (1643–1679). Oxford, 1674. Alembic Club, Edinburgh (reprinted 1957).

McIlroy, M.B. (1958). Dyspnea and the work of breathing in diseases of the heart and lungs. Prog. Cardiovasc. Dis. 1:284–297.

Meakins, J.M. (1923). The cause and treatment of dyspnea in cardiovascular disease. B.M.J. 1:1043–1045.

Means, J.H. (1924). Dyspnoea. Med. Monogr. 5:309–416.

Miescher-Rüsch, F. (1885). Bemerkungen zur Lehre von den Atembewegungen. Arch. Anat. Physiol. (Leipzig) 6:355–380.

Morgagni, G. (1989). The seats and causes of disease investigated by anatomy. De Sedibus et Causis Morborum per Anatomen Indagatis (1682–1771). In: Excerpts in Doctors, the Biography of Medicine. Edited by S.B. Nuland. Knopf, New York, pp. 145–170.

Noble, M.I.M., Eisele, J.H., Trenchard, D., and Guz, A. (1970). Effect of selective peripheral nerve blocks on respiratory sensations. In: Breathing: Hering-Breuer Centenary Symposium. Edited by R. Porter. Churchill (CIBA Found. Symp.), London, pp. 233–246.

Noble, M.I.M., Frankel, H.L., Else, W., and Guz, A. (1972). The sensation produced by threshold resistive loads to breathing. Eur. J. Clin. Invest. 2:72–77.

Otis, A.B. (1986). History of Respiratory Mechanics. In: Handbook of Physiology. Section III: The Respiratory System, Vol. III. Edited by A.P. Fishman, P.T. Macklem, J. Mead, and S.R. Geiger. American Physiological Society, Bethesda, MD, pp. 1–12.

Otis, A.B., Fenn, W.O., and Rahn, H. (1950). Mechanics of breathing in man. J. Appl. Physiol. 2:592–607.

Pflüger, E. (1868). On the causes of respiratory movement, and of dyspnea and apnea. Über die Ursache der Atembewegungen, sowie der Dyspnoe und Apnoe. Pflüger's Arch. Ges. Physiol. 1868; 1:61–106. Reprinted in West, J.B. (Editor). Translations in Respiratory Physiology, Dowden, Hutchinson & Ross, Stroudsburg, PA, 1975, pp. 404–434.

Richards, D.W., Jr. (1953). The nature of cardiac and of pulmonary dyspnea. The Lewis A. Conner Memorial Lecture. Circulation 7:15–29.

Rohrer, F. (1916). The correlation of respiratory forces and their dependence upon the state of expansion of the respiratory organs. Der Zusammenhang der Atemkrafte und ihre Abhangigkeit vom Dehnungszustand der Atmungsorgane. Pflüger's Arch. Ges. Physiol. 165:419–444, 1916. Reprinted in West, J.B. (Editor). Translations in Respiratory Physiology. Dowden, Hutchinson & Ross, Stroudsburg, PA, 1975, pp. 67–88.

Rohrer, F. (1925). The physiology of respiratory movements. Physiologie der Atembewegung. Handbuch der Normalen und Path. Physiol., A.T.J. Bethe, et al. (Editors). Berlin, Springer, Vol. 2, pp. 70–127, 1925. Reprinted in West, J.B. (Editor). Translations in Respiratory Physiology. Dowden, Hutchinson & Ross, Stroudsburg, PA, 1975, pp. 93–170.

Schwartzstein, R.M., LaHive, K., Pope, A., Steinbrook, R.A., Leith, D.E., Weiss, J.W., Fencl, V., and Weinberger, S.E. (1987). Detection of hypercapnia by normal subjects. Clin. Sci. 73:333–335.

Schwartzstein, R.M., Simon, P.M., Weiss, J.W., Fencl, V., and Weinberger, S.E. (1989). Breathlessness induced by dissociation between ventilation and chemical drive. Am. Rev. Respir. Dis. 139:1231–1237.

Simon, P.M., Schwartzstein, R.M., Weiss, J.W., Lattive, K., Fencl, V., Teghtsoonian, M., and Weinberg, S.E. (1989). Distinguishable sensations of breathlessness induced in normal volunteers. Am. Rev. Respir. Dis. 140:1021–1027.

Singer, C. (1957). A Short History of Anatomy and Physiology from the Greeks to Harvey. Dover, New York.

Singer, C. (1959). A Short History of Scientific Ideas to 1900. London, Oxford.

Stevens, S.S. (1975). Psychophysics. Introduction to its Perceptual, Neural, and Social Prospects. Edited by G. Stevens. John Wiley & Sons, New York.

Stubbing, D.G., Killian, K.J., and Campbell, E.J.M. (1981). The quantification of respiratory sensations by normal subjects. Respir. Physiol. 44:251–260.

Stubbing, D.G., Ramsdale, E.H., Killian, D.J., and Campbell, E.J.M. (1983). Psychophysics of inspiratory muscle force. J. Appl. Physiol. 54:1216–1221.

Virchow, R. (1978). Cellular Pathology as Based upon Physiological and Pathological Histology. Leslie B. Adams Jr., Birmingham, AL.

Von Neergaard, K., and Wirz, K. (1927). Method for measuring lung elasticity in living human subjects, especially in emphysema. Uber eine Methode zur Messung der Lungenelastizitat am lebenden Menschen, insbesondere beim Emphysem, Z. Klin. Med. 105:35–50, 1927. Reprinted in West, J.B. (Editor). Translations in Respiratory Physiology. Dowden, Hutchinson & Ross, Stroudsburg, PA, 1975, pp. 227–269.

Winterstein, H. (1911). The regulation of breathing by the blood. Die Regulierung der Atmung durch das Blut. Pflugers Arch. Ges. Physiol. 138:167–184, 1911. Reprinted in West, J.B. (Editor). Translations in Respiratory Physiology. Dowden, Hutchinson & Ross, Stroudsburg, PA, 1975, pp. 529–542.

Winterstein, H. (1921). The reaction theory of respiratory regulation. Die Reaktionstheorie der Atmungs-regulation. Pflugers Arch. Ges. Physiol. 187:293–298, 1921. Reprinted in West, J.B. (Editor). Translations in Respiratory Physiology. Dowden, Hutchinson & Ross, Stroudsburg, PA, 1975, pp. 543–548.

Wirz, K. (1923). Changes in the pleural pressure during respiration, and causes of its variability. Das Verhalten des Druckes in Pleuraraum bei der Atmung und die Ursachen seiner Veranderlichkeit. Pflugers Arch. Ges. Physiol. 199:1–56, 1923. Reprinted in West, J.B. (Editor). Translations in Respiratory Physiology. Dowden, Hutchinson & Ross, Stroudsburg, PA, 1975, pp. 174–226.

Wolkove, N., Altose, M.D., Kelsen, S.G., Konapalli, P.G., and Cherniack, N.S. (1981). Perception of changes in breathing in normal human subjects. J. Appl. Physiol. 50: 78–83.

Wright, G.W., and Branscomb, B.V. (1954). Origin of the sensation of dyspnea. Trans. Am. Clin. Climatol. Assoc. 66:116–125.

Zechman, F.W., Jr., and Wiley, R.L. (1986). Afferent inputs to breathing: respiratory sensation. In: Handbook of Physiology, Section 3, The Respiratory System, Vol. II, Part I. Edited by S.R. Geiger, J.G. Widdicombe, N.S. Cherniack, and A.P. Fishman. American Physiological Society, Williams & Wilkins, Bethesda, MD, pp. 449–474.

Zechman, F.W., O'Neill, R., and Shannon, R. (1967). Effect of low cervical spinal cord lesions on detection of increased airflow resistance in man. Physiologist 10:356.

2

Respiratory Sensation
A Neurophysiological Perspective

FREDERIC L. ELDRIDGE and ZIBIN CHEN

University of North Carolina
Chapel Hill, North Carolina

I. Introduction

Numerous sensations associated with the respiratory tract and breathing reach the level of consciousness. Some are these are not unpleasant; others are clearly unpleasant. One can classify the sensations into two main groups. The former include the same kind of somatic sensations, mostly not unpleasant, that have been studied more extensively in relation to limb movement and skeletal muscle activity, that is, position, passive movement or displacement, active movement, resistance to movement or load, and a sense of muscular tension, but pain would have to be included. In respiratory terms, such sensations might include the perception of volume, magnitude of tidal ventilation, frequency, pressure, mechanical load, and a sense of respiratory muscular tension, as well as pain from respiratory structures.

The other important sensations associated with breathing are unpleasant and come under the rubric of the terms "respiratory distress" or "dyspnea," a precise definition for which is difficult to make because both normal subjects (Simon et al., 1989) and patients with cardiorespiratory disease (Simon et al., 1989, 1990; Elliott et al., 1991) use, even when conditions are apparently about the same, a variety of different terms, such as breathlessness, shortness of breath, "air hunger," "tightness in chest," "suffocating," and others, to express what they are feeling. It is probable that several different sensations are actually being experienced (Simon et al., 1989, 1990; Elliott et al., 1991). These unpleasant sensations are discussed in detail in Chaps. 5 and 16.

It has been suggested that dyspnea is somewhat analogous to a diffuse visceral type of pain (Simon et al., 1990; Elliott et al., 1991). Both are subjective phenomena arising through a variety of neural mechanisms, which can include signals from peripheral receptors and probably medulla in breathing, with transmission and complex processing of these signals in pons, midbrain, thalamus, and sensory cortex before reaching conscious perception.

The respiratory sensations that involve perception of position, volume, frequency, pressure, and a sense of tension or effort are of course important for proper functioning of respiration as well as maintenance of posture. However, dyspnea in all its forms has, because of the clinical importance of the symptom, received the major share of attention of those studying respiratory sensation. This can be readily seen in the coverage of this volume, in which the majority of chapters relate primarily to dyspnea rather than to the first group of mostly not unpleasant sensations.

II. Control of Respiration

Consideration of the neurophysiology of respiratory sensation requires first a discussion of the control of breathing. We propose to divide our discussion into three parts: first, the respiratory controller, a rhythm and central pattern generator in the medulla; then the outputs, the motor or efferent components of the system; and, finally, the inputs, mostly the traditional peripheral sensory or afferent mechanisms but also other inputs that cannot be so classified. Because no part of the brain above the medulla and pons is essential to the generation of regular respiratory rhythm and maintenance of relatively normal levels of blood gases and pH, much of the discussion uses findings obtained in the reduced control system, extensively studied in anesthetized and decerebrate animals.

A. Respiratory Controller: Rhythm Generation

The respiratory controller's rhythm generator, or oscillator, is located in the medulla (see Feldman, 1986 for review). Its mechanism is not certain (see Selverston and Moulins, 1985, for discussion of types of oscillator networks). Over some decades, the idea that the oscillator involved a pacemaker had changed to the likelihood that neural networks with appropriate inhibitory and excitatory connections were responsible. More recently, studies in the in vitro neonatal rat brain preparation have reraised the possibility of endogenous burster neurons, that is, an intrinsic pacemaker, in the medulla (Onimaru et al., 1987). A current plausible proposal is that, in intact adults at least, the respiratory oscillator involves a hybrid form in which that the oscillatory pattern is generated by both conditional burster neurons, conditional because neural inputs or humoral agents are necessary to cause the oscillatory behavior, and network interactions that are involved in both the generation of the rhythm and the shaping of the neural motor output that ultimately causes respiratory muscles to contract (Smith et al., 1991). It has been pointed out that because each mechanism tends to reinforce the other, such an oscillator would be more robust and reliable than one with only a single mechanism (Selverston and Moulins, 1985), of clear value for the respiratory oscillator on which life depends.

Several important observations should be made about the respiratory central pattern generator's operation.

First, it can generate the oscillating motor programs without phasic peripheral feedback. On the other hand, sufficient tonic neural input is required to keep it above a firing/oscillating threshold; apnea develops, of course, when inputs fall to too low a level. It is traditional to think of the central chemoreceptors—responsive to the CO_2/H^+ stimulus in brain extracellular fluid—as the main source of this input. However, in many situations other neural inputs may be more important and can take the place of central CO_2, in part or in whole, in keeping the controller system above its threshold (so-called apneic threshold) for maintenance of rhythmic breathing. The threshold is thus related to properties of the oscillator rather than to dependence upon a specific input, and no specific level of P_{CO_2} acting on the central chemoreceptors can be considered necessary for breathing. One example can be found in the reduced preparation, in which breathing that has been caused to cease by induced hypocapnia can be made to resume by input from the carotid body without a change in P_{CO_2}. A second example is found in the intact subject, in whom the loss during sleep of what appears to be a strong neural "wakefulness" input from reticular formation or higher brain structures leads to a greater dependence on chemoreceptor input and requires P_{CO_2} to increase about 5–6 mm Hg to maintain a lesser amount of ventilation (Phillipson and Bowes, 1986). Finally, some persons with little or no ventilatory responsiveness to either central or peripheral chemoreceptor inputs and with often severe hypoventilation during sleep (so-called Ondine's curse), which can occur congenitally or in some patients with medullary disease, nevertheless may have relatively normal ventilation when they have the wakefulness input and have a normal or even exaggerated ventilatory response to the inputs associated with exercise (Shea et al., 1993a; Heywood et al., 1993).

Second, many central pattern generators produce not only the efferent motor output that goes to its primary effector, in our case respiratory muscles, but also send a copy or copies (called efferent copies or corollary discharges) to other neural structures (Pinsker and Ayers, 1983). The information so sent may influence and cause entrainment or coordination with other motor programs, such as chewing, swallowing, and sympathetic activity. A good example is the corollary discharge from locomotor circuits in the spinal cord, studied in fictively locomoting, paralyzed animals, that go to distant limbs, to the respiratory controller, and even to higher in the brain (Arshavsky et al., 1988).

Finally, we believe (also suggested by Feldman et al., 1987) that the respiratory central pattern generator can be viewed as analogous to the spinal oscillators that subserve the motor programs of locomotion. Because respiration involves a specialized oscillator, there are some obvious differences, such as the bilaterally common function of the respiratory controller (although it can be separated into two independently functioning halves by splitting the medulla and cervical spinal cord) (Eldridge and Paydarfar, 1989), the potential backup of a pacemaker-like mechanism, and a lower threshold for oscillation. There are, nevertheless, a number of similarities: the locomotor system does not oscillate spontaneously, it requires a neural input to produce oscillation, the pattern is affected by phasic feedback inputs, and it sends signals by efferent copy or corollary discharge to distant sites, probably having both motor and sensory actions.

B. Outputs from the Controller

Rhythmic motor output from the respiratory controller, that is, waxing and waning excitatory synaptic drive or central respiratory drive potential (CRDP), goes via the spinal cord to the motoneurons of those muscles (diaphragm, inspiratory intercostal, scalene, and sternocleidomastoid) directly involved in expanding the chest and lungs during inspiration and to those involved in producing an expiratory action (expiratory intercostal and abdominal muscles). It also goes directly from medulla via cranial nerves (7, 9, 10, and 12) to innervate nasal, tongue, pharyngeal, and laryngeal muscles, which participate in opening or stiffening the upper airway during inspiration, to innervate and set the tone of bronchopulmonary airway smooth muscle, and to control the rate of airflow during expiration (see review by Bartlett, 1986, for details of upper airway mechanisms). In addition, the rhythmic respiratory activity can affect sympathetic activity (Preiss et al., 1975).

From the standpoint of sensory feedback that may have an impact on sensation, it is important to note that there are two motoneuronal systems in the spinal cord. One is the α-motor system, whose neurons send α fibers that innervate the main muscle fibers. The second is the γ-motor system whose neurons send smaller fusimotor, γ fibers, to intrafusal muscles that act on associated muscle spindles, sensory organs that act as stretch receptors. Both motor systems probably receive similar synaptic input (CRDP) from the controller (Sears, 1964a; Corda et al., 1966).

Finally, it should be noted that outputs almost certainly project to more rostral regions of the brain. There are anatomical connections from medulla to diencephalon that support this conclusion (Bayev et al., 1988) and electrophysiological evidence that a neural output related to respiratory magnitude is sent from the controller, presumably as a corollary discharge, to midbrain and thalamus (Chen et al., 1991, 1992) and probably to cortex (see Sec. IV.A).

C. Inputs to the Controller

The central generator neurons and interneurons receive inputs from many sources, and there are many different effects on the controller: stimulation or inhibition of respiration, change in form or magnitude of individual breaths, setting or resetting of respiratory rhythm and rate, and activation of respiratory memory-like processes. The inputs include not only those that are traditionally thought of as "sensory" and "afferent," such as chemoreceptor-mediated input from the carotid body or mechanoreceptor-mediated input from the lungs, but also others that are not traditionally thought of as "sensory," including mechanisms intrinsic to the medulla and those that emanate from regions of the brain rostral to the controller.

Because this overview has to do primarily with the neurophysiology of respiratory sensation, rather than respiratory control, we do not intend to go into the details of individual input mechanisms as they affect respiratory control, for they are well reviewed elsewhere, but present some major categories. It is difficult to make other than an arbitrary classification, but we have chosen to consider them in terms of those from the periphery, those intrinsic to the medulla, and those from supramedullary brain.

Peripheral Inputs

Inputs from the periphery are a large group. Their receptors are of various types and include chemoreceptors, mechanoreceptors, and thermoreceptors. They can be phasic, tonic, or tonic with phasic components (Jammes, 1988). It goes almost without saying that efferent signals from a controller change the state of the controlled object, in our case the respiratory muscles and airflow, and in consequence there is a change in afferent input from receptors in the controlled object. When the receptor activation is associated with the effects of breathing, the inputs are termed respiratory-related feedback mechanisms. Some represent classic negative respiratory feedback: a change in motor output leads to increased or decreased stimulation of receptors that in turn leads to changes in motor output in the opposite direction. Others produce a positive feedback, in that the change in receptor activity leads to a further change in controller output in the same direction. A number of peripheral inputs whose receptors are not activated by breathing nevertheless affect the respiratory controller and its motor output. They can be termed non–respiratory-related inputs; some can be considered nonrespiratory feedback mechanisms, such as impulses from leg muscles during locomotion.

Respiratory-Related Inputs

Peripheral Chemoreceptors. Inputs from peripheral chemoreceptors (carotid bodies and aortic bodies) respond with increased activity when exposed to increased arterial P_{CO_2}/H^+ and/or decreased P_{O_2}, the two having a multiplicative effect on the receptors, and also to increased arterial concentration of K^+. The activity from these receptors is basically tonic, but there is a clear phasic component, related primarily to the oscillation of blood P_{CO_2} that occurs with each breath (Eldridge and Millhorn, 1986). This input represents one of the classic negative respiratory feedback mechanisms, for example, decreased ventilation $\rightarrow$ increased stimulation of chemoreceptors $\rightarrow$ increased ventilation, and is undoubtedly responsible to a large extent for the rapid and fairly tight control of arterial blood gases in normal subjects (see review by Fitzgerald and Lahiri, 1986).

Lower Airways and Lungs. There are several types of input (see review by Coleridge and Coleridge, 1986 and Chap. 6). One involves the slowly adapting receptors (SAR or pulmonary stretch receptors) that are activated by increasing volume of the lungs and whose impulses travel to the medulla via the vagus nerves. A point of interest is that SAR in the lung are also further stimulated by hypocapnia (Bradley et al., 1976; Nilsestuen et al., 1981). SAR input has an inhibitory effect on inspiratory neurons and is responsible for the negative feedback Hering-Breuer inspiration-terminating reflex but also probably has an excitatory effect on expiratory neurons (Bartoli et al., 1973), as well as causing relaxation of tracheobronchial smooth muscle.

A second type of input comes from rapidly adapting receptors (RAR or "irritant" receptors), which occur in both mucosa and smooth muscle of extra- and intrapulmonary airways. They are activated by changes in conformation of airways during high ventilatory flow rates, by morphological changes in airways, such as congestion or bronchoconstriction, by certain chemicals, and by particulants. From a functional standpoint the RAR, unlike SAR, have generally facilitatory effects on the controller. They are primarily responsible for the tachypnea and increased peak phrenic activity that occur during deflation of a lung (the deflation reflex). Evidence in animals indicates that, because of excitatory effects on the controller even during normal tidal inspirations, RAR make a contribution to the patterning of inspiration even during eupnea (Pack et al., 1981). They can also trigger coughing and augmented breaths or sighs.

Finally, there are large numbers of receptors in bronchial and pulmonary airways and near alveolar capillaries in the lungs (called J receptors) whose impulses are carried in unmyelinated C fibers in the vagus nerves. These receptors appear to respond to mechanical deformation and to chemicals, such as phenyl diguanide, capsaicin, and prostaglandins in the lungs and, in addition, to histamine and bradykinin in the airways. In experimental situations, activation of these receptors leads to apnea or rapid shallow breathing (Green et al., 1984), airway constriction, and increased secretion from mucous glands. They may be involved in triggering cough as well as conscious sensations, such as tickling and even pain from the lower airway (Morton et al., 1950).

Upper Airways. There are a great number of receptors in nasal passages, pharynx, and larynx whose impulses have an effect on the respiratory controller. They include mechanoreceptors sensitive to pressure and to flow of gas, those sensitive to irritants, chemoreceptors, thermoreceptors, and nociceptors (see review by Widdicombe, 1986). Their afferent pathways include three cranial nerves (5, 9, and 10). Inputs from the nose are involved in generation of apnea, sneezing, and mucous secretion. Pharyngeal inputs can also lead to inhibition of respiration as well as swallowing and sniffing. More information is available about laryngeal inputs, partly because it and its nerves are readily accessible for study but also because of its important inhibitory effects on respiration. Many of the inputs have both respiratory and cardiovascular effects. It has generally proved to be difficult to study many of the upper airway inputs in isolation, so relatively little is known about specific pathways or about integrations of inputs from various regions.

Respiratory Muscles, Tendons, and Thoracic Joints. There are three main types of mechanoreceptors whose impulses travel in the spinal cord to the controller (see review by Shannon, 1986; also Chap. 4).

The muscle spindles, which are length or stretch receptors, are linked to intrafusal muscle fibers and the γ-motor system (see Sec. II.B). Because the main muscle (α system) and intrafusal fibers (γ system) are arranged in parallel, an equivalent shortening of each, as in normal breathing, should not cause much change in length of the spindle and little change in its firing. On the other hand, a contraction of intrafusal muscles not matched by appropriate shortening of the main muscle, such as tracheal occlusion, loaded breathing, or when the main muscles are weak, can cause lengthening of the spindle and thus its stimulation. Passive lengthening by, for example, a ventilator does the same. This mechanism is probably most important for thoracic muscles, because the diaphragm contains relatively few spindles (Corda et al., 1965). The generated signals return to the spinal cord to produce additional (stretch reflex) activation of α motoneurons but of course have the potential for more rostral distribution.

Tendon organs are force receptors that have a higher threshold for activation than spindles. Costovertebral joint or movement receptors have been minimally studied.

At the segmental level, spindle input has facilitatory effects on the same segment's muscles, as well as those of other spinal segments, and has been shown to be responsible for the intercostal to phrenic facilitatory reflex that can be seen in spinalized animals (Decima et al., 1967). Tendon organ input has an inhibitory effect on α motoneurons of the same segment, but not much is known about its spread (Sears, 1964b). From a functional standpoint, it has been suggested by von Euler (1973) that these segmental feedbacks are primarily involved in adjustments of the strength of respiratory muscle contraction to various loads and conditions and by Jung-Calliol and Duron (1976) that the thoracic muscles are primarily postural muscles, their proprioceptors having little influence on the controller under normal conditions.

Nevertheless, spindle input (Remmers, 1976), tendon organ input (Bolser et al., 1983), and costovertebral joint movement (Shannon, 1980) all have inhibitory effects at the level of the central controller and the ability to cause respiratory rhythm changes.

There are probably some other inputs. Respiratory muscles, including the diaphragm, almost certainly contain other kinds of pressure-sensitive, chemosensitive, and noci-sensitive receptors, some with free nerve endings, whose impulses are carried in thin-fiber myelinated and unmyelinated afferents. For example, Jammes et al. (1986) have shown that nonmyelinated afferents from the diaphragm are stimulated by lactic acid and by hyperosmotic NaCl. They have suggested that inputs in these small afferents may contribute to ventilatory changes during sustained diaphragmatic work.

Non–Respiratory-Related Inputs

Peripheral input to the controller that is not directly related to respiratory activity also encompasses a number of mechanisms. The responses occur in anesthetized or decerebrate animals, so they do not necessarily require cortical mechanisms or consciousness. They include inputs from nonrespiratory skeletal muscles, via stretch receptors and chemosensitive and pressure-sensitive receptors with thin-fiber and unmyelinated afferents (thought to be a factor in the ventilatory response to exercise), from cardiac structures, from carotid sinus baroreceptors, and from thermal and nociceptors in the skin and muscle. There is probably an input from the spinal circuitry involved in rhythmic limb movements (locomotion) that is a result of a corollary discharge and that therefore occurs even in the absence of muscular contraction and limb movement in the paralyzed preparation.

Inputs Intrinsic to Medulla

Central Chemoreceptors

It has been known for over a century that the medulla contains structures that are chemosensitive, that respond to increased partial pressure of CO_2 and concentration of H^+ ions, and that stimulate the respiratory controller. These chemoreceptors represent a negative feedback that probably plays some role in the maintenance of stable ventilation and blood gases in the normal awake person. At times it becomes a more important source of input, certainly during sleep, when the loss of neural input associated with wakefulness requires more chemoreceptor input to maintain an adequate level of breathing, and also during breath holding, smothering, and the breathing of increased concentrations of CO_2 (often iatrogenic, of course).

The location of the central chemoreceptors is still not certain. Studies 30 years ago led to a widely accepted idea that these receptors were located exclusively just beneath the surface of the ventrolateral medulla and that they responded to changes in cerebrospinal fluid (CSF) pH. However, studies from other laboratories have yielded results not consistent with this view (see review by Millhorn and Eldridge, 1986); for example, the respiratory response is much more closely related to extracellular fluid (ECF) pH than to CSF (Kiley et al., 1985), and the respiratory responses to acidosis of the ECF pH evoked by carbon dioxide are not the same as those evoked by metabolic ECF acidosis of the same degree (Eldridge et al., 1985a; Harada et al., 1985). There are also newer studies that support a view that true chemosensitive neurons are much more widely dispersed in the medulla. For example, Dean et al. (1990), using medullary slices, found that there were CO_2-excitable neurons in the nucleus tractus solitarius of the dorsal medulla that retained their responsiveness during high-Mg^{2+}/low Ca^{2+} synaptic blockade.

It is also not certain whether the chemosensitive neurons, wherever they are, are part of the rhythm-generating system or separate and requiring synaptic connections to the controller neurons for their effect. Supporting the latter are (1) studies of the relationships of carotid sinus nerve and central chemoreceptor inputs to respiratory output in cats that indicate the existence in the medulla of a common neuronal pathway for the two inputs before they have reached the controller (Eldridge et al., 1981), and (2) the aforementioned patients with "Ondine's curse" who have little or no respiratory response to either peripheral or central input but who may breathe relatively normally when awake and can increase ventilation normally during exercise (Shea et al., 1993a).

Short-Term Potentiation

This mechanism is not an input in the traditional sense but rather an autogenous mechanism that still makes an important contribution to overall activity of the controller. Associated with inputs that cause respiration to increase is the gradual activation of a central neuronal mechanism, probably involving changes in the synaptic terminal's membrane, that potentiates the respiratory response to the same continuing input (Wagner and Eldridge, 1991). The gradual increase is called short-term potentiation, which, acting as a short-term memory, is responsible after the input stops for what has been termed a respiratory afterdischarge, increased output that slowly declines to the original level as the potentiation decays over some minutes. The potentiation is facilitatory with facilitatory inputs but can be seen as an inhibitory potentiation in inputs with inhibitory effects on respiration, such as stimulation of larynx or superior laryngeal nerve (see review by Eldridge and Millhorn, 1986). Short-term potentiation is probably an important mechanism involved in the stabilization of respiration and prevention of periodic breathing.

Inputs from Higher Brain

Inputs from regions above the medulla, pons and mesencephalon, diencephalon and telencephalon, including the cortex, have a number of important effects on the respiratory controller (see review by Hugelin, 1986). Although these input mechanisms are often termed behavioral, to contrast with the so-called metabolic or automatic mechanisms often attributed to the brain stem, many of them are *not* "voluntary," that is, requiring conscious direction by cortical mechanisms, but are also completely automatic. For example, rhythmical finger tapping, a voluntary activity, is accompanied by entrainment of respiratory rhythm, probably an involuntary automatic neural mechanism (Wilke et al., 1975).

One can show with electrical stimulation in animals that various respiratory responses, facilitatory or inhibitory to either magnitude or frequency of breathing, or both, can come from most parts of the supramedullary brain; specific findings depend upon the exact location of the stimulus and other factors, such as depth of anesthesia. Although it is difficult to relate the findings to the normal physiological situation, such studies have provided evidence of termination of these inputs on medullary controller neurons. In some cases, the inputs appear to go directly to and terminate on respiratory motoneurons in the spinal cord, bypassing the medullary controller.

Midbrain and Pons

The midbrain includes the reticular formation whose activation is clearly involved in arousal responses and in the state of wakefulness and is depressed in sleep (Huttenlocher, 1961) and anesthesia (Syka et al., 1977). Because the reticular formation is a neural network widely distributed up and down the neuraxis without clearly delineated pathways (see review by Brodal, 1981), it is unlikely that only the mesencephalon is responsible for the facilitatory input to breathing. As noted earlier, this is a powerful input because its loss during sleep must be replaced by a large increase in chemoreceptor input.

Respiratory responses to auditory inputs have been demonstrated. Gautier (1972) showed that there were immediate effects on the pattern of breaths, which depended on time in the cycle that the stimulus occurred and more delayed effects, which he believed were consistent with activation of reticular system. Haas et al. (1986) showed that rhythmic auditory signals (music) could act as a zeitgeber with ability to entrain respiratory rhythm. Probably some of these responses involve consciousness and cortical processing of input before the effect on respiration. On the other hand, several studies suggest a direct pathway from auditory system to the medulla: in one, auditory input caused modulation of activity of dorsal cuneate nucleus in decerebrate, decerebellate animals (Saade et al., 1989); in the other, high- or low-frequency auditory input in decerebrate cats caused both resetting of respiratory rhythm with single short stimuli and entrainment of respiration with repeated rhythmic stimuli (Eldridge et al., 1990).

Diencephalon

Although the diencephalic reticular formation must be involved in the mechanism of wakefulness, the hypothalamus is the other important source of input to the controller. One such input comes from the small paraventricular locomotor region. These neurons, when activated spontaneously in decorticate animals or by electrical or chemical stimulation, lead even in an absence of the cortex to locomotion and respiratory and circulatory responses that slightly precede the onset of locomotion (Eldridge et al., 1985b). Because the same responses occur in the paralyzed preparation, that is, in the absence of respiratory or nonrespiratory feedback, it is believed that the hypothalamic signals travel in parallel to the medullary controller and the spinal locomotor generators. Appropriate anatomical connections through midbrain and pons to solitary tract nuclei and nucleus ambiguus, as well as connections into the spinal cord, have been demonstrated (Luiten et al., 1985). It is probable that the input contributes an important part of the increased respiratory drive during exercise (Eldridge and Waldrop, 1991).

A second type of input comes from the thermally sensitive (both warm and cold) receptors in the preoptic and supraoptic areas of the hypothalamus. Warming leads to increased ventilation and often marked increase in frequency (thermal panting in animals) when temperature increases.

Cortex

Everyday observation assures us that the cortex must be involved in voluntary breathing changes, such as deep breathing, deliberate hyperventilation, breath holding, singing, and speaking. Even nonvoluntary cortical activities associated with mental activity and emotions have effects on breathing, although the mechanisms are probably not very specific and may involve reticular formation activity, as previously described. Hugelin (1986) adduces evidence that there may, in addition, be inhibitory influences that act tonically on lower centers.

Nevertheless, there appear to be more specific pathways, involving paucisynaptic pathways. Single-shock stimulations of the cortex can lead to complex bilateral short-latency excitation or inhibition of medullary respiratory units (Bassal et al., 1981), as well as short-latency responses to spinal intercostal respiratory motoneurons (Aminoff and Sears, 1971). Evidence that such direct pathways exist for phrenic motoneurons and diaphragm comes from (1) both retrograde (Rickard-Bell et al., 1985) and antegrade (Cheema et al., 1984) tracer studies, (2) the finding of short-latency activation of phrenic motoneurons from the sensorimotor cortex (Lipski et al., 1986), and (3) activation of the diaphragm by cranial percutaneous (Gandevia and Rothwell, 1987) and transcranial magnetic stimulation (Corfield et al., 1993) in human beings.

Thus, cortical activation, voluntary and nonvoluntary, has three potential ways of affecting respiration: (1) by a nonspecific action on the reticular arousal mechanism; (2) by direct action on the medullary controller—the resetting of rhythm by cortical stimulation supports this view (Bassal and Bianchi, 1982); and (3) by pathways that go directly to cervical and thoracic respiratory motoneurons. The latter mechanism is of potential interest, as will be seen, because it represents a way in which breathing can be increased without engaging the medullary controller.

D. Summary

This overview of the respiratory control system should make it abundantly clear that it is a very complex apparatus. Most of the outputs can be incorporated into traditional thinking about the respiratory system. One, however, the rostrally directed corollary discharge from medulla, is different and represents an output that may have important implications for development of sensation. It is also apparent that there are many and varied inputs to the system; some of these fall under the usual rubric of respiratory "control," but many others do not.

Our approach to the question assured that all inputs had effects on the controller. Although many are in the traditional "afferent" and "sensory" category, it does not necessarily follow that they all have direct access to cortical structures or that they contribute directly to conscious respiratory sensation. It is probable that some contribute indirectly to conscious sensation by effects on the controller, which sends its own corollary discharge signals to the higher brain, that others have direct ascending pathways to higher brain and cortex, and that some do both. As will be shown (see Sec. IV.A), some of the latter may have opposing effects, such as inhibition by laryngeal input of the controller but excitation of a direct pathway.

III. Insights from Psychophysics

Psychophysics is the study of the relationship between a physical change (stimulus) and the conscious sensation evoked by that change. A number of techniques, involving threshold discrimination and scaling of the sensory experience, have been used to study what we have called the mainly not unpleasant somatic respiratory sensations (see review by Zechman and Wiley, 1986), as well as the sensations of dyspnea (Adams and Guz, 1991).

A. Somatic Sensations

Human beings have the ability to detect, quantify, and discriminate between different loads (resistive and elastic) and to detect alterations of ventilation and changes in flows, volumes, and durations of breathing. A number of different receptors and mechanisms have been suggested as contributing to these detections and include most of those already discussed, upper airway, vagally mediated pulmonary receptors, thoracic muscle and chest wall receptors, and the central respiratory drive mechanism we have discussed as a medullary corollary discharge [also called motor command (Zechman and Wiley, 1986; Gandevia et al.,

1981), central respiratory command (Adams and Guz, 1991), and efferent copy (Killian and Campbell, 1991; Manning et al., 1992)].

The very fact that the sensations are appreciated at a conscious level means that there are pathways for information from receptors and other sources to be processed centrally and to reach the cortex. Nevertheless, as Zechman and Wiley (1986) noted, "the neurophysiological mechanisms subserving the sensory experiences arising when the ventilatory pump generates changes of flow, volume or pressure or when the pump is impeded by loads are poorly understood." One psychophysical study that has a bearing on this question tested the ability of tracheostomized, high-level quadriplegics (C1–3) to detect changes (inspiratory duration held constant) in tidal volumes delivered by a ventilator (Banzett et al., 1987). The quadriplegics could detect changes as small as 100 ml, about the same as a group of normal subjects. The study is of importance in that the absence of inputs from upper airway, chest, and respiratory muscles did not impair the ability to detect volume changes. The authors appropriately concluded that vagally mediated afferent information from lungs and/or lower airway was responsible for their findings. No implications could be made about central nervous system pathways or mechanisms.

B. Dyspnea

The situation is not greatly different for the unpleasant sensations of dyspnea, for which there are also good scaling techniques (see Chap. 3) and many clinical and psychophysical studies. Many of the studies are primarily descriptive, showing the relation between level of distressful sensation and one or several measurable variables, such as level of exercise, degree of fitness, magnitude of ventilation, work of breathing, duration of breath holding, diaphragmatic contraction, arterial P_{CO_2} or P_{O_2}, and the effects of disease. These studies have provided useful information and correlations of magnitude of dyspnea with the associated factors in both normal subjects and patients with disease. Again, the experiencing of the sensation means that neural information from receptors or other sources has reached the cortex. However, the problem with many such studies is that the methods used to elicit the sensation, such as hypercapnia, hypoxia, exercise, respiratory loads, weakened respiratory muscles, and breath holding, have the potential to activate a number of receptor-mediated and other neural inputs at the same time and so are not helpful in elucidating neurophysiological pathways or central processing mechanisms.

Nevertheless, there are studies that provide at least some insights into the importance, or unimportance, of the mechanisms potentially involved in the production of dyspnea. It is these we propose to discuss here, although not in depth, because they are discussed in a number of chapters in this volume and recent reviews on the subject (Adams and Guz, 1991; Tobin, 1990; Schwartzstein et al., 1990; Killian and Campbell, 1991). Five main categories of inputs and mechanisms have been proposed as important in the genesis of dyspnea: (1) a signal related to magnitude of central respiratory neural drive, the rostrally directed medullary corollary discharge we discussed earlier (Secs. II.A and B); (2) input from chemoreceptors; (3) inputs from respiratory muscle and chest wall receptors; (4) inputs from the lungs; and (5) inputs from upper airways.

Central Respiratory Neural Drive

In recent years there has been increasing acceptance of a view that the level of central (medullary) respiratory activity or drive is an important (Altose et al., 1985), perhaps the most important (Adams and Guz, 1991), component of the mechanisms that lead to the sensation of "breathlessness." There is no way to measure respiratory neural drive directly, however. The level of drive is often inferred from some mechanical output variable, such as ventilation or work of breathing, or from respiratory muscle activity. This is not really satisfactory because abnormalities of mechanics of lungs and chest or problems with muscular function, neuromuscular transmission, or neural transmission in the spinal cord cause a dissociation between actually measured output and what is needed, the central neural drive.

A number of definitive studies have in fact relied on this dissociation to show the importance of the central drive mechanism. With this indirect approach, a stimulus is given, for example hypercapnia or exercise, that is known to increase respiratory neural drive, muscular activation, and ventilation under usual conditions. If there are inherent, acquired, or investigator-induced abnormalities of mechanical, muscular, or peripheral neural function in the subject, the resulting actual ventilation, muscular contraction, or even neural activation of the muscles is less than expected for the presumed level of central neural drive. Conversely, the presumed level of drive and resulting magnitude of sensation are greater than expected for the amount of ventilation or muscle contraction.

Examples of studies that showed this dissociation include an increase in sensation during the reduction of respiratory muscle performance by fatigue (Gandevia et al., 1981) or curarization (Campbell et al., 1980) or by reduced effectiveness of shortened inspiratory muscles at high lung volumes (Killian et al., 1984). Even more impressive examples include the development, during hypercapnia, of the "air hunger" form of dyspnea (1) in normal subjects paralyzed by a neuromuscular blocking agent and ventilated via an endotracheal tube (Banzett et al., 1990) and (2) in tracheostomized, ventilated, high-level (C1–3) quadriplegics (Banzett et al., 1989). These studies showed that feedback associated with muscular contraction and chest movement and with feedback from the upper airway is not essential for the development of dyspnea under these conditions. The studies left only two possibilities: (1) increased medullary corollary discharge to the cortex, and (2) pathways for afferent input from peripheral and central chemoreceptors that go directly to supramedullary brain and cortex, bypassing the medullary controller. A recent study by the same group (Shea et al., 1993b) of children with the congenital central hypoventilation syndrome (Ondine's curse) showed that they did not develop dyspnea when given CO_2 to breathe—their ventilation, of course, did not increase—but did when exercise led to an increase in ventilation. The findings suggest that there is no direct pathway for chemoreceptor inputs to reach the higher brain and supports the importance of the medullary drive mechanism, although the authors cautiously raised an alternative possibility that there might be "direct projections of limb afferents or locomotor center activity" to explain the sensation during exercise.

Further support for the central drive mechanism comes from studies in which ventilation was caused to increase in different ways: one was by automatic mechanisms (hypercapnia or exercise), both presumably causing an increase in central respiratory drive, the other involving isocapnic voluntary hyperpnea with the same levels of ventilation. In both normal subjects and patients with chronic obstructive pulmonary disease, breathlessness was less during voluntary isocapnic hyperpnea than during hypercapnically induced hyperpnea (Adams et al., 1985; Freedman et al., 1987; Chonan et al., 1990b) or the hyperpnea associated with exercise (Lane et al., 1987; Altose et al., 1988). Although one of these studies (Chonan et al., 1990b) did not find the difference between exercise-induced and voluntary hyperpneas, the weight of the evidence supports a conclusion that the automatic mechanisms, which certainly activate the medullary controller, are associated with more breathlessness than voluntary hyperpnea, which may not activate the controller as much. If one accepts the idea that motor activity from the cortex can go directly to spinal motoneurons and bypass the medullary controller (see Sec. II.C), then it is not difficult to accept that for the same level of ventilation, voluntary breathing may cause less engagement of the controller and thus less of the rostrally directed corollary discharge that causes the sensation.

Chemoreceptors

No one would question the clear association between dyspnea and the hypercapnic stimulation of central chemoreceptors or the hypoxic and hypercapnic stimulation of peripheral chemoreceptors. However, both inputs cause an increase in central respiratory neural activity and in consequence an increase in the corollary discharge mechanism. The question is thus whether these inputs have an additional "dyspnogenic" effect by direct neural pathways that bypass the medullary controller.

In hypercapnia and input from central and peripheral chemoreceptors, most studies have not been definitive because of difficulties in obtaining an accurate value of medullary P_{CO_2} from end-tidal or arterial P_{CO_2} and in obtaining a satisfactory index of central respiratory drive from levels of ventilation alone (for example, subjects with quadriplegia or respiratory muscle paralysis *must* have an increase in central drive when made hypercapnic but have no or a reduced expression in mechanical output). Several studies support a lack of direct effect of hypercapnically increased chemoreceptor input. In two (Ward and Whipp, 1989; Lane et al., 1990), the exercise stimulus was given alone or a lesser exercise was combined with hypercapnia to yield the same indirect index of central drive, that is, ventilation. It was found that there was no difference in the intensity of breathlessness in the two conditions. Even more convincing that the direct effect of CO_2 input is not important is the study quoted earlier (Shea et al., 1993b) in which children with congenital absence of respiratory response to hypercapnia (Ondine's curse syndrome), who have a response to and develop breathlessness with exercise, do not develop breathlessness with hypercapnia.

In contrast to hypercapnia, there is a little more evidence that hypoxia-stimulated inputs from the carotid bodies have a direct action in producing dyspnea that is independent of the level of central drive. Ward and Whipp (1989) found that hypoxia during exercise produced more of a sensation of "respiratory difficulty" than exercise alone, even though the level of ventilation was the same. Chronos et al. (1988) found in some heavily exercising normal subjects that after a change from breathing of air to 15% O_2 there was an increase in breathlessness before the consequent increase in ventilation, and presumably central drive, occurred. These findings support the idea of a direct effect from the carotid bodies. Nevertheless, there is a problem with the conclusion—that the carotid body receptors are responsive to both hypoxia and hypercapnia and that the signals travel to the brain in the same nerve fibers. Thus, one expects a direct effect from both stimuli or no such effect from either.

Respiratory Muscles and Chest Wall

Inputs from chest and respiratory muscles, especially those from stretch receptors (spindles), have for many years been proposed as important in signaling abnormalities, or mismatches, of the relation between muscular contraction and mechanical movement, and thus important in generating dyspnea. It is probable that these signals lead to the not unpleasant conscious perception of posture and loads (Gottfried et al., 1984), but there is less solid evidence that they contribute much to dyspnea.

In one study (Homma et al., 1984) that addressed this question, alternating vibrations of the chest wall (expiratory in timing in upper chest and inspiratory in lower) were evaluated for an effect on "breathlessness" measured on a three-point scale. The vibrations led to an increase in breathlessness, but it was associated with an almost 40% increase in respiratory frequency and some increase in tidal volume, suggesting that the respiratory controller had also been activated. A second study (Manning et al., 1991), using a more rigorous psychophysical technique, determined the effect of vibration of the upper chest wall in subjects in whom breathlessness had already been induced by a combination of hypercapnia and inspiratory resistive loading, with ventilation and end-tidal P_{CO_2} kept constant. This study found a modest reduction in the sensation of breathlessness, the opposite of the Homma study. Although the investigators speculated that the effect was through stimulation of receptors in the "chest wall," it is also possible that mechanoreceptors stimulated by transmitted vibrations in the lungs and upper airways were also involved.

The most important studies are those of Banzett et al. (1989, 1990) in which paralysis of respiratory muscles because of blocking agents or quadriplegia did not prevent the development of air hunger during stimulation of central neural respiratory drive by hypercapnia. Although these studies eliminate input from chest wall (or upper airways) as essential to the development of the sensation, they by no means rule out a contribution from the chest wall or muscles in the intact individual.

Lungs and Lower Airways

Inputs originating here have also long been proposed as sources of signals that cause dyspnea, but again much of the evidence is equivocal, because the study procedures usually change more than one input variable. Even in the lung, that there are three types of receptors, with potentially different actions, makes for uncertainties in interpreting results.

Some studies show that these inputs are not important in generating the sensation. For example, patients with heart-lung transplants who have lost all of their pulmonary and most of their lower airway receptors have a normal ventilatory response and normal perception of breathlessness during maximal exercise (Banner et al., 1989; Kimoff et al., 1990).

In other studies, the breathlessness of normal individuals (Winning et al., 1985) and patients with interstitial disease (Winning et al., 1988) that developed during exercise or hypercapnia was not consistently affected by aerosol anesthesia of the airways, although in laryngectomized subjects such anesthesia led to greater breathlessness for the same level of ventilation (Hamilton et al., 1987). Taguchi et al. (1991) reported that, during isocapnic voluntary hyperpnea, histamine-induced bronchoconstriction led to increased dyspnea; this was decreased by inhaled lidocaine, even though ventilation was kept constant. The authors concluded that vagal nerve activity, "specifically the irritant one, may increase the sensation of dyspnea"; however, their use of voluntary hyperpnea as the index of medullary respiratory neural drive makes the conclusion problematical.

Two studies provide more convincing evidence that pulmonary receptors have an important and specific effect, that is, an inhibitory modulation of the sensation by input from pulmonary stretch receptors. Manning et al. (1992) induced with hypercapnia a modest level of air hunger in high-level ventilated quadriplegics. By increasing or decreasing the ventilator's tidal volume but keeping end-tidal P_{CO_2} constant, the investigators could cause the magnitude of the sensation to change; there was an inverse relation between tidal volume and the sensation. Thus, for the same level of central drive, there was a clear effect from lung inflation. The investigators concluded that afferent information from the lungs was responsible; although specific receptors and mechanisms could not be further identified, pulmonary stretch receptor input was a good candidate. The second study (Flume et al., 1993) used the respiratory distress (air hunger) of breath holding and its relief by rebreathing a gas that did not improve blood gases (Fowler, 1954; Flume et al., 1994). Patients who had undergone bilateral lung transplants, and who had lost about half of their pulmonary receptors, were compared with normal subjects. The normals experienced immediate relief of the breath-holding distress with the first breath of rebreathing, but the patients experienced less relief, which was of slower onset. The investigators concluded that the difference was caused by a loss of the inhibitory effect of pulmonary stretch receptor input on neurons involved in generating the sensation.

Upper Airways

In addition to effects on the controller, many inputs from receptors in the upper airway are perceived at a conscious level. There remains only the question of whether they make a contribution to the sensation of dyspnea that is independent of the level of central respiratory neural drive.

Cold air directed at the face has an inhibitory effect on controller activity during breath holding (McBride and Whitelaw, 1981). In one study (Schwartzstein et al., 1987), cold air seemed to lead to a very modest reduction of breathlessness induced by massive inspiratory resistive load (63 cm H_2O/L/s) and/or marked hypercapnia. With only hypercapnia (60 mm Hg) ventilation was slightly but significantly less during the cold exposure, whereas during loading and loading plus hypercapnia there was no significant difference in ventilation between control and cold exposure. To reach a valid conclusion that cold receptors led *directly* to a reduction of perception of breathlessness would require an equivalency of ventilation and central neural respiratory drive not clearly accomplished in these experiments. Spence et al. (1993) showed that exercise-induced breathlessness in patients with chronic obstructive pulmonary disease was reduced during breathing of cold air, but it was accompanied by a reduction of ventilation; there was no difference in breathlessness at equivalent levels of ventilation. The findings do not support a direct, independent effect of input from cold receptors on the sensation.

Other

The finding that intensities of breathlessness were similar in control subjects and patients with heart or heart-lung transplants (Banner et al., 1989; Kimoff et al.,

1990), whose cardiopulmonary responses to dynamic exercise were similar, excludes input from cardiac receptors as important to the sensation induced by increased central respiratory neural drive but of course does not rule out a small contribution in the intact individual.

C. Summary

Psychophysical studies clearly show that a variety of functions of the respiratory system can be sensed and perceived at the cortical level, although pathways and mechanisms are not well understood. Clinically the most important is the sensation of dyspnea, for which a number of mechanisms have been proposed over the years.

One has to be impressed with a feature that stands out in almost all the psychophysical studies of factors, other than the magnitude of central neural respiratory activity, that have been proposed as involved in causation of dyspnea or breathlessness. It is that the studies are performed in subjects who have already been made breathless by a mechanism that increases central drive, that is, by hypercapnia or exercise. Only when this has been accomplished does it appear to be possible to study the effects of the other inputs, suggesting that they are less strong and of less importance. Thus, one must conclude that an increase in central neural respiratory drive, with transmission to higher brain of the magnitude of medullary activity via corollary discharge, is the sine qua non for development of dyspnea and that the other proposed factors are modifiers of the sensation.

The idea is depicted in Fig. 1, which shows the relation between central neural drive (as an arbitrary index) and a rating of dyspnea. One must assume that neuronal mechanisms subserving the dyspneic sensation are well below threshold at rest. As central drive increases, the activity of some neuronal pathways also increases, but until a threshold level is exceeded is not able to excite all steps in the pathway and reach the cortex and perception. That there is such a threshold is supported by the findings of Banzett et al. (1989) in quadriplegics, in whom P_{CO_2} had to increase by at least 7 mm Hg before air hunger developed. Also, it is a common observation that moderate increases in ventilation and central neural drive during exercise do not cause dyspnea to develop; it appears only when the threshold level is passed.

Let us also assume that we add other inputs (positive or negative effects, shown by arrows in Fig. 1) that have relatively small effects on dyspnea. At subthreshold levels of central drive (as in box A), this input would have no effect on dyspnea even though it has an effect on neurons subserving the sensation. If the central drive were at threshold for the sensation (box B), a facilitatory input would cause the dyspnea to appear (arrow) but an inhibitory input would have no effect. In the midrange of dyspnea (box C), both facilitatory and inhibitory inputs would affect its magnitude. If dyspnea were already at its maximal saturated level (box D), only an inhibitory input would affect the rating of dyspnea.

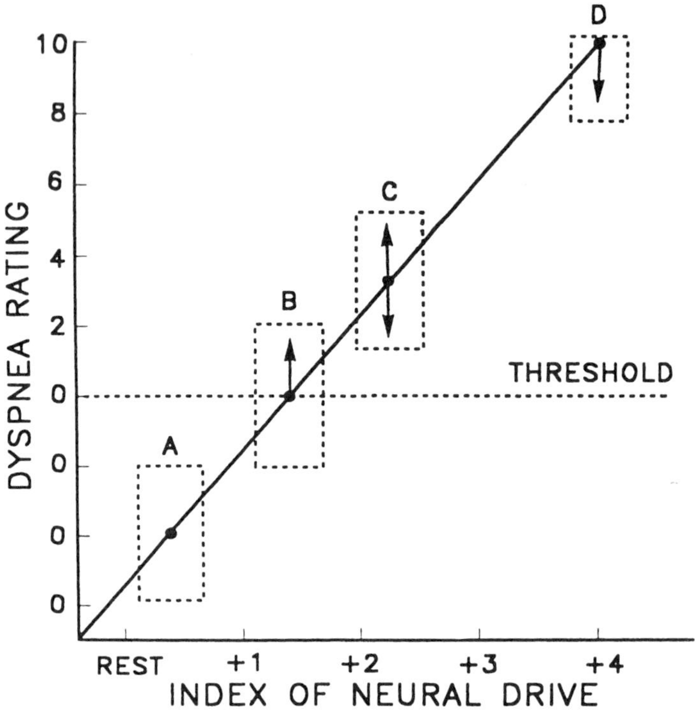

Figure 1 Relation (diagonal line) between index of medullary neural respiratory drive and the rating of dyspnea. At rest in normal subjects, drive level is below threshold for evoking dyspnea. As central drive increases, the activity of neuronal pathways subserving the sensation may increase, but only after a threshold level is exceeded does actual dyspnea develop and increase progressively as drive further increases. If other weak neural inputs (facilitatory or inhibitory) that act on the neuronal pathways but that do not affect respiratory drive are added, they have the effects on dyspnea shown by arrows (see text).

IV. Neurophysiology

There is a very limited amount of work on the neurophysiology of respiratory sensation in general and dyspnea in particular. What there is can be considered in two categories, one the studies of unit activity of single neurons and the second studies of cortical potentials.

A. Neurons

The studies in this section are mainly from our laboratory. We present evidence that the neurons reported are sensory, that is, involved in the transmission of respiratory information to supramedullary brain and that they may have relevance to the sensation of dyspnea. The studies involved the recording of phrenic nerve activities and single-unit firing of neurons in the rostral pons (Chen and Eldridge, 1992), mesencephalon (Chen et al., 1991), and thalamus (Chen et al., 1992) of unanesthetized, decerebrated, paralyzed, and ventilated cats in which vagi and carotid sinus nerves had been ablated. The lack of anesthesia, and consequently the decerebration, were essential because the neuronal activity could not be found in the presence of anesthesia. The discussion involves the categories of input mechanisms that were used in the previous section.

Central Respiratory Neural Drive

Mesencephalon

Measurements of neuronal firing were made first at low levels of respiratory neural drive, indexed by phrenic activity and associated with normal P_{CO_2} levels, and then during increased drive produced by hypercapnia acting on the central chemoreceptors or by stimulation of a carotid sinus nerve (CSN) to mimic input to the controller from the carotid body.

At least a quarter of the studied neurons in the mesencephalic reticular formation (central tegmental field; Fig. 2), which were silent or irregularly tonic at low levels of respiratory drive, developed a rhythmic change in firing associated with each respiration when drive was increased. Although a small number (9%) showed a rhythmic decrease in firing, 91% showed an increase. The change in firing usually began during late inspiration and always persisted into the post-inspiratory period. Figure 3 shows an example of a mesencephalic neuron that increased its firing during hypercapnia and Fig. 4 an example with CSN stimulation (Chen et al., 1991).

In mesencephalic neurons, there appeared to be a threshold at about 50% of maximum respiratory activity below which the rhythmic firing did not occur; this was true whether or not the neuron had been silent (Fig. 5B) at low levels of drive or had been firing tonically with no discernible respiratory rhythm (Fig. 5A). Above this level, the neuronal firing increased progressively during both inspiration and expiration as respiratory drive increased.

The graded increase in firing with increased respiratory neural drive can be easily seen in Fig. 6, which shows a mesencephalic neuron and phrenic activity averaged over a number of consecutive breaths at each of four levels of drive. At the lowest level of drive (P_{CO_2} = 29 mm Hg), which is not shown, the neuron was silent. When drive was increased a little by CSN stimulation, the neuron began to fire irregularly with suggestion of a rhythmic component (Fig. 6A). As stimulation and drive were progressively increased, the magnitude of rhythmic activity of the neuron also progressively increased (Fig. 6B, C, and D).

To show that the neuronal rhythm was coming from the medulla, not from

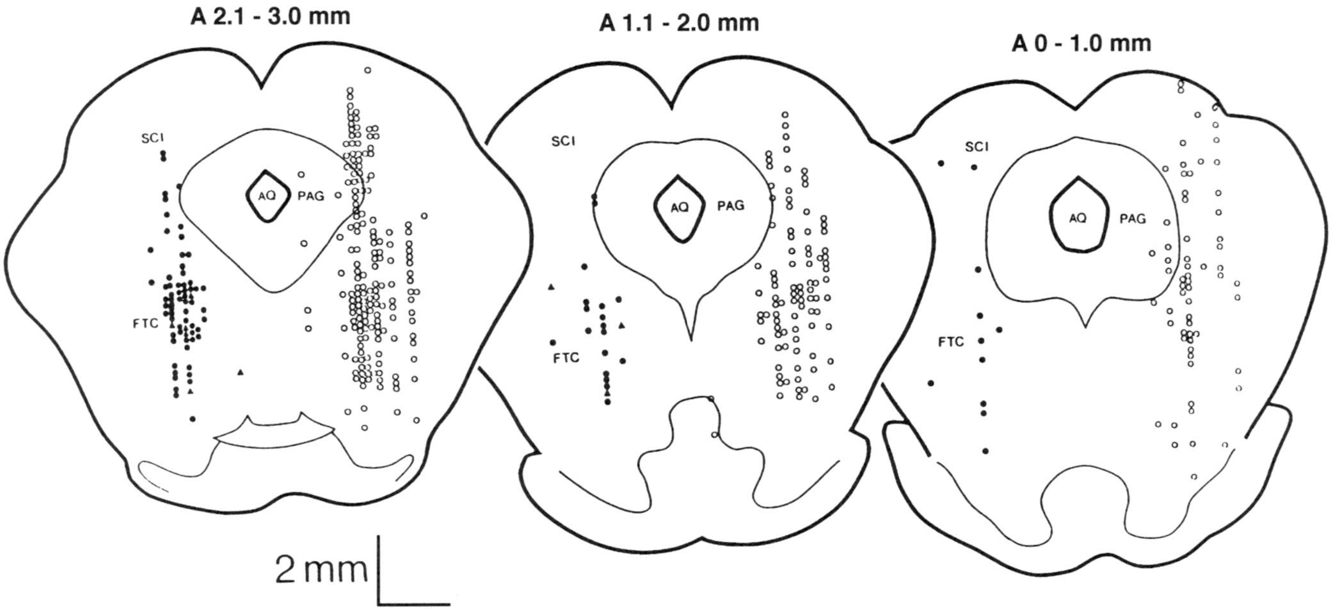

Figure 2 Locations of 354 mesencephalic neurons in 21 cats. Transverse stereotaxic planes from 0 to 3 mm anterior are represented. Right sides (open circles): locations of neurons that did not develop respiratory-associated changes in firing. Left sides: locations of neurons that developed respiratory rhythmic firing pattern during increased respiratory drive: (closed circles) neurons that increased activity (91%); (triangles) neurons that decreased activity (9%). AQ = aqueduct; PAG = periaqueductal gray; SCI = superior colliculus; FTC = central tegmental field. (Reprinted from Chen et al., 1991.)

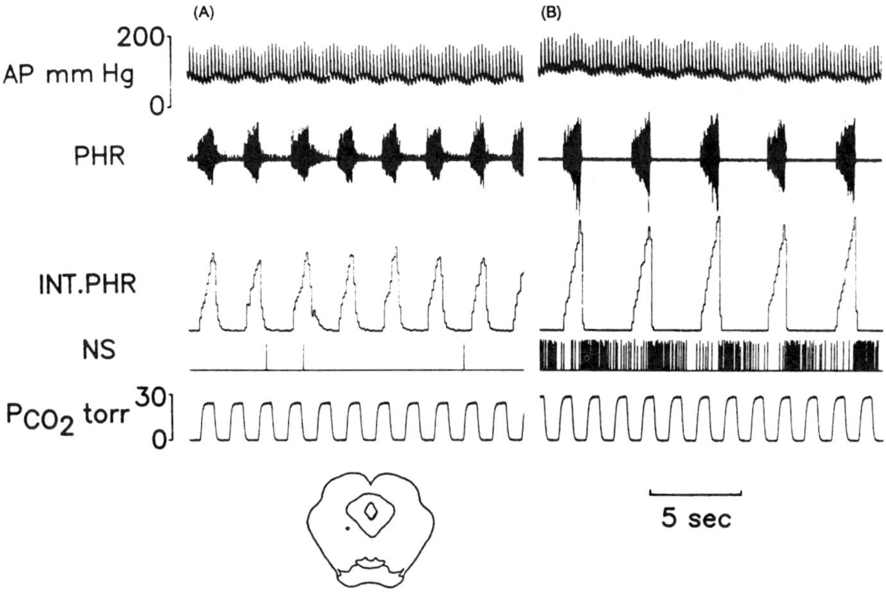

Figure 3 (A) Recording of arterial pressure (AP), phrenic nerve and integrated phrenic activity, spikes from a mesencephalic neuron (location on diagram) at end-tidal P_{CO_2} of 27.5 mm Hg. Neuron's activity is irregular and minimal. (B) Recording during increased respiratory drive to P_{CO_2} of 32.4 mm Hg. Neuron has regular respiratory-associated rhythmic firing pattern. (Reprinted from Chen et al., 1991.)

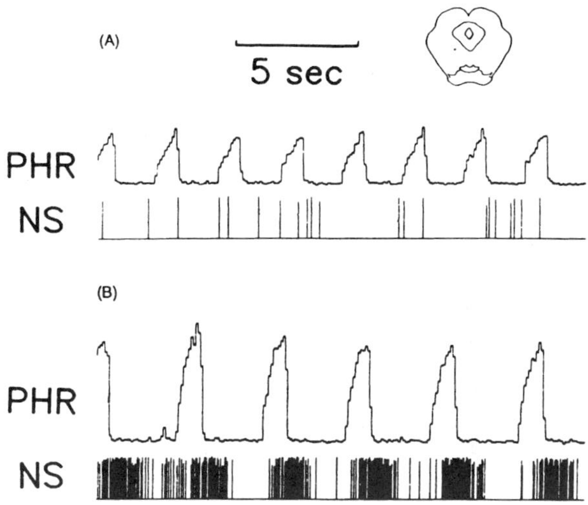

Figure 4 Integrated phrenic activity and mesencephalic neuron spike (NS) responses to carotid sinus nerve (CSN) stimulation at constant P_{CO_2} (A) before and (B) during CSN stimulation, which causes respiratory drive to increase and respiratory-associated neuronal activity to develop. (Adapted from Chen et al., 1991.)

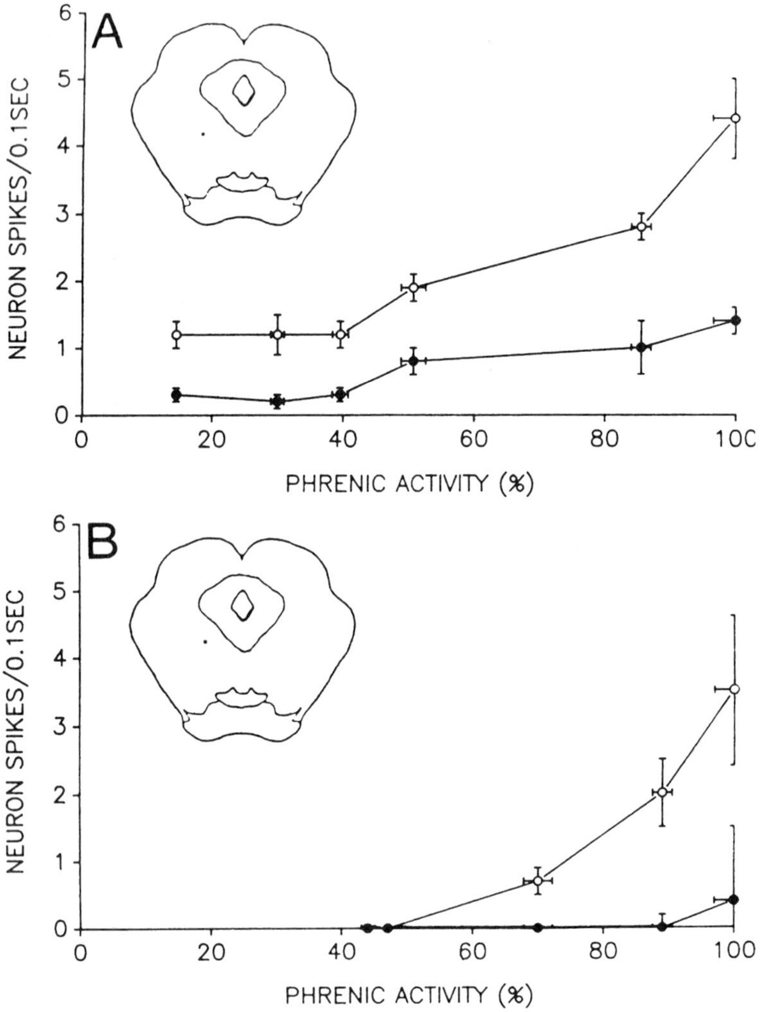

Figure 5 Relations between average spike rate and phrenic activity, shown as percentage of its maximum response to stimulation, in two mesencephalic neurons. (open circles) Maximal firing rate within a respiratory cycle; (closed circles) minimal firing rate. Both are means ± standard error of the mean. Neither of the neurons, one of which is tonic at low phrenic activity (A), the other silent at low phrenic activity (B), showed a respiratory-associated increase in activity until respiratory activity had increased to more than 50% of its maximum. (Reprinted from Chen et al., 1991.)

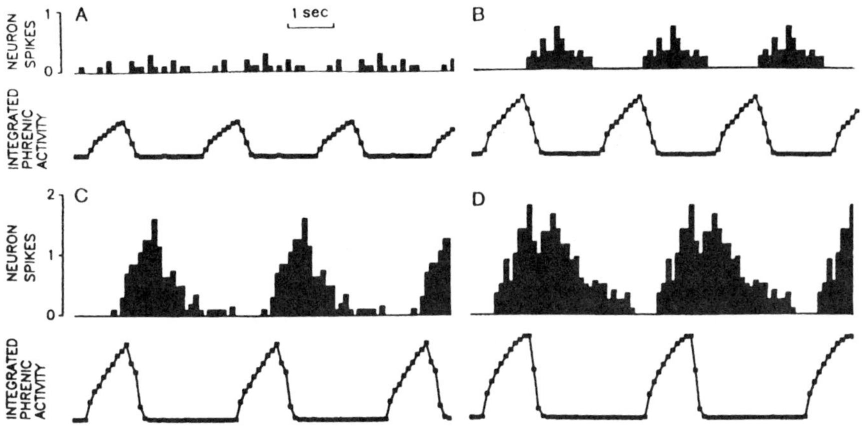

Figure 6 Histograms of mesencephalic neuron's firing rate (spikes/0.1 s) and phrenic activity averaged over 6–10 breaths, showing the effect of increasing central respiratory drive by CSN stimulation at constant P_{CO_2} of 29 mm Hg. Without CSN stimulation the neuron was silent. (A) Irregular firing during weak CSN stimulation. (B–D) Increasing phrenic activity and rhythmic neuronal firing evoked by progressive stronger CSN stimulation. Note that here and in Figs. 7, 9, 11, and 12, the repeats of rhythmic events in each panel are replottings of the same data. (Reprinted in part from Chen et al., 1991.)

phrenic motoneuron pools or other peripheral spinal inputs, animals were studied before and after spinal transection at the C1–2 level. The example in Fig. 7A1 shows a mesencephalic neuron that was tonic at low respiratory drive (P_{CO_2} = 22 mm Hg) and developed rhythmic activity related to respiration during CSN stimulation (Fig. 7A2). The cutting of the spinal cord led to loss of phrenic activity, but the medulla continued to generate rhythmic respiration, as evidenced by hypoglossal nerve (12) activity, and to activate the respiratory-associated rhythm in the neuron (Fig. 7B). The neurons continued to show graded increases in magnitude of rhythmic activity as respiratory drive, now reflected by hypoglossal activity, was increased either by stimulation of CSN or by hypercapnia. The findings show that feedback from the spinal cord is not necessary for development of the neuronal rhythmic activity.

The potential involvement of the rhythmic mesencephalic neurons in modulation of respiratory rhythm itself was tested by using low doses of a short-lasting anesthetic, Saffan, to reduce or eliminate the respiratory-associated neuronal activity. An example is shown in Fig. 8, where the control shows phrenic activity and associated firing of the mesencephalic neuron. During infusion of Saffan, neuronal firing was almost abolished but there was no change in phrenic activity or pattern. The neuronal firing had returned 10 minutes into recovery, with still no change in the respiratory pattern. The top panel shows that there were no signifi-

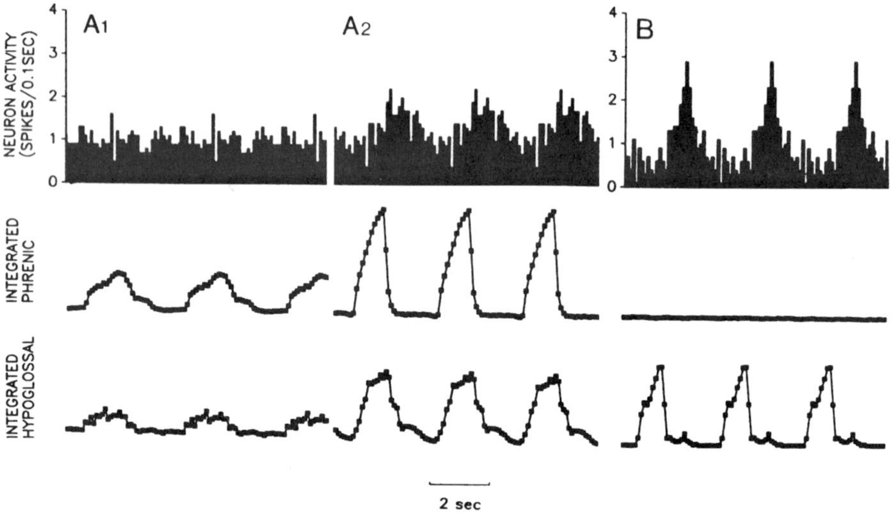

Figure 7 (A1) Tonic firing of mesencephalic neuron at low level of respiratory drive (P_{CO_2} of 22 mm Hg), indexed by integrated phrenic and hypoglossal activities. (A2) Respiratory-associated rhythm that occurred when respiratory drive had been increased by CSN stimulation. (B) Same cat after transection of spinal cord at C1–2, showing disappearance of phrenic activity but continuing hypoglossal nerve activity representing respiration and continuing respiratory-associated rhythmic activity in the mesencephalic neuron. (Reprinted from Chen et al., 1991.)

cant changes in respiratory period or durations of inspiration and expiration and indicates that the mesencephalic rhythmic firing does not produce significant modulation of respiratory rhythm.

Thalamus

Some thalamic neurons (14% of 545 neurons tested) showed behavior similar to that of the mesencephalic neurons (Chen et al., 1992), that is, rhythmic activity related to respiration and graded in magnitude according to level of neural respiratory drive (Fig. 9). The locations of these neurons are shown in Fig. 10; they are in regions of the thalamus where the so-called nonspecific thalamocortical system is said to be located (Hobson and Steriade, 1986). That the respiratory-associated rhythm is similar in both mesencephalic and thalamic neurons is shown in Fig. 11, which has four pairs of simultaneously recorded neurons. The main differences are that the thalamic firing occurs slightly later than mesencephalic (consistent with a downstream position in the pathway) and that there is a higher threshold for activation (at 70% of maximum respiratory activity) than for mesencephalic neurons (50% of maximum).

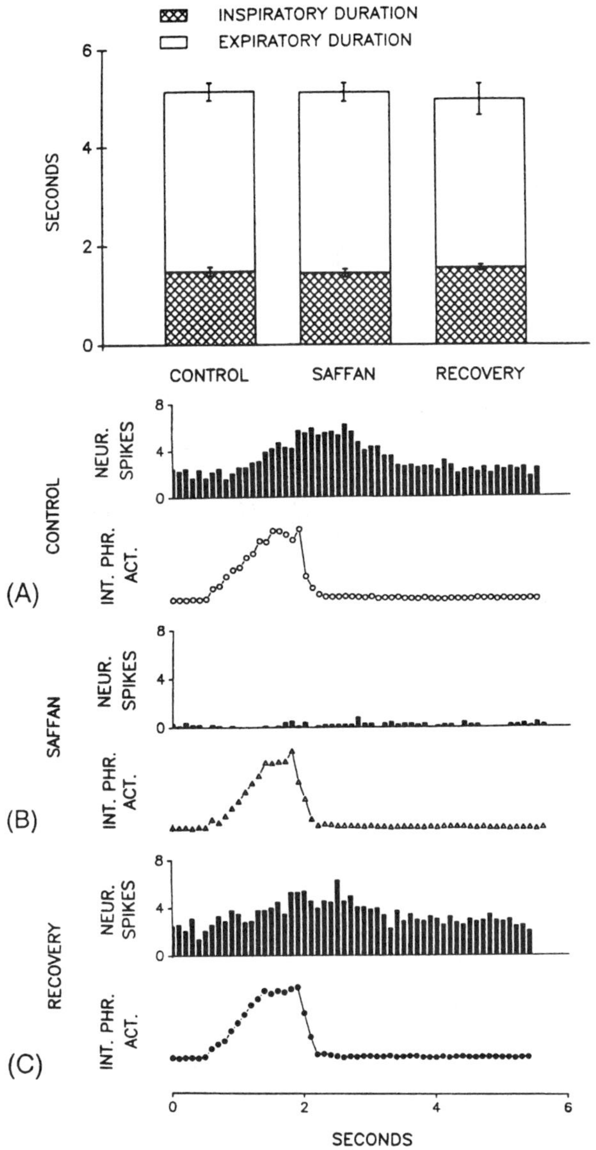

Figure 8 Effect of short-lasting anesthetic agent, Saffan, on respiratory-associated rhythmic firing of mesencephalic neuron and on phrenic activity: (A) control at P_{CO_2} of 40 mm Hg; (B) several minutes after intravenous infusion of Saffan; (C) 10 minutes after cessation of Saffan infusion. The anesthesia caused rhythmic neuronal firing to disappear and loss of almost of all firing but little change in phrenic activity or in its various periods.

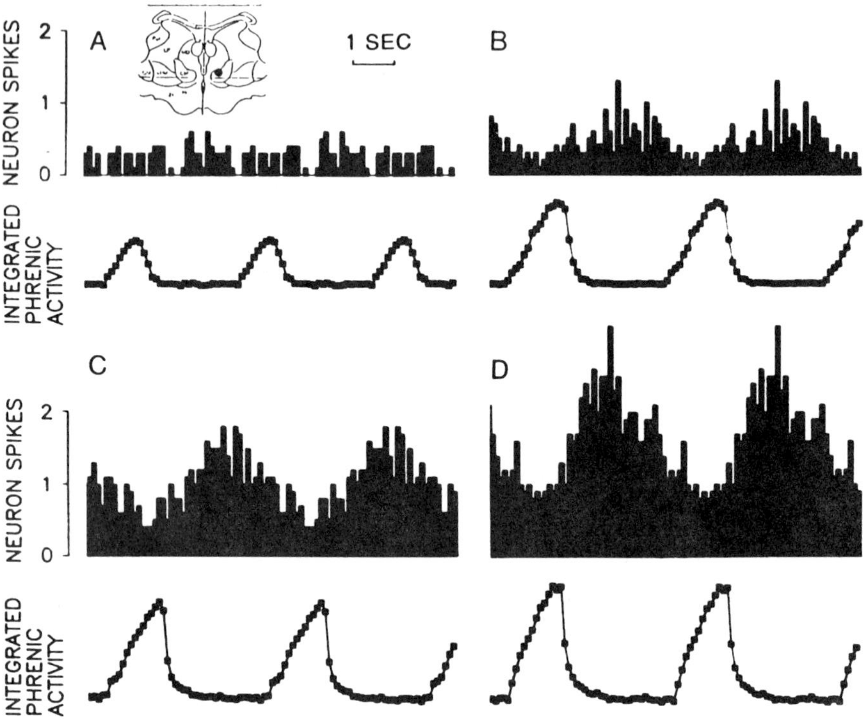

Figure 9 Histograms of thalamic neuron firing rate (neuron spikes per 0.1 s) and integrated phrenic activity averaged over 8–10 breaths: (A) irregular tonic firing at P_{CO_2} of 28 mm Hg; (B) P_{CO_2} of 33 mm Hg; (C and D) with additional stimulation of carotid sinus nerve. Firing of the neuron increases progressively as respiratory drive (phrenic) increases.

Pons

Finally, we have recorded rostral pontine neurons (Chen and Eldridge, 1992) that also develop respiratory-associated rhythmic firing of the same type, that is, in late inspiration and early expiration, and graded in amplitude according to the level of respiratory drive. Figure 12 shows an example of simultaneous recording of one of these pontine neurons and a mesencephalic neuron; those in the pons fire earlier than those in the mesencephalon, consistent with an upstream position in the pathway. Furthermore, respiratory-associated mesencephalic activity was depressed by electrolytic lesions of, or lidocaine injections into the rostral pons.

Thus, these neurons in pons, mesencephalon, and thalamus appear to have an input from the medulla that is related to magnitude of central neural respiratory drive and to have relatively high thresholds for activity that are consistent with the

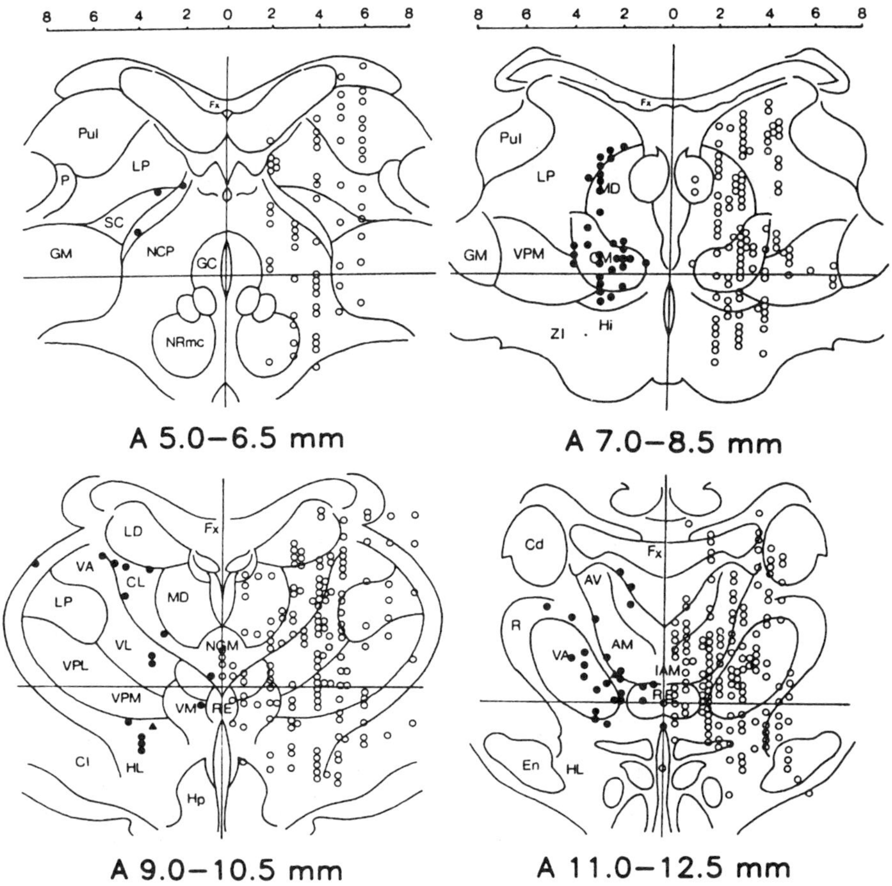

Figure 10 Locations of 545 thalamic neurons in 16 cats. Transverse stereotaxic planes from A5.0 to A12.5 mm. Right sides (open circles) show locations of 469 neurons that did not develop respiratory-associated changes in firing. Left sides (closed circles) show locations of 76 neurons that developed respiratory-associated rhythmic firing at high levels of respiratory drive; 2 neurons (triangles) showed decreases in firing. Abbreviations represent standard nomenclature for thalamic regions.

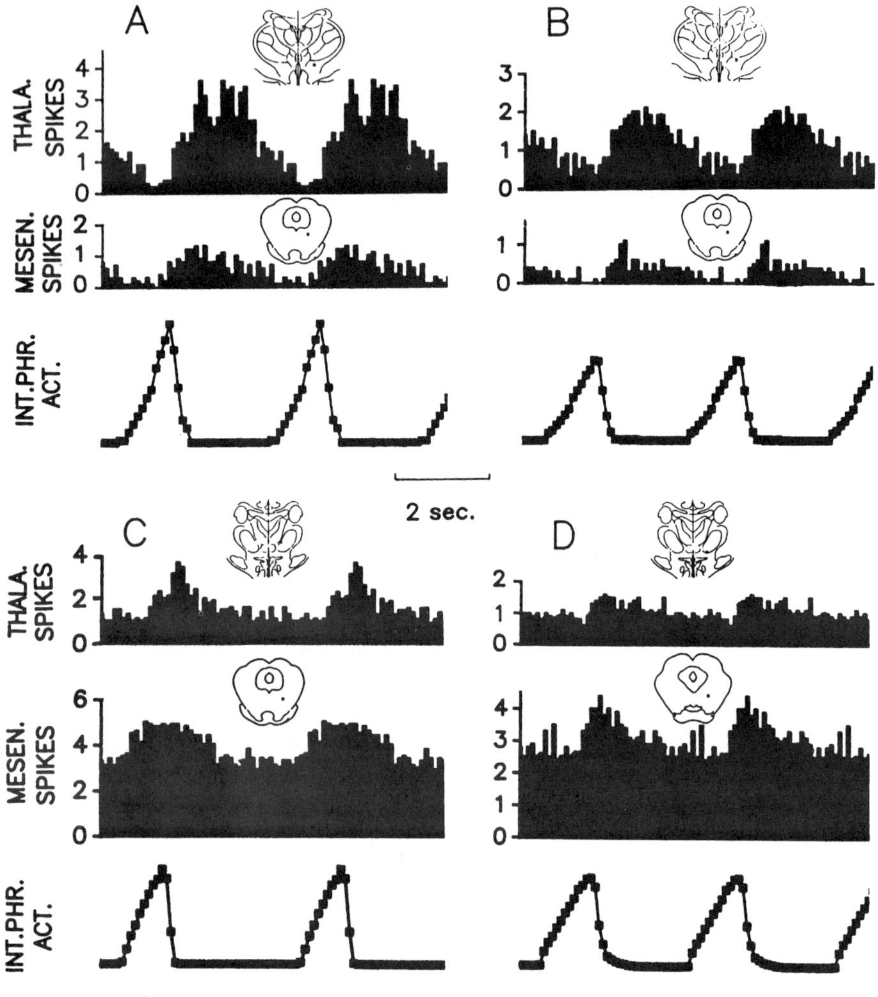

Figure 11 Histograms of firing rate (spikes per 0.1 s) of four different simultaneously recorded thalamic and mesencephalic neuron pairs and integrated phrenic activity (int.phr.act.) at high respiratory drive levels (P_{CO_2} = 46 mm Hg in A, 52 in B, 42 in C, and 43 in D) in three cats. Both neurons show respiratory-associated rhythms in all examples, but onsets and peaks of rhythmic firing occur earlier in mesencephalic than in thalamic neurons. (Reprinted in modified form from Chen et al., 1992.)

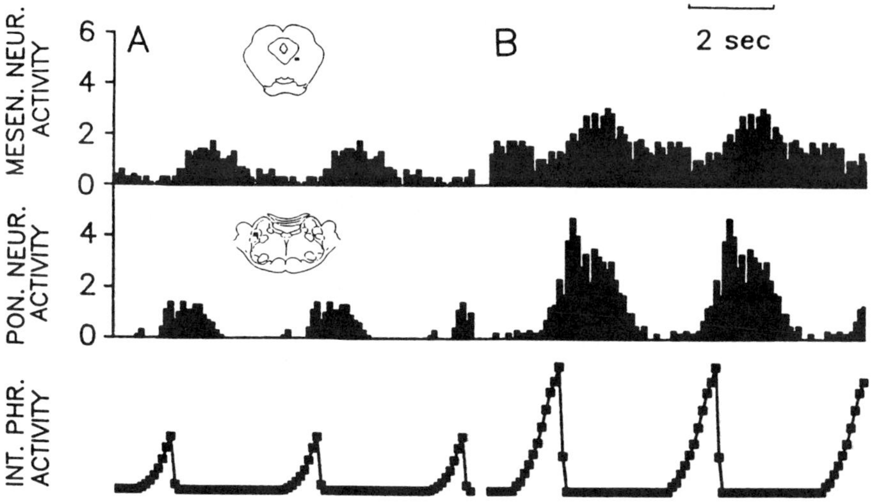

Figure 12 Histograms of averaged (7 breaths) spike rates (neur. activity per 0.1 s) and integrated phrenic activity (int. phr) of simultaneously recorded mesencephalic and rostral pontine neurons. Respiratory-associated rhythmic activity was present in both neurons at P_{CO_2} of 40 mm Hg, respiratory activity of 40% of maximum, and was increased in both neurons when respiratory activity was increased to 82% of maximum by hypercapnia (P_{CO_2} of 65 mm Hg).

findings from psychophysical studies, for example, Banzett et al. (1989). We suggest that they represent the neural substrate for transmission of this information to the cortex in graded form.

Lungs and Lower Airway

The preceding studies were performed in the absence of input from vagally mediated pulmonary receptors. To determine their effects, studies were performed in paralyzed, ventilated animals with intact vagi but with spinal cords transected at C7–T1 to eliminate input from chest wall and muscles (Eldridge and Chen, 1992).

Pulmonary Stretch Receptors

After mesencephalic neurons with the central respiratory-associated rhythm were found, we tested the effects of changing pulmonary stretch receptor input by (1) stopping and starting the ventilator, (2) changing the ventilator's tidal volume, and (3) vagal section. The essential finding is shown in Fig. 13, where a mesencephalic neuron that was silent, despite a high respiratory drive (P_{CO_2} = 44 mm Hg), when the ventilator was on and causing pulmonary stretch receptor input, developed a respiratory-associated rhythm when it was turned off. The reintroduc-

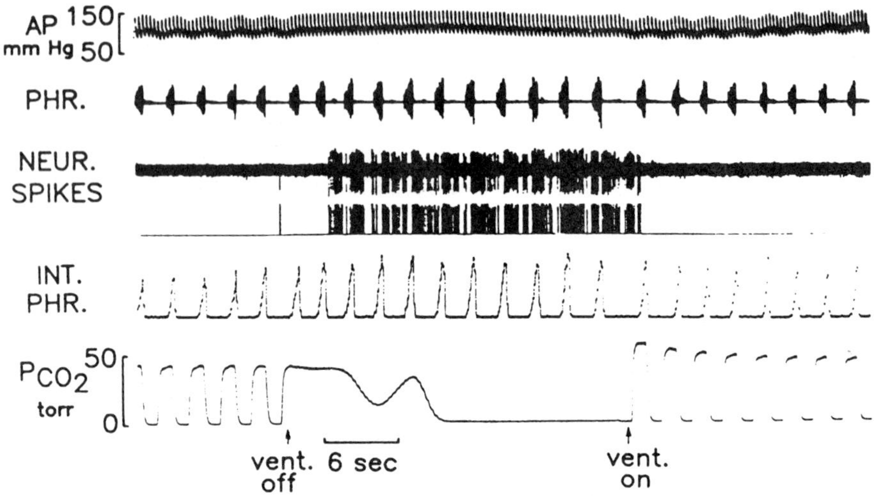

Figure 13 Effects on mesencephalic neuron spikes (neur. spikes; upper = raw, lower = window discriminated) of stopping and restarting ventilator in animal with intact vagi but transected (C7–T1) spinal cord. Phrenic (phr.) and integrated phrenic (int. phr) activity reflects a high level of respiratory neural drive (P_{CO_2} = 44 mm Hg). Note that respiratory-associated mesencephalic activity appears when ventilator is turned off (vent. off) and disappears promptly when ventilator is turned back on (vent. on), even though P_{CO_2} was increased. AP = arterial pressure.

tion of expansion of the lungs led to immediate disappearance of the mesencephalic rhythm, even though P_{CO_2} and respiratory drive increased during the period of apnea. Large ventilator-produced tidal volumes had a greater effect than small. Vagal section abolished the effect. Differential cooling of the vagi showed that the important fibers were of the large myelinated type.

All methods of testing thus showed that vagally mediated input, probably from pulmonary stretch receptors, tonically inhibits in a graded manner the respirator-associated firing of the mesencephalic neurons.

Rapidly Adapting (Irritant) Receptors

The effects of rapid adapting airway receptors were studied in animals with intact vagi and with thoracic input ablated by spinal cord (C7–T1) section. Mesencephalic neurons that had already been shown to develop the respiratory-associated rhythm at high levels of respiratory drive were studied during mechanical stimulation of RAR (scratching tracheal mucosa with a thin wire loop). The uniform response was a short-latency stimulation of the mesencephalic neuron (Fig. 14). This was true whether respiratory drive was above threshold for the

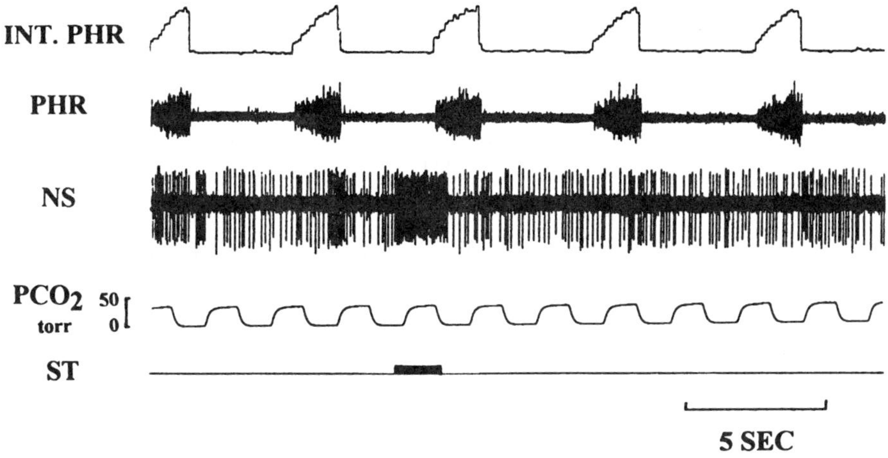

Figure 14 Effect on neuronal spikes (NS) in a mesencephalic neuron, known to develop a respiratory-associated rhythm at high drive, of a mechanical stimulus (ST, bar) of rapidly adapting receptors in trachea of cat with intact vagi and transection of spinal cord at C7–T1. There is a short-latency facilitatory response in the neuron.

centrally generated respiratory-associated rhythm, as in Fig. 14, or below that threshold. The effect waned fairly rapidly, even with continued stimulation, so there must have been either or both adaptation of the receptor response or accommodation of central neural pathways.

Thorax and Respiratory Muscle

Chen et al. (1991, 1992) found in animals with cut vagi but intact spinal cords that there were neurons in the mesencephalon, thalamus, and also rostral pons (unpublished data), which increased their firing each time the thorax was expanded by the ventilator. The firing did not occur when the ventilator was off. An example in a mesencephalic neuron is shown in Fig. 15; this neuron did not exhibit the respiratory-associated rhythm at any time but developed only the ventilator-related rhythm; it is representative of 27 of 44 tested neurons. The latency of the response (indexed by fall in airway P_{CO_2}) is relatively short (around 100 ms). A total of 17 neurons, however, developed both the centrally generated respiratory-associated rhythm and the ventilator-related rhythm at the same time (Fig. 16). The difference in latencies for the two rhythms is apparent (short for the ventilator related and long for the centrally generated). Some thalamic neurons showed the same behavior.

In summary, some neurons in pons, mesencephalon, and thalamus clearly respond to an input from respiratory muscles or chest wall associated with

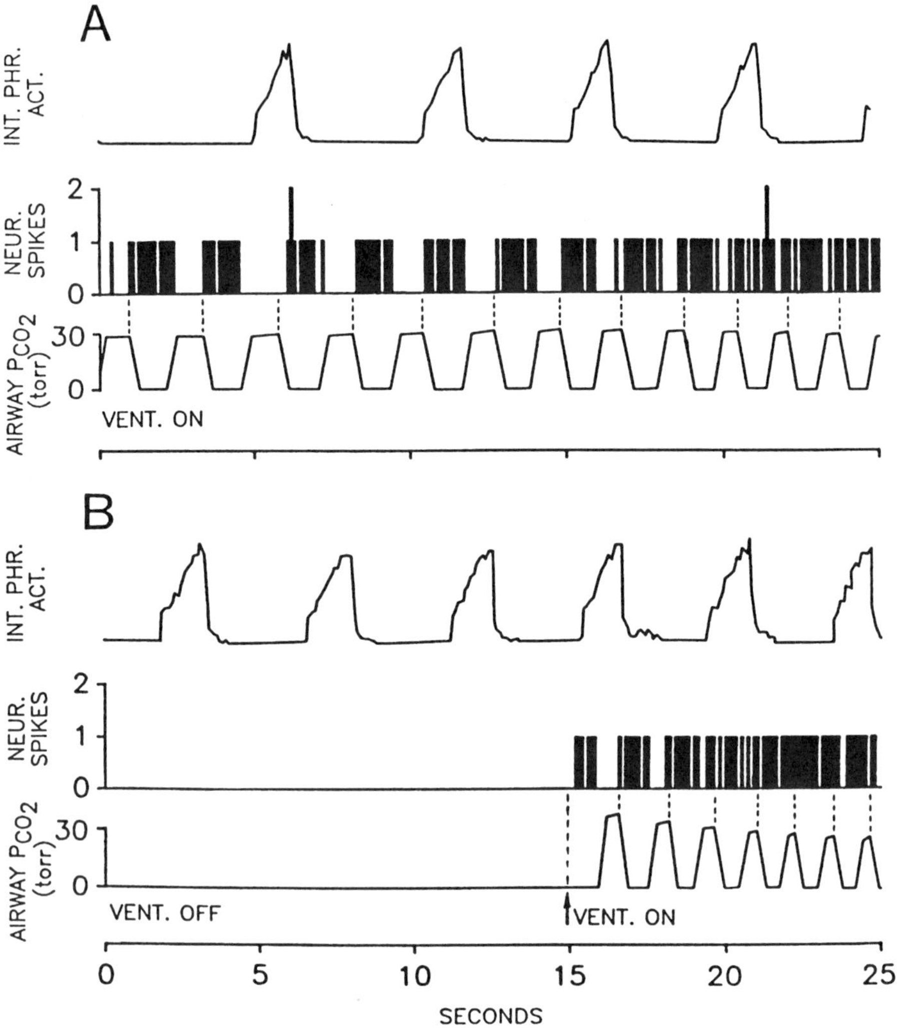

Figure 15 Rhythmic firing of mesencephalic neuron (neur. spikes) related to expansion of the chest by ventilator (A). Cat with cut vagi. When ventilator is off (B), firing disappears, to return as soon as it is restarted. There was no centrally generated respiratory-associated activity in this neuron. Int. phr. act = integrated phrenic activity. (Reprinted from Chen et al., 1991.)

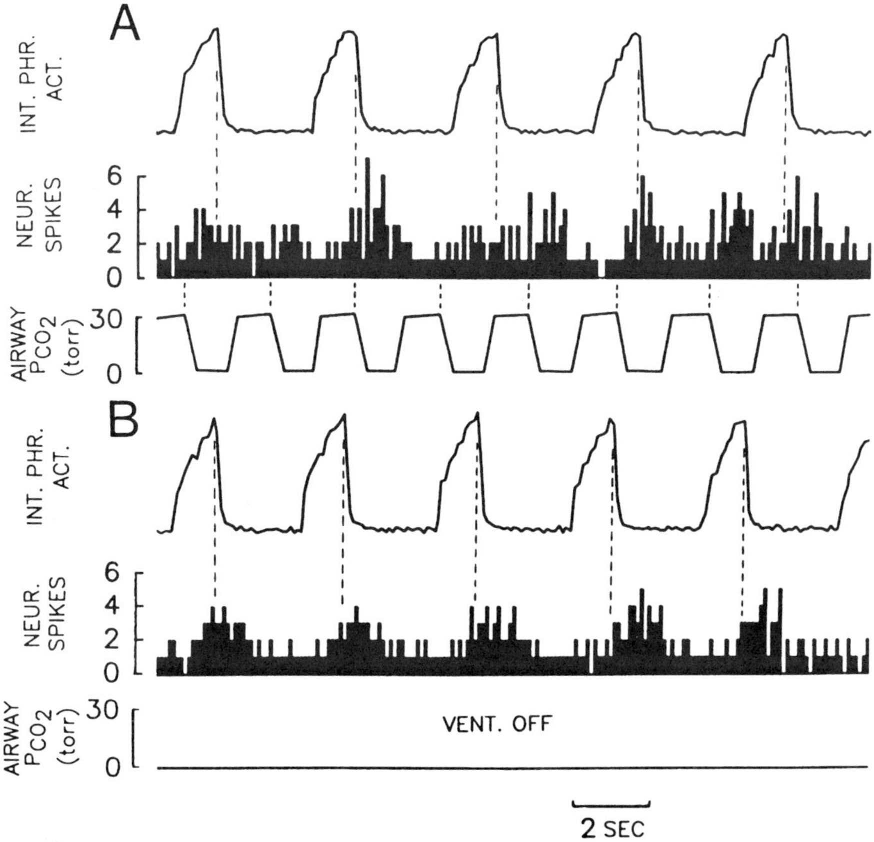

Figure 16 Mesencephalic neuron (neur. spikes) in cat with cut vagi, which shows both centrally generated respiratory-associated increases in firing and those related to expansion of chest by the ventilator (A). When the ventilator was turned off, only the respiratory associated rhythmic firing remained (B). Int. phr. act = integrated phrenic activity. (Reprinted from Chen et al., 1991.)

expansion of the thorax. Some of the same neurons also respond to the centrally generated respiratory signal. The latter thus provide some integration of the information from the two inputs even at as low a level as the mesencephalon.

Upper Airway

Input from upper airways was studied by mechanical stimulation of nasal mucosa, pharynx, and larynx and electrical stimulation of glossopharyngeal and superior laryngeal nerves (Chen and Eldridge, 1993). All mesencephalic neurons studied were first shown to develop the centrally generated respiratory-associated rhythm at high levels of respiratory drive but were often studied when respiratory drive was low enough not to evoke the rhythmic firing. The inputs all produced stimulation of the mesencephalic neurons. Figure 17 shows the increased firing of a neuron that resulted from mechanical stimulation of the nose. Figure 18A shows a facilitation resulting from electrical stimulation of nerve 9 from the pharynx and Fig. 18B a similar effect from stimulation of the superior laryngeal nerve; mechanical stimulation by inflation of balloons in pharynx or larynx had the same effects. It is noteworthy that all three inputs led to a dissociation between activity of the neuron (facilitated) and central neural respiratory drive (inhibited, reflected by loss of phrenic activity and resetting of respiratory rhythm).

Chemoreceptors

Input from carotid body chemoreceptors was mimicked by brief electrical stimulations of the carotid sinus nerve. Evidence was found that this input could rapidly affect mesencephalic, as well as thalamic, neuronal firing without apparent stimulation of medullary respiratory neural drive. An example is given in Fig. 19, in which a CSN stimulation given during expiration led to a prolongation of expiration and resetting of rhythm, typical of such expiratory stimulations (Eldridge, 1976), but also to a marked increase in firing of the mesencephalic neuron. The

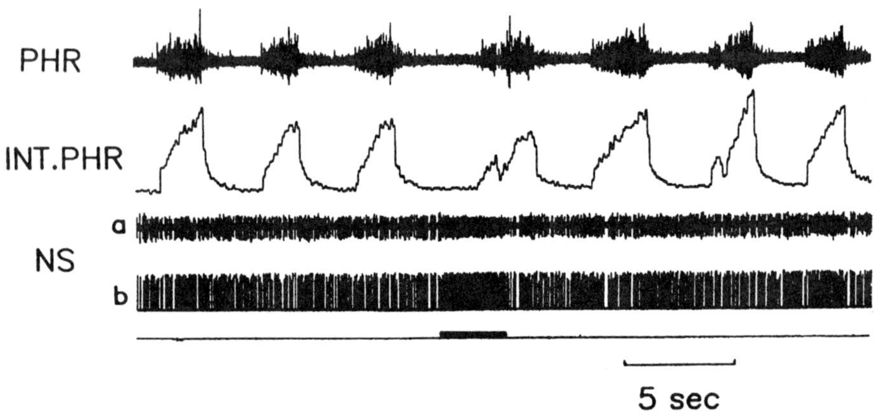

Figure 17 Effect of mechanical stimulation of nasal mucosa just inside nostril on neuronal spikes (NS; a = raw, b = window discriminated) of mesencephalic neuron that had already been shown to develop respiratory-associated rhythm when respiratory drive was high. The excitation of the neuron was accompanied by an inhibition of phrenic (phr., int.phr.) activity and resetting of respiratory rhythm.

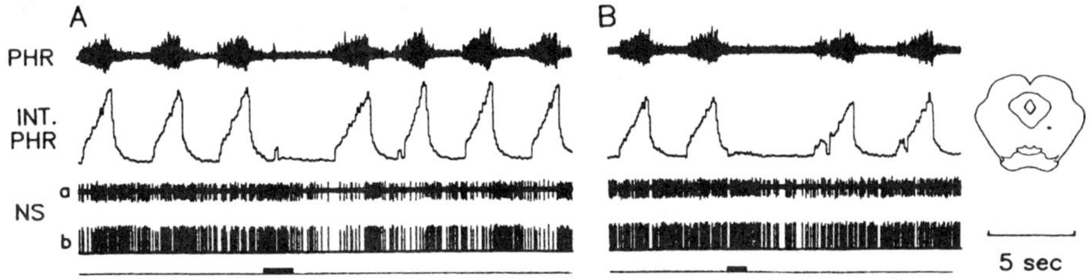

Figure 18 Effect of electrical stimulation of ninth nerve distal to insertion of CSN (A) and superior laryngeal nerve (B) on spikes of mesencephalic neuron (NS; a = raw, b = window discriminated) that had respiratory-associated rhythm. Both inputs led to an excitatory response in the neuron while inhibiting phrenic (phr., int. phr.) activity.

finding suggests that information from the carotid bodies about both CO_2 and O_2 stimulation is able to access the supramedullary brain without a necessary facilitatory effect on medullary respiratory drive.

B. Cortex

Evoked Potentials

Sensations related to stimulation of mechanical receptors in the respiratory system obviously can be perceived at the cortical level; they were discussed briefly earlier and are detailed in Chap. 4.

The transmission of these inputs to the somatosensory cortex has been demonstrated by the recording and averaging over a number of trials of cortical electrical potentials that are evoked by various events, such as occlusion of the airway (Davenport et al., 1986), resistive loads (Bloch et al., 1990), and electrical stimulation of low-threshold afferents (Group I and II) from intercostal muscles (Gandevia and Macefield, 1989) in awake human subjects.

The latency of the cortical evoked responses (CEP) in the first two reports was longer than in comparable studies involving mechanical stimulation of limbs, perhaps because of slower activation of respiratory receptors. The study of Gandevia and Macefield (1989), however, which used a precisely timed stimulus to afferent respiratory nerves, yielded responses that were consistent with a short-latency projection to the human cerebral cortex.

Revelette and Davenport (1990) found that the latency of the CEP became shorter and its magnitude greater if airway occlusion were performed at mid-inspiration rather than at the onset of inspiration. Latency of the CEP is also shorter at increased levels of central respiratory drive, expressed as the $P_{0.1}$ occlusion pressure (Davenport et al., 1986), or produced by increased P_{CO_2} (Davenport et al., 1993a). The findings are consistent with activation by central respiratory drive (corollary discharge) of neurons in the sensory pathway, so that

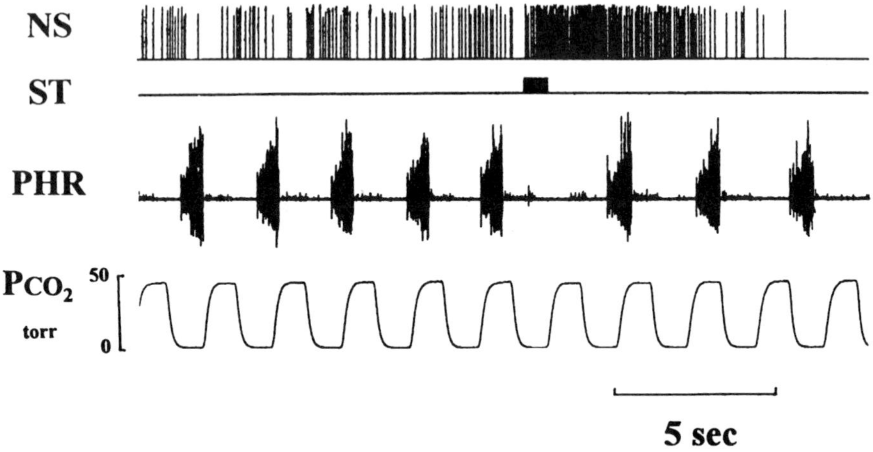

Figure 19 Nerve spikes (NS) in mesencephalic respiratory-associated neuron before and after brief (<1 s) electrical stimulation (ST) of carotid sinus nerve. Note rapid excitatory response in neuron along with prolongation of expiration and resetting of phrenic (phr) rhythm.

they are closer to a threshold for transmission of the mechanical inputs to the cortex.

There are also reports of cortical potentials or changes in the electroencephalogram (EEG) evoked in anesthetized animals by mechanical and electrical stimulation of intercostal muscles (Davenport et al., 1993b), by electrical stimulation of vagus nerves (O'Brien et al., 1971; Balzamo et al., 1990) and chemical (pheylydiguanide) stimulation of thin-fiber pulmonary receptors (Balzamo and Jammes, 1989), by electrical stimulation of phrenic nerve afferents (Davenport et al., 1985), and by electrical stimulation of tongue, face, and superior laryngeal nerves (O'Brien et al., 1971). The latter authors even showed that some individual neurons in the sensory cortex could be excited by traction of the tongue or electrical stimulation of vocal cords.

Respiratory-Associated Potentials

The only studies of cortical potentials that show a convincing relation to respiration itself are those of Kumagai et al. (1966) performed in unanesthetized but paralyzed cats. These investigators reported EEG responses in midbrain and sensory cortex with each respiration, as indexed by phrenic activity. The timing of the response, late inspiratory/postinspiratory, was similar to those neurons reported by Chen et al. (see Sec. IV.B) in midbrain and thalamus that responded to centrally generated respiratory drive. The findings are plausible because of the absence of general anesthesia and a probable high-level respiratory neural drive following multiple surgical procedures and support a conclusion that the medullary collateral discharge related to respiration has access to the cortex.

There are other reports in human beings of changes in EEG associated with breathing (Darrow et al., 1953; Fenyö and Hazsnos, 1964; Lehman and Knauss, 1964; Grözinger et al., 1974). Several are very brief reports. The studies were performed in resting subjects with unstressed respiration. A perusal of the published findings leaves one less than convinced of their validity.

C. Summary

The neurophysiological studies show that there are pathways in pons, mesencephalon, and thalamus whose neurons develop firing with each respiratory burst, once a level of medullary respiratory neural drive exceeds a certain threshold. This information appears to be transmitted to the cortex. At the same time, it is clear that most of the other neural inputs from the respiratory system (from upper airways, lungs and lower airways, respiratory muscles and thorax, and peripheral chemoreceptors) that have been postulated as important in respiratory sensation also activate some neurons in pons, mesencephalon, and thalamus; this information can also be transmitted to the cortex. Most of the inputs are primarily excitatory to the neurons, with the exception of the inhibitory effect of pulmonary stretch receptors, and have relatively short latencies.

Some of the neurons may subserve only one modality, for example the neurons in our experiments that developed a ventilator-related firing from chest movement but not the firing related to centrally generated respiratory drive. Others are clearly multimodal; that is, the longer latency response to medullary drive input and the shorter latency responses to other inputs occur in the same neuron. If these neurons are, as postulated, involved in respiratory sensation and dyspnea, then they provide beginning integration of the inputs at a level of the brain at least as low as the pons and mesencephalon.

V. An Integration

Both neurophysiological and some psychophysical studies suggest that it is possible for the effects of a single input to reach the cortex and consciousness as nondyspneic somatic sensations. It is likely that some of this input is transmitted by single-modality neurons and pathways, as in specific pain mechanisms (Cervero and Laird, 1991), although combinations of inputs may still be required for perceptions of common respiratory sensations, such as position, movement, volume changes, and muscular tension. As for the unpleasant diffuse sensation of dyspnea, it is more likely to be associated with multiple inputs, like some kinds of pain.

We have already noted our belief that the medullary respiratory neural drive signal (corollary discharge) is the most important of the various inputs; it probably leads to the air hunger kind of sensation so clearly demonstrated in ventilated quadriplegics (Banzett et al., 1989). It seems to be a basic requirement for the development of dyspnea in most of the settings in which it occurs. In this regard, it is important that there is a neural threshold for increased central drive below which the sensation is not generated. This would explain the lack of dyspnea in normal subjects with moderately increased respiratory activity during exercise and also the ready development of dyspnea in patients with impaired respiratory function and increased drive at rest.

How then does one explain the apparently different sensations of dyspnea reported by Simon et al. (1989, 1990) and Elliott et al. (1991)? Although we stated earlier that inputs other than central respiratory drive are modifiers of effects of drive, we believe that a broader view is required. In addition to the modality-specific pathways, there are clearly multimodal neurons and nonspecific pathways that receive not only the corollary discharge from the medulla but also inputs from most areas of the respiratory system, and others, such as the face. Stein and Meridith (1993) note that neurons in the brain that are capable of receiving more than one input are widespread; they point out that there must be integration of different inputs at the level of single neurons and that multimodal stimulation is likely to be associated with the same event. The ultimate result is that the sensory perception is a function of spatial and temporal patterns of activation of non-specific pathways, as well as of the effects of specific pathways, to and in the cortex.

These considerations apply to the sensation of dyspnea. It is likely that all of the inputs shown to activate neurons that are also activated by central drive make a contribution to the sensation once the neurons are above their threshold. Although it might be thought that most of the respiratory inputs occur simultaneously, for example during inspiration, this is probably not correct; there will be, because of subtly different times of activation of receptors and different latencies to central neurons, differences in patterns and magnitudes of the various inputs, especially with disease. We suggest that it is these differences that account for the different sensory experiences.

In concluding this perspective, we would add two additional comments on potential effects of respiratory sensory input to the cortex.

One is that the complex processing of cortical inputs that leads to conscious perception of the sensations, especially the distressful sensations, also leads, by a long feedback loop to the respiratory controller, to a modification of breathing patterns to minimize the distress and sense of respiratory effort (Chonan et al., 1990a). Such a response is clearly behavioral and perhaps even learned. One must question whether it is "voluntary" in a strict sense of the term. (See Chap. 9 for further discussion.)

The second is the possibility that the mechanisms activating neurons in mesencephalon and thalamus not merely lead to a sensory experience but also have a role in causing arousals from sleep, such as occur in periodic breathing, for example Cheyne-Stokes breathing or obstructive sleep apnea. It has been reported that arousals during sleep apnea are related not to the level of chemical stimulation per se but rather to the level of respiratory neural drive (Gleeson et al., 1990). The neurophysiological findings provide a mechanistic basis for such information reaching the thalamus and/or cortex to cause such arousals.

Acknowledgments

The authors' experiments reviewed here and the review itself were supported by U.S. Public Health Service Merit Award Grant HL-17689.

References

Adams, L., and Guz, A. (1991). Dyspnea on exertion. In: Exercise: Pulmonary Physiology and Pathophysiology. Edited by B.J. Whipp and K. Wasserman. Dekker, New York, pp. 449–494.

Adams, L., Lane, R., Shea, S.A., Cockcroft, A., and Guz, A. (1985). Breathlessness during different forms of ventilatory stimulation: a study of mechanisms in normal subjects and respiratory patients. Clin. Sci. 69:663–672.

Altose, M., Cherniack, N., and Fishman, A.P. (1985). Respiratory sensations and dyspnea. J. Appl. Physiol. 58:1051–1054.

Altose, M., Chonan, T., and Mulholland, M.B. (1988). Comparison of the sensation of effort of breathing and shortness of breath during exercise and voluntary hyperventilation. Am. Rev. Respir. Dis. 137:387.

Aminoff, M.J., and Sears, T.A. (1971). Spinal integration of segmental, cortical and breathing inputs to thoracic respiratory motoneurones. J. Physiol. (Lond.) 215: 557–575.

Arshavsky, Y.I., Orlovski, G.N., and Perret, C. (1988). Activity of rubrospinal neurons during locomotion and scratching in the cat. Behav. Brain Res. 28:193–199.

Balzamo, E., and Jammes, Y. (1989). Vagal afferents and EEG rhythms in the SI area in anesthetized cats: similarities between responses to electrical and chemical (phenyldiguanide) stimulations. Arch. Int. Physiol. Biochim. 979:483–492.

Balzamo, E., Gayan-Ramirez, G., and Jammes, Y. (1990). Pulmonary vagal afferents and spontaneous EEG rhythms in the cat sensorimotor cortex. J. Autom. Nerv. Sys. 30: 149–158.

Banner, N.R., Lloyd, M.H., Hamilton, R.D., Innes, J.A., Guz, A., and Yacoub, M. (1989). Cardiopulmonary response to dynamic exercise after heart and combined heart-lung transplantation. Br. Heart J. 61:215–223.

Banzell, R.B., Lansing, R.W., and Brown, R. (1987). High-level quadriplegics perceive lung volume changes. J. Appl. Physiol. 62:567–573.

Banzett, R.B., Lansing, R.W., Reid, M.B., Adams, L., and Brown, L. (1989). "Air hunger" arising from increased P_{CO_2} in mechanically ventilated quadriplegics. Respir. Physiol. 76:53–68.

Banzett, R.B., Lansing, R.W., Brown, R., Topulos, G.P., Yager, D., Steele, S.M., Londoño, B., Loring, S.H., Reid, M.B., Adams, L., and Nations, C.S. (1990). "Air hunger" from increased P_{CO_2} persists after complete neuromuscular block in humans. Respir. Physiol. 81:1–18.

Bartlett, D., Jr. (1986). Upper airway motor systems. In: Handbook of Physiology. Section 3. The Respiratory System, Vol. II, Control of Breathing, Part 2. Edited by N.S. Cherniack and J.G. Widdicombe. American Physiological Society, Bethesda, MD, pp. 223–245.

Bartoli, A., Bystrzycka, E., Guz, A., Jain, S.K., Noble, M.I.M., and Trenchard, D. (1973). Studies of the pulmonary vagal control of central respiratory rhythm in the absence of breathing movements. J. Physiol. (Lond.) 230:449–465.

Bassal, M., and Bianchi, A.L. (1982). Inspiratory onset or termination induced by electrical stimulation of the brain. Respir. Physiol. 50:23–40.

Bassal, M., Bianchi, A.L., and Dussardier, M. (1981). Effets de la stimulation des structures nerveuses centrales sur l'activité des neurones respiratoires chez le chat. J. Physiol. (Paris) 77:779–795.

Bayev, K.V., Beresovskii, V.K., Kebkalo, T.G., and Savoskina, L.A. (1988). Afferent and efferent connections of brainstem locomotor regions: study by means of horseradish peroxidase transport technique. Neuroscience 26:871–891.

Bloch, E., Harver, A., and Squires, N.K. (1990). Event-related potentials elicited by resistive loads in normal subjects. Am. Rev. Respir. Dis. 141:A308.

Bolser, D.C., Lindsey, B.G., and Shannon, R. (1983). Inhibition of medullary inspiratory drive by intercostal muscle tendon organs. Soc. Neurosci. Abstr. 9:1160.

Bradley, G.W., Noble, M.I.M., and Trenchard, D. (1976). The direct effect on pulmonary stretch receptor discharge produced by changing lung carbon dioxide concentration in dogs on cardiopulmonary bypass and its action on breathing. J. Physiol. (Lond.) 261:359–373.

Brodal, A. (1981). The reticular formation and some related nuclei. In: Neurological Anatomy in Relation to Clinical Medicine, 3rd edition. Oxford University Press, New York, pp. 394–447.

Campbell, E.J.M., Gandevia, S.C., Killian, K.J., Mahutte, C.K., and Rigg, J.R.A. (1980). Changes in the perception of inspiratory resistive loads during partial curarization. J. Physiol. (Lond.) 309:93–100.

Cervero, F., and Laird, J.M.A (1991). One pain or many pains? A new look at pain mechanisms. NIPS 6:268–273.

Cheema, S.S., Rustioni, A., and Whitsel, B.L. (1984). Light and electron microscopic evidence for direct corticospinal projection to superficial laminae of the dorsal horn in cats and monkeys. J. Comp. Neurol. 225:276–290.

Chen, Z., and Eldridge, F.L. (1992). Relations of respiratory-associated (R-A) rhythmic activities of neurons in pons and midbrain. FASEB J. 6:A1828.

Chen, Z., and Eldridge, F.L. (1993). Upper airway and facial inputs stimulate midbrain neurons with respiratory-associated firing. FASEB J. 7:A459.

Chen, Z., Eldridge, F.L., and Wagner, P.G. (1991). Respiratory-associated rhythmic firing of midbrain neurones in cats: relation to level of respiratory drive. J. Physiol. (Lond.) 437:305–325.

Chen, Z., Eldridge, F.L., and Wagner, P.G. (1992). Respiratory-associated thalamic activity is related to level of respiratory drive. Respir. Physiol. 90:99–113.

Chonan, T., Mulholland, M.B., Altose, M.D., and Cherniack, N.S. (1990a). Effects of changes in level and pattern of breathing on the sensation of dyspnea. J. Appl. Physiol. 69:1290–1295.

Chonan, T., Mulholland, M.B., Leitner, J., Altose, M.D., and Cherniack, N.S. (1990b). Sensation of dyspnea during hypercapnia, exercise, and voluntary hyperventilation. J. Appl. Physiol. 68:2100–2106.

Chronos, N., Adams, L., and Guz, A. (1988). Effect of hyperoxia and hypoxia on exercise-induced breathlessness in normal subjects. Clin. Sci. 74:531–537.

Coleridge, H.M., and Coleridge, J.C.G. (1986). Reflexes evoked from tracheo-bronchial tree and lungs. In: Handbook of Physiology. Section 3. The Respiratory System, Vol. II, Control of Breathing, Part 2. Edited by N.S. Cherniack and J.G. Widdicombe, American Physiological Society, Bethesda, MD, pp. 395–429.

Corda, M., von Euler, C., and Lennerstrand, G. (1965). Proprioceptive innervation of the diaphragm. J. Physiol. (Lond.) 178:161–177.

Corda, M., von Euler, C., and Lennerstrand, G. (1966). Reflex and cerebellar influences on α and on "rhythmic" and "tonic" γ activity in the intercostal muscle. J. Physiol. (Lond.) 184:898–923.

Corfield, D.R., Murphy, K., and Guz, A. (1993). Does cortical activation of the human diaphragm act via brainstem respiratory centres? J. Physiol. (Lond.) 467:17P.

Darrow, C.W., Stroup, M., Kris, C., Arnott, G.P., Brudo, C., and Ginsburg, N. (1953). Cyclic respiratory and cardiac changes in EEG. Electroenceph. Clin. Neurophysiol. Suppl. 3:44.

Davenport, P.W., Thompson, F.J., Reep, R.L., and Freed, A.N. (1985). Projection of phrenic nerve afferents to cat sensorimotor cortex. Brain Res. 328:150–153.

Davenport, P.W., Friedman, W.A., Thompson, F.J., and Franzén, O. (1986). Respiratory-related cortical potentials evoked by inspiratory occlusion in humans. J. Appl. Physiol. 60:1843–1848.

Davenport, P.W., Holt, G.A., and Hill, P.M. (1993a). The effect of increased inspiratory drive on the sensory activation of the cerebral cortex by inspiratory occlusion. In: Respiratory Control: Central and Peripheral Mechanisms. Edited by D.F. Speck, M.S. Dekin, W.R. Revelette, and D.T. Frazier. University Press of Kentucky, Lexington, pp. 216–221.

Davenport, P.W., Shannon, R., Mercak, A., Reep, R.L., and Lindsey, B.G. (1993b). Cerebral cortical evoked potentials elicited by cat intercostal muscle mechanoreceptors. J. Appl. Physiol. 74:799–804.

Dean, J.B., Bayliss, D.A., Erickson, J.T., Lawing, W.L., and Millhorn, D.E. (1990). Depolarization and stimulation of neurons in nucleus tractus solitarii by carbon dioxide does not require chemical synaptic input. Neuroscience 36:207–216.

Decima, E.E., von Euler, C., and Thoden, U. (1967). Spinal intercostal-phrenic reflexes. Nature 215:312–313.

Eldridge, F.L. (1976). Expiratory effects of brief carotid sinus nerve and carotid body stimulations. Respir. Physiol. 26:395–410.

Eldridge, F.L., and Chen, Z. (1992). Respiratory-associated rhythmic firing of midbrain neurons is modulated by vagal input. Respir. Physiol. 90:31–46.

Eldridge, F.L., and Millhorn, D.E. (1986). Oscillation, gating, and memory in the respiratory control system. In: Handbook of Physiology. Section 3. The Respiratory System, Vol. II, Control of Breathing, Part 2. Edited by N.S. Cherniack and J.G. Widdicombe, American Physiological Society, Bethesda, MD, pp. 93–114.

Eldridge, F.L., and Paydarfar, D. (1989). Desynchronized respiratory rhythms and their interactions in cats with split brain stems. J. Physiol. (Lond.) 410:513–532.

Eldridge, F.L., and Waldrop, T.G. (1991). Neural control of breathing during exercise. In: Exercise: Pulmonary Physiology and Pathophysiology. Edited by B.J. Whipp and K. Wasserman. Dekker, New York, pp. 309–370.

Eldridge, F.L., Gill-Kumar, P., and Millhorn, D.E. (1981). Input-output relationships of central neural circuits involved in respiration in cats. J. Physiol. (Lond.) 311:81–95.

Eldridge, F.L., Kiley, J.P., and Millhorn, D.E. (1985a). Respiratory responses to medullary hydrogen ion changes in cats: different effects of respiratory and metabolic acidoses. J. Physiol. (Lond.) 358:285–297.

Eldridge, F.L., Millhorn, D.E., Kiley, J.P., and Waldrop, T.G. (1985b). Stimulation by central command of locomotion, respiration and circulation during exercise. Respir. Physiol. 59:313–337.

Eldridge, F.L., Sinclair, J.D., and Wagner, P.G. (1990). Phase resetting of the respiratory cycle by auditory stimuli demonstrated in decerebrate cats. J. Physiol. (Lond.) 423:28P.

Elliott, M.K., Adams, L., Cockcroft, A., Macrae, K.D., Murphy, K., and Guz, A. (1991). The language of breathlessness. Am. Rev. Respir. Dis. 144:826–832.

Feldman, J.L. (1986). Neurophysiology of breathing in mammals. In Handbook of Physiology. The Nervous System, Vol. IV, Intrinsic Regulatory Systems of the Brain. Edited by F.E. Bloom. American Physiological Society, Bethesda, MD, pp. 463–524.

Feldman, J.L., McCrimmon, D.R., Smith, J.C., Ellenberger, H.H., and Speck, D.D. (1987). Respiratory pattern generation in mammals. In: Neurobiology of the Control of Breathing. Edited by C. von Euler and H. Lagercrantz. Raven Press, New York, pp. 157–164.

Fenyö, E., and Hasznos, T. (1964). Periodic EEG complexes in subacute panencephalitis: reactivity, response to drugs and respiratory relationships. Electorenceph. Clin. Neurophysiol. 16:446–458.

Fitzgerald, R.S., and Lahiri, S. (1986). Reflex responses to chemoreceptor stimulation. In: Handbook of Physiology. Section 3. The Respiratory System, Vol. II, Control of Breathing, Part 2. Edited by N.S. Cherniack and J.G. Widdicombe. American Physiological Society, Bethesda, MD, pp. 313–362.

Flume, P.A., Eldridge, F.L., and Edwards, L.J. (1993). Role of vagal input in the relief of the distress of breathholding: normals vs. pts. with double lung transplants. Am. Rev. Respir. Dis. 147:A550.

Flume, P.A., Eldridge, F.L., Edwards, L.J., and Houser, L.M. (1994). The Fowler breath-holding study revisited: continuous rating of respiratory sensation. Respir. Physiol. 95:53–66.

Fowler, W.S. (1954). Breaking point of breath-holding. J. Appl. Physiol. 6:539–545.
Freedman, S., Lane, R., and Guz, A. (1987). Breathlessness and respiratory mechanics during reflex or voluntary hyperventilation in patients with chronic airflow limitation. Clin. Sci. 73:311–318.
Gandevia, S.C., and Macefield, G. (1989). Projection of low-threshold afferents from human intercostal muscles to the cerebral cortex. Respir. Physiol. 77:203–214.
Gandevia, S.C., and Rothwell, J.C. (1987). Activation of the human diaphragm from the motor cortex. J. Physiol. (Lond.) 384:109–118.
Gandevia, S.C., Killian, K.J., and Campbell, E.J.M. (1981). The effect of respiratory muscle fatigue on respiratory sensations. Clin. Sci. 60:463–466.
Gautier, H. (1972). Respiratory and heart rate responses to auditory stimulation. Physiol. Behav. 8:327–332.
Gleeson, K., Zwillich, C.W., and White, D.P. (1990). The influence of increasing ventilatory effort on arousal from sleep. Am. Rev. Respir. Dis. 142:295–300.
Gottfried, S.B., Leech, I., DiMarco, A.F., Zaccardelli, W., and Altose, M.D. (1984). Sensation of respiratory force following low cervical spinal cord transection. J. Appl. Physiol. 57:989–994.
Green, J.F., Schmidt, N.D., Schultz, H.D., Roberts, A.M., Coleridge, H.M., and Coleridge, J.C.G. (1984). Pulmonary C-fibers evoke both apnea and tachypnea of pulmonary chemoreflex. J. Appl. Physiol. 57:562–567.
Grözinger, B., Kriebel, J., and Kornhuber, H.H. (1974). Respiration correlated brain potentials. J. Interdiscipl. Cycle Res. 5:287–294.
Haas, F., Distenfeld, S., and Axen, K. (1986). Effects of perceived musical rhythm on respiratory pattern. J. Appl. Physiol. 61:1185–1191.
Hamilton, R.D., Winning, A.J., Perry, A., and Guz, A. (1987). Aerosol anesthesia increases hypercapnic ventilation and breathlessness in laryngectomized humans. J. Appl. Physiol. 63:2286–2292.
Harada, Y., Kuno, M., and Wang, Y.Z. (1985). Differential effects of carbon dioxide and pH on central chemoreceptors in the rat respiratory center in vitro. J. Physiol. (Lond.) 368:679–693.
Heywood, P., Morell, M.J., Moosavi, S., Stevens, J., and Guz, A. (1993). Ventilatory control awake, asleep and during exercise in man with unilateral rostral ventrolateral medullary lesions. Abstr. XXXII Cong. Int. Union Physiol. Sci., Glasgow, p. 191.
Hobson, J.A., and Steriade, M. (1986). Neuronal basis of behavioral state control. In: Handbook of Physiology. Section I. The Nervous System, Vol. IV. Intrinsic Regulatory Systems of the Brain. Edited by F.E. Bloom. American Physiological Society, Bethesda, MD, pp. 701–823.
Homma, I., Obata, T., Sibuya, M., and Uchida, M. (1984). Gate mechanism in breathlessness caused by chest wall vibration in humans. J. Appl. Physiol. 56:8–11.
Hugelin, A. (1986). Forebrain and midbrain influence on respiration. In: Handbook of Physiology. Section 3. The Respiratory System, Vol. II, Control of Breathing, Part 2, Edited by N.S. Cherniack and J.G. Widdicombe. American Physiological Society, Bethesda, MD, pp. 69–91.
Huttenlocher, P.R. (1961). Evoked and spontaneous activity of single units of medial brain stem during natural sleep and waking. J. Neurophysiol. 24:451–468.

Jammes, Y. (1988). Tonic sensory pathways of the respiratory system. Eur. Respir. J. 1: 176–183.
Jammes, Y., Buchler, B., Delpierre, S., Rasidakis, A., Grimaud, C., and Rousos, C. (1986). Phrenic afferents and their role in inspiratory control. J. Appl. Physiol. 60:854–860.
Jung-Calliol, M.C., and Duron, B. (1976). Number of neuromuscular spindles and electrical activity of respiratory muscles. In: Respiratory Centres and Afferent Systems. Edited by B. Duron. INSERM, Paris, Vol. 59, pp. 165–174.
Kiley, J.P., Eldridge, F.L., and Millhorn, D.E. (1985). The roles of medullary extracellular and cerebrospinal fluid pH in control of respiration. Respir. Physiol. 59:117–130.
Killian, K.J., and Campbell, E.J.M. (1991). Dyspnea. In: The Lung: Scientific Foundations. Edited by R.G. Crystal and J.B. West. Raven Press, New York, pp. 1433–1443.
Killian, K.J., Gandevia, S.C., Summers, E., and Campbell, E.J.M. (1984). Effect of increased lung volume on perception of breathlessness, effort and tension. J. Appl. Physiol. 57:686–691.
Kimoff, R.J., Cheong, T.H., Cosio, M.G., Guerraty, A., and Levy, R.D. (1990). Pulmonary denervation in humans. Effects on dyspnea and ventilatory pattern during exercise. Am. Rev. Respir. Dis. 142:1034–1040.
Kumagai, H., Sakai, F., Sakuma, A., and Hukuhara, T. (1966). Relationship between activity of respiratory center and EEG. Prog. Brain Res. 21:98–111.
Lane, R., Cockcroft, A., and Guz, A. (1987). Voluntary isocapnic hyperventilation and breathlessness during exercise in normal subjects. Clin. Sci. 73:519–523.
Lane, R., Adams, L., and Guz, A. (1990). The effects of hypoxia and hypercapnia of perceived breathlessness during exercise in humans. J. Physiol. (Lond.) 428:579–593
Lehman, D., and Knauss, T.A. (1964). Relations between EEG patterns and phases of the respiratory cycle. Electroenceph. Clin. Neurophysiol. 17:714.
Lipski, J., Bektas, A., and Porter, R. (1986). Short latency inputs to phrenic motoneurones from the sensorimotor cortex in the cat. Exp. Brain. Res. 61:280–290.
Luiten, P.G.M., ter Horst, G.J., Karst, H., and Steffens, A.B. (1985). The course of paraventricular hypothalamic efferents to autonomic structures in medulla and spinal cord. Brain Res. 329:374–378.
Manning, H.L., Basner, R., Ringler, J., Rand, C., Fencl, V., Weinberger, S.E., Weiss, J.W., and Schwartzstein, R.M. (1991). Effect of chest wall vibration on breathlessness in normal subjects. J. Appl. Physiol. 71:175–181.
Manning, H.L., Shea, S.A., Schwartzstein, R.M., Lansing, R.W., Brown, R., and Banzett, R.B. (1992). Reduced tidal volume increases "air hunger" at fixed P_{CO_2} in ventilated quadriplegics. Respir. Physiol. 90:19–30.
McBride, B., and Whitelaw, W.A. (1981). A physiological stimulus to upper airway receptors in humans. J. Appl. Physiol. 51:1189–1197.
Millhorn, D.E., and Eldridge, F.L. (1986). Role of ventrolateral medulla in regulation of respiratory and cardiovascular systems. J. Appl. Physiol. 61:1249–1263.
Morton, D.R., Klassen, K.P., and Curtis, G.M. (1950). The clinical physiology of the human bronchi. I. Pain of tracheobronchial origin. Surgery 28:699–704.
Nilsestuen, J.O., Coon, R.L., Woods, M., and Kampine, J.P. (1981). Location of lung receptors mediating the breathing frequency response to pulmonary CO_2. Respir. Physiol. 45:343–355.

O'Brien, J.H., Pimpaneau, A., and Albe-Fessard, D. (1971). Evoked cortical responses to vagal, laryngeal and facial afferents in monkeys under chloralose anaesthesia. Electroenceph. Clin. Neurophysiol. 31:7–20.

Onimaru, H., Arata, A., and Homma, I. (1987). Localization of respiratory rhythm-generating neurons in the medulla of brainstem-spinal cord preparations from newborn rats. Neurosci. Lett. 78:151–155.

Pack, A.I., Delaney, R.G., and Fishman, A.P. (1981). Augmentation of phrenic neural activity by increased rates of lung inflation. J. Appl. Physiol. 50:149–161.

Phillipson, E.A., and Bowes, G. (1986). Control of breathing during sleep. In: Handbook of Physiology. Section 3. The Respiratory System, Vol. II, Control of Breathing, Part 2. Edited by N.S. Cherniack and J.G. Widdicombe. American Physiological Society, Bethesda, MD, pp. 649–689.

Pinsker, H.M., and Ayers, J. (1983). Neuronal oscillators. In: The Clinical Neurosciences. Vol. V, Neurobiology. Edited by W.D. Willis, Jr. Churchill Livingston, New York, pp. V203–V266.

Preiss, G., Kirchner, F., and Polosa, C. (1975). Patterning of sympathetic preganglionic neuron firing by the central respiratory drive. Brain Res. 87:363–374.

Remmers, J.E. (1976). Functional role of the inspiratory terminating reflex from intercostal muscle spindles. In: Respiratory Centres and Afferent Systems. Edited by B. Duron. INSERM, Paris, Vol. 59, pp. 181–191.

Revelette, W.R., and Davenport, P.W. (1990). Effects of timing of inspiratory occlusion on cerebral evoked potentials in humans. J. Appl. Physiol. 68:282–288.

Rickard-Bell, G.C., Bystrzycka, E.K., and Nail, B.S. (1985). Cells of origin of corticospinal projections to phrenic and thoracic respiratory motoneurones in the cat as shown by retrograde transport of HRP. Brain Res. Bull. 14:39–47.

Saade, N., Bassim, Y.R., Atweh, S.F., and Jabbur, S.J. (1989). Auditory influences via cochlear nucleus on cuneate neurons in decerebrate-decerebellate cats. Brain Res. 486:403–406.

Schwartzstein, R.M., Lahive, K., Pope, A., Weinberger, S.E., and Weiss, J.W. (1987). Cold facial stimulation reduces breathlessness induced in normal subjects. Am. Rev. Respir. Dis. 136:58–61.

Schwartzstein, R.M., Manning, H.L., Weiss, J.W., and Weinberger, S.T. (1990). Dyspnea: A sensory experience. Lung 168:185–199.

Sears, T.A. (1964a). Efferent discharges in alpha and fusimotor fibres of intercostal nerves of the cat. J. Physiol. (Lond.) 174:295–313.

Sears, T.A. (1964b). Some properties and reflex connexions of respiratory motoneurones of the cat's thoracic spinal cord. J. Physiol. (Lond.) 175:386–403.

Selverston, A.I., and Moulins, M. (1985). Oscillatory neural networks. Annu. Rev. Physiol. 47:29–48.

Shannon, R. (1980). Respiratory pattern changes during costovertebral joint movement. J. Appl. Physiol. 48:862–867.

Shannon, R. (1986). Reflexes from respiratory muscles and costovertebral joints. In: Handbook of Physiology. Section 3. The Respiratory System, Vol. II, Control of Breathing, Part 2. Edited by N.S. Cherniack and J.G. Widdicombe. American Physiological Society, Bethesda, MD, pp. 431–447.

Shea, S.A., Andres, L.P., Shannon, D.C., and Banzett, R.B. (1993a). Ventilatory responses to exercise in humans lacking ventilatory chemosensitivity. J. Physiol. (Lond.) 468:623–640.

Shea, S.A., Andres, L.P., Shannon, D.C., Guz, A., and Banzett, R.B. (1993b). Respiratory sensations in subjects who lack a ventilatory response to CO_2. Respir. Physiol. 93:203–219.

Simon, P.M., Schwartzstein, R.M., Weiss, J.W., Lahive, K., Fencl, V., Teghtsoonian, M., and Weinberger, S.E. (1989). Distinguishable sensations of breathlessness in normal volunteers. Am. Rev. Respir. Dis. 140:1021–1027.

Simon, P.M., Schwartzstein, R.M., Weiss, J.W., Fencl, V., Teghtsoonian, M., and Weinberger, S.E. (1990). Distinguishable types of dyspnea in patients with shortness of breath. Am. Rev. Respir. Dis. 142:1009–1014.

Smith, J.C., Ellenberger, H.H., Ballanyi, K., Richter, D.W., and Feldman, J.L. (1991). Pre-Botzinger complex: a brainstem region that may generate respiratory rhythm in mammals. Science 254:726–729.

Spence, D.P.S., Graham, D.R., Ahmed, J., Rees, K., Pearson, M.G., and Calverley, P.M.A. (1993). Does cold air affect exercise capacity and dyspnea in stable chronic obstructive pulmonary disease? Chest 103:693–696.

Stein, B.E., and Meridith, M.A. (1993). The Merging of the Senses. MIT Press, Cambridge, MA.

Syka, J., Popelar, J., and Radil-Weiss, T. (1977). Comparison of spontaneous activity of mesencephalic reticular neurones in the waking state and during pentobarbital anaesthesia. Physiol. Bohemoslov. 26:21–30.

Taguchi, O., Kikuchi, Y., Hida, W., Iwase, N., Satoh, M., Chonan, T., and Takishima, T. (1991). Effects of bronchoconstriction and external resistive loading on the sensation of dyspnea. J. Appl. Physiol. 71:2183–2190.

Tobin, M.J. (1990). Dyspnea. Pathophysiologic basis, clinical presentation and management. Arch. Intern. Med. 150:1604–1613.

von Euler, C. (1973). The role of proprioceptive afferents in the control of respiratory muscles. Acta Neurobiol. Exp. (Warsz) 33:329–341.

Wagner, P.G., and Eldridge, F.L. (1991). Development of short-term potentiation of respiration. Respir. Physiol. 83:129–140.

Ward, S.A., and Whipp, B.J. (1989). Effects of peripheral and central chemoreflex activation on the isopnoeic rating of breathing in exercising humans. J. Physiol. (Lond.) 411:27–43.

Widdicombe, J.G. (1986). Reflexes from the upper respiratory tract. In: Handbook of Physiology. Section 3. The Respiratory System, Vol. II, Control of Breathing, Part 2. Edited by N.S. Cherniack and J.G. Widdicombe. American Physiological Society, Bethesda, MD, pp. 363–394.

Wilke, J.T., Lansing, R.W., and Rogers, C.A. (1975). Entrainment of respiration to repetitive finger tapping. Physiol. Psychol. 3:345–349.

Winning, A.J., Hamilton, R.D., Shea, S.A., Knott, C., and Guz, A. (1985). The effect of airway anaesthesia on the control of breathing and the sensation of breathlessness in man. Clin. Sci. 68:215–225.

Winning, A.J., Hamilton, R.D., and Guz, A. (1988). Ventilation and breathlessness on maximal exercise in patients with interstitial lung disease after local anaesthetic aerosol inhalation. Clin. Sci. 74:275–281.

Zechman, F.W., Jr., and Wiley, F.W., Jr., (1986). Afferent inputs to breathing: respiratory sensation. In: Handbook of Physiology. Section 3. The Respiratory System, Vol. II, Control of Breathing, Part 2. Edited by N.S. Cherniack and J.G. Widdicombe, American Physiological Society, Bethesda, MD, pp. 449–474.

3

Psychophysical Methods in the Study of Respiratory Sensation

ROBERT W. LANSING

University of Arizona
Tucson, Arizona

ROBERT B. BANZETT

Harvard School of Public Health
and Harvard Medical School
Boston, Massachusetts

I. Introduction

The aim of psychophysics is to quantify the relationship between sensory experiences and the physical stimuli that evoke them. The importance of being able to express our knowledge of any natural phenomenon numerically, at least for scientific purposes, was expressed by Kelvin (1891):

> When you can measure what you are speaking about, and express it in numbers, you know something about it; but when you cannot measure it, when you cannot express it in numbers, your knowledge is of a meager and unsatisfactory kind: it may be the beginning of knowledge, but you have scarcely, in your thoughts, advanced to the stage of science.

The quantification of perceptual phenomena can contribute to our understanding of sensory processing in several ways. (1) It establishes that subjective responses can be reliably measured and that they have an orderly relationship to physical changes. (2) It describes the perceptual performance of a particular sense modality in response to its adequate stimuli. These descriptions document the natural operating characteristics of that modality and can lead to the formulation of general laws of sensory function. (3) It enables the assessment of effects of various physiological interventions and clinical states on sensory function; the underlying mechanisms for these effects can then be studied. (4) It facilitates investigation of afferent pathways responsible for different sensory experiences, particularly when these paths can be isolated and stimulated independently. Neural processing at different stages along the pathway can also be studied in relation to the final perception.

Psychophysical methods comprise a set of generally accepted rules for the orderly presentation of physical stimuli and for the measurement of their sensory effects. The success of these methods in quantifying human sensory performance accounts for their continued use in both laboratory and clinical studies for more than a century. The most extensive information on sensory processing has been assembled for vision and hearing, in which stimuli can be controlled with great precision. The psychophysical study of respiratory sensations began relatively recently with the pioneering work of Campbell (Campbell et al., 1961) and Bakers and Tenney (1970). Respiratory studies present difficult problems of stimulus control and the selective activation of specific sensory pathways. Nevertheless, psychophysical measurement has provided us with a wealth of quantitative data on human sensitivity to various respiratory changes and has contributed to the testing of hypotheses about the neural origin of various breathing sensations. That large volume of work is summarized in other chapters of this volume, as well as in several recent reviews (Harver and Mahler, 1990; Katz-Salamon, 1988; Zechman and Wiley, 1986).

II. Psychophysics: An Overview

A. Psychophysical Experiment

Imagine that you are a subject in a psychophysical experiment. Your experience will be nearly the same as it would have been in the nineteenth century. You understand that the purpose of the study is to test your ability to detect (or rate) simple stimulus changes, usually changes in a single physical dimension, such as the intensity of a sound. You will be seated in a quiet room, isolated as much as possible from outside distractions, and confronted with an apparatus for delivering the stimuli you are to judge. The experimenter explains the "rules" for the testing session: how to position yourself, what kinds of stimuli you will be given, the timing of stimulus presentations, and the specific way you must report your sensation (for example, yes or no answers, a rating number, or a simple manual adjustment). You may be given a preview of the stimulus and allowed practice trials to familiarize yourself with the testing procedure. Stimuli will be presented to you according to a schedule (unknown to you) specifying their order, timing, and frequency of repetition. To overcome the effects of moment-to-moment changes in external or internal conditions, each stimulus is repeated as many times as practical. Despite the careful instruction and practice, you may still be uncertain about your perceptual task and, unbeknownst to the experimenter, decide on your own how you should respond.

In some laboratories you would be excluded from the study if you were inconsistent in your judgments and failed to improve with further instruction or training. If this is done, the experimenter should set the criteria for excluding you before the study is begun and should report such exclusions when publishing the data (see Revelette et al., 1984 as an example of this procedure). The practice of excluding subjects who are inconsistent in their judgments is acceptable for study of basic perceptual laws and the limits of human perception, but not for clinical or population studies. The knowledge that some individuals are inconsistent in making judgments may be important in assessing a patient's report of symptoms, for instance.

Psychophysical testing sessions are necessarily long and tedious, and there are no formally prescribed procedures for assuring constant high levels of motivation and attention. This is not surprising considering the diverse personalities of subjects studied and the degree to which their enthusiasm for the task depends on their personal interactions with the experimenter. The procedures used to deal with these "personal variables" differ widely among laboratories and unfortunately are rarely described in detail in published reports. Sensory performance is improved if subjects are informed when a stimulus is delivered, if there are suitable rest periods, and if subjects are motivated by words of encouragement and other inducements.

The constrained stimulus environment and the simple sensory tasks of the laboratory are rarely encountered in everyday life (there are exceptions, including wine tasters and sonar operators). It is important to bear this in mind when relating psychophysical results to the experiences of subjects in other circumstances. In the natural environment a person's attention would rarely be focused on a single stimulus change, and in most cases such a change might occur infrequently, unpredictably, or in a situation in which it was of little importance. Perceptual performance should therefore be better in the psychophysical laboratory. Does a person notice a change in breathing as readily while jogging in a park as when jogging on a laboratory treadmill with instructions to scale the amount of breathlessness? On the other hand, an urgent need or extended practice sometimes improves perceptual discrimination; a man worried about his heart may come to notice small changes in his chest sensations, and a blind woman may become especially attentive to things she hears and touches.

The use of a formal psychophysical protocol with precise stimulus control cannot remove the influence of life experiences and personality traits. The impact of emotional states and personal traits on breathing sensations is well documented (reviewed by Aitken et al., 1970). For example, patients with symptoms of depression or anxiety experienced breathlessness disproportionately to the severity of their pulmonary disease (Burns and Howell, 1969).

Protocols for psychophysical testing provide an operational definition of a sensation being studied, allowing one to duplicate the experiment of others or to compare results among similar studies. The importance of providing such operational definitions in measurement was recognized first in physics (Bridgman, 1927) and later by experimental psychologists. It is particularly important for psychological studies of perception in which there is greater ambiguity about the phenomena being measured. In concluding that a certain group of subjects were more "breathless" than another group, the advantage of defining breathlessness in terms of the procedures used to measure it are apparent.

B. Special Features of Respiratory Psychophysics

Psychophysical studies have shown that normal subjects can detect and rate many respiratory changes: tidal volume, absolute lung volume, minute ventilation, airway pressure, external resistance, respiratory muscle tension, and sense of exerted effort. The consistency with which this perceptual data can be obtained from individuals or groups of subjects has permitted the study of how sensory performance is affected by many experimental manipulations and clinical conditions (e.g., external loading, exercise, blood gas changes, and respiratory muscle fatigue).

The respiratory motor system is similar to other skeletal motor systems in its elemental structures and the neural pathways controlling movement (bones, joints, skeletal muscle, tendons, muscle receptors, afferent nerves, and central pathways). Respiratory and limb movements are similar in that several types of receptors and afferent pathways are stimulated with each movement, producing natural perceptions that are a mixture of these sensory signals. Both respiratory and limb muscles can be brought under exquisite voluntary control with a high level of conscious sensory processing of proprioceptive signals; the two systems might then be expected to have comparable sensitivities to force and motion. The accuracy with which a tidal volume and an arm position can be reproduced are similar, about 2% of the full range of motion (Plassman and Lansing, 1990; Martenuik et al., 1972). The slope of the curve relating volume size to perceived volume is similar to that relating the extent of arm movement to perceived movement (Bakers and Tenney, 1970; Martenuik and Ryan, 1972). Too strict a comparison is probably not justified because even for limb movements these values are influenced greatly by the rate, extent, duration, and force of the movement, the muscle strategies used, and the relative contribution of muscle, joint, and tactile afferents (Dickinson, 1976).

The respiratory system differs in several important ways from other somatomotor systems, and these must be taken into account in psychophysical studies:

1. With each breath afferent signals from the lungs, upper airways, and abdominal viscera project to the brain via cranial nerves. The mechanical linkage of rib cage and lungs assures that somatic and visceral mechanoreceptors are simultaneously stimulated during breathing movements. This large number of simultaneous afferent sources makes it difficult to assess the unique contribution of each to the perception, especially when changes in respiratory variables (pressure, volume, and flow) bring these afferent sources into play in various combinations. A similar problem, but to a lesser degree, was faced in attempts to identify the afferent sources of limb "position sense"; after more than 100 years of speculation and experimentation only recently has progress been made in identifying these (Matthews, 1977). The physiological dissociation of separate peripheral afferent paths by selectively stimulating or inactivating them is necessary to resolve these questions, but for the deep-lying muscles and visceral structures of the respiratory system this is especially difficult.
2. Psychophysical experiments on other sensory systems often present hundreds of stimuli to obtain the most sensitive and reliable measures of perceptual discrimination. The timing of respiratory variables is slow, so most kinds of stimuli can be presented no more frequently than 20 times per minute (once per breath). To avoid hypo- or hyperventilation, periods of normal breathing must be interspersed with the test trials, thus further limiting the presentation rate. Changes in blood gas stimuli take many seconds or even minutes to equilibrate, and thus presentations must be made at an even lower rate.
3. Respiratory muscles are under both automatic and behavioral control. Many psychophysical studies require voluntary breathing movements; the extrapolation of these results to normal automatic breathing must be done with caution, because the origin of motor command is quite different.
4. Sensations of respiratory discomfort have much in common with pain because of their powerful noxious quality and their consequent potency for eliciting behavioral responses. The afferent sources of these feelings are poorly understood, preventing the precise manipulation of the adequate stimulus. (See Chap. 6.) As for pain, the language available to a subject to describe these experiences is much less precise than that for vision or hearing. This can lead to confusion about what is actually measured in a psychophysical study.
5. Most people pay less attention to breathing than to body movements,

which are less automatic and are under visual guidance (excepting those whose performances require attention to breathing, such as singers, wind instrument players, and yoga practitioners). Training may optimize judgment of respiratory stimuli.

6. The blood gas manipulations introduced intentionally or otherwise in a psychophysical experiment can produce nonrespiratory effects that can complicate the subject's task of reporting respiratory sensations (e.g., the flushing, sweating, dizziness, and clouding of consciousness that may accompany hypercapnia).

C. Which Aspects of Perception Can Psychophysical Tests Measure?

Are Quantities or Qualities Measured?

Psychophysical procedures can be used to answer questions not only of how much, but of what kind. They have been used successfully to measure many kinds of subjective, often complex, experience (e.g., emotional state, pain, and esthetic quality) and can be used to assess quality as well as intensity of breathing experiences. Differences among the quality of sensations have been quantified by having subjects judge them two at a time and report if they are different, or by asking subjects to rate their degree of similarity numerically (for example, the taste of different substances). Such psychophysical judgments need not require verbal reports even though the subject or experimenter may apply labels to unique sensations identified by this procedure (for example, "sweet," "sour," "salty," or "bitter"). Psychophysical judgments of similarity have been used to derive "spatial maps" representing different qualities of pain (Clark, 1984), taste and smell (Bartoshuk, 1977; Shiffman and Erickson, 1971), and respiratory sensation (Harver et al., 1988). The measurement of affective components of breathing discomfort is of interest because these feelings can lead to changes in breathing pattern and often motivate efforts to seek clinical help.

The limitation imposed by language in the study of sensory quality is evidenced by the fact that people can apparently discriminate over 7 million different hues in psychophysical tests but can consistently identify only 7–11 hues by name (Geldard, 1953; Ratliff, 1976). Universal color systems, such as the Munsell system, are based on physically determined combinations of wavelength and intensity, not on color language; we have insufficient shared experience and language to give us confidence to select a "dusky peach" to paint our walls without looking at a sample chip. "Breathlessness" is used to describe a variety of qualitatively different breathing sensations; Howell (1970) has pointed out:

> Patients with pulmonary disease experience a number of sensations which relate to breathing, or to a disturbance of breathing. They tend to describe all of them as breathlessness, probably because of the way in which the inquiry is made by their

doctors. But when asked to describe in detail what they feel, two things become apparent: first, patients experience great difficulty in describing their sensations and, second, there is more than one sensation which may be experienced.

Melzack and Torgerson (1971) dealt systematically with the language people use to describe pain. The many words used by physicians, patients, and healthy people were clustered to obtain measures that reflected different dimensions of painful experience (intensity, location, temporal quality, emotional quality, and others). The resulting McGill pain questionnaire (Melzack, 1975) formalized the procedure for obtaining the verbal reports and quantifying different aspects of pain. This questionnaire is now widely used in clinics and laboratories to assess pain.

Using a similar approach, several groups have begun to study the language of breathing (Chap. 5). They are developing a lexicon of those breathing sensations that vary systematically with various respiratory stimuli and clinical conditions (Simon et al., 1989, 1990; Banzett et al., 1989; Elliot et al., 1991). Simple counting of the frequency with which subjects associate descriptive words with particular breathing experiences can provide a quantitative measure of differences in the perceived quality of those experiences. Such an approach is especially informative when verbal descriptors selected are subjected to appropriate statistical treatments, such as cluster analysis.

A frequent but mistaken assumption is that quantitative psychophysical studies are independent of language. Even studies yielding numerical values for thresholds or magnitude usually depend heavily on language. This is particularly true for a respiratory event with many different attributes to which the subject might attend. The experimenter's verbal instructions must enable the subject to focus on the sensory aspect of interest and assume that the subject and experimenter share a common background of perceptual experience and words to describe it. Harver and Mahler (1990) have pointed out that when asked to scale magnitude a subject may attend to only one aspect of a complex stimulus or may merge several dimensions of the experience into the dimension requested by the experimenter. For example, subjects asked to rate the size of a resistive airway load might be attending and reporting sensations of exerted effort, muscle tension, changes in airway pressure, or some mixture of these. A further complication is that as a stimulus event grows in size, for example increasing lung volume, new afferent paths may be activated, evoking a different kind of sensation. Is the experience of the last 200 ml of a vital capacity maneuver the same as the comparable volume change in mid-range? Lack of attention to real differences in quality among respiratory sensations has no doubt led experimenters in different laboratories to assume that they were measuring the same sensation when in fact they were not. Judging from the different situations in which subjects have been asked to rate breathlessness (exercise, hypercapnia, hypoventilation, and various pulmonary disorders), it is unlikely that subjects were judging the same qualitative experience (see Chap. 5).

Are Conscious or Unconscious Processes Measured?

Any stimulus that activates afferent pathways evokes responses in many regions of the brain and can influence a variety of perceptual, cognitive, and behavioral systems often without our being aware of these effects. Which aspects of the central nervous response are reflected in a subject's response to psychophysical stimuli?

If we accept the conventional usage, "conscious awareness" of an event is indicated by a person's ability to remember and describe it. Using this definition, there is now extensive experimental evidence of "perception without awareness." Stimuli of which a subject is not aware, by all ordinary standards, can be responded to, cause a shift in attention, be stored in memory, and influence thought and emotional state (Bornstein and Pittman, 1992; Dixon, 1981; Marcel, 1983). Common observation tells us that well-learned tasks can be guided by stimuli to which we do not attend and cannot recall; while thinking about this chapter, the authors have at times driven several miles through Boston traffic without remembering details of the route taken or stops at traffic lights, for example. Ordinarily, one can become aware of such stimuli by adequately focusing attention. However, there are cases in which stimuli that are not brought to awareness even with focused attention can nonetheless guide voluntary responses, as demonstrated by the "blind sight" experiments in which patients who are apparently blind to objects presented in a portion of their visual field can localize them by pointing if forced to do so (Weiskrantz, 1986). The conscious discrimination of stimuli in a psychophysical experiment thus provides only limited information about the availability of afferent signals for various types of behavioral control. If a stimulus is available to conscious awareness, it can be used in behavioral control; other stimuli that are registered and analyzed in "preconscious" central stages but not admitted to conscious perception may also be available.

Subjects typically have little confidence in their reports of stimuli near threshold. It has been repeatedly demonstrated that when forced to guess, subjects correctly discriminate stimulus changes at better than a chance level even when they claim to be unaware of them. Pierce and Jastrow (1884), in the first experiment ever performed in a psychology laboratory in the United States, found that even when their own confidence ratings were 0, they judged difference in weights correctly 61–70% of the time, and the proportion of correct choices varied with the actual differences in weight. In our own experiments with tidal volume perception using a two-alternative forced choice procedure, we found that often we and our subjects were correct in over 80% of the trials with no awareness of a stimulus change (unpublished observations). Riggs (1987) expressed the impressions of many psychologists who have served as subjects in psychophysical experiments.

> As a subject, one develops the feeing that the whole procedure is going on automatically: pairs of intervals (time) are judged, the percentages of correct choices are far above chance, and the subject is not aware of the stimuli. Could it be that some lower center of the brain is used for making such judgments so that conscious awareness is somehow bypassed?

There has been a continuing debate about "subliminal perception" and the meaning of "threshold" (summarized by Cheesman and Merikle, 1986; Dixon, 1981; Kihlstrom et al., 1992). It is now clear that we should distinguish among the thresholds obtained with different response measures and should not assume that the subject was consciously aware of the stimulus unless other evidence is provided. Thresholds obtained by different psychophysical methods, by recording evoked cortical potentials, or by triggered behaviors, such as simple reaction times, can be quite different. This suggests that the same afferent signals project to different cerebral areas and may be utilized independently by different behavioral systems. It has been shown that visual stimuli below the psychophysical threshold, determined by the sensitive forced choice method, can trigger prepared motor programs in a reaction time experiment (Taylor and McCloskey, 1990). If such effects are found for respiratory stimuli, we would have to abandon the assumption that stimuli below the conscious psychophysical threshold cannot be processed at a cortical level or participate in the behavioral control of breathing. Adjustments to various perturbations of breathing might be detected and responded to by an intermediate-level motor control system operating below the level of awareness.

A behavioral approach not based on language and conscious experience may allow a comparison of animal and human discriminations of respiratory sensory processes. There is now an extensive experimental literature in "animal psychophysics" describing the visual, auditory, and tactile discriminations of which animals are capable using behavioral conditioning procedures (Stebbins et al., 1984). Thresholds and power functions comparable to those obtained for humans have been reported (LaMotte and Mountcastle, 1975). Only a few studies have applied this approach to respiratory sensation (Davenport et al., 1991; Arieli, 1990), but it holds promise for studies of neural mechanisms of sensation that cannot be done in humans.

Are Single Sensory Attributes or Complex Perceptions Measured?

The traditional psychophysical experiment examines the change in a single sensation evoked by one type of stimulus change. Are natural perceptions simply compounds of such elemental sensory experiences? Can these sensory elements be discovered by conscious introspection? To be specific, is my perception of a ball made up of independent sensations of its size, color, shape, and brightness, each identifiable by introspection and measurable with psychophysical procedures? Can my perception of tidal volume be broken down into component sensations of chest wall motion, lung expansion, inspiratory muscle contraction, and airflow through the upper airway, and can each component be identified and quantified by introspection? These questions were the center of theoretical debates in the early half of this century, but the weight of experimental evidence suggests that the answer to all these questions is "no" (see Boring, 1950; Teuber, 1960; and Hochberg, 1984 for the history and current status of this problem). The yellow and blue lights that mix to produce the perception of gray could never be identified by introspection, but their role as cues can still be studied by experimental manipulation of wavelength and intensity. A subject may be capable of noticing the several different cues for depth perception, but the immediate compelling recognition of depth occurs without conscious analysis of the relative contribution of these (psychologists have had to identify these cues by experiment even though they personally have been relying on them for a lifetime). It has also been established that a sensation associated with a particular stimulus dimension (sound frequency) can alter the perception of another physical dimension (sound intensity) (see Teuber, 1960; Marks, 1974). These multidimensional effects make it unlikely that the investigation of the psychophysical properties of individual sensory attributes can be used to reconstruct adequately the complex perceptions that result from their combination. This does not preclude the systematic study of the effects of stimulus context or of the perceptual laws governing stimulus combinations (Marks, 1986). It is also still useful to search for the afferent paths and stimuli responsible for perception, because these must underlie complex perceptions even though the whole may not be a simple sum of the parts. Quantitative measurements of sensation when various afferent paths are interrupted or stimulated independently are effective in ascertaining which afferent pathways reach consciousness (see Chap. 6).

III. Psychophysical Measurement

A. Background

Classic psychophysics, with its origins in the work of Weber and Fechner in the nineteenth century (reviewed by Boring, 1950), was devoted primarily to determining the limits of sensory performance, that is, the least amount of stimulus energy that can be detected (absolute threshold), or the smallest change in a stimulus that can be perceived (difference threshold). The observer's simple "yes" or "no" judgments were used to measure thresholds. A systematic relationship of perceptual judgments to stimulus intensity was found: as intensities increased a larger stimulus change was necessary for them to be perceived (difference threshold). This could be expressed mathematically by the proportional relation of the difference threshold to the initial stimulus intensity (Weber's law) or by a logarithmic function (Fechner's law). Over the years these laws were found to have many exceptions, or loopholes, yet they remain useful today. Although it has been seriously questioned whether the power function can be regarded as a universal "psychophysical law" applicable to all situations and all stimuli (Uttal, 1973; Marks, 1974), there is no doubt that these functions provide a convenient metric to describe and compare sensory performance.

In the 1930s and 1940s, sensory psychologists were finding that sensations of stimulus magnitude could be estimated directly by subjects and assigned to a numerical scale rather than by determining difference thresholds; the relationship between physical and sensory intensity could best be described by a power rather than a logarithmic (Fechnerian) function (see Marks, 1974). Stevens developed the method of magnitude estimation for the direct scaling of sensations and showed that a power function, with a suitable exponent, best describes the growth of sensation with the growth of stimulus intensity regardless of the sensory modality studied (Stevens, 1956; 1961; 1975). As the result of this work, several types of direct scaling techniques are now widely used and provide convenient, sensitive measures of a subject's ability to judge the physical intensity of stimuli. These functions describe the nonlinear sensory compression that allows perception of stimuli over a wide range of physical intensities or, in other cases, expansion, which allows great sensitivity over a narrow range of stimulus intensities. Some qualifications in the interpretation of magnitude estimation data are discussed later.

A second development, signal detection theory (Green and Swets, 1966; Tanner and Swets, 1954), called into question the meaning of sensory "thresholds" as derived using classic methods and demonstrated that nonstimulus factors internal to the subject (attention, motivation, and response bias) can affect the response to a stimulus. The concepts and mathematical procedures used in this approach were derived from work on engineering problems in communication systems with electronic signals in a background of noise and were then applied to the problem of how an observer in a psychophysical experiment judged that a stimulus change had occurred. The outcome of this work was threefold: it provided a new theoretical framework for interpreting psychophysical data; it focused attention on the importance of subject variables in determining sensory judgments; and it provided a method for estimating the contribution of these nonstimulus variables. (For examples of this approach and comparisons of the results obtained with classic versus signal detection methods, see Narbed et al., 1983; Sekular et al., 1973.) The traditional procedures for determining sensory thresholds are still widely used, but the interpretation of these thresholds must take into account nonstimulus influences on the subject's judgments.

A more recent approach, which has been called cognitive psychophysics or integration psychophysics, attempts to deal with complex determinants of an observer's response to stimuli that were often neglected in traditional psychophysics (see Algom, 1992; Geissler, 1990). This approach analyzes sensory experience to simple or complex stimuli in relation to stimulus context, memory, the history of stimulation, and stimulus meaning in relation to the behavioral situation of the subject. The conventional distinction between perception and thought is rejected as an artificial partitioning of the information processing system. Perception is seen as the result of a number of unconscious operations that are inferred from the results of various experimental manipulations or from theoretical models ("computational models").

B. Some Specific Procedures: What Do the Numbers Mean?

Threshold Measures

The *absolute threshold*, the least physical stimulation a person can detect, and the *difference threshold*, the smallest stimulus change a person can detect, are expressed in physical units. The threshold is a statistical average based on repeated presentations of a range of stimulus intensities. In finding the absolute threshold, for example, strong stimuli are always perceived, weak are never perceived, and those between them are perceived only some of the time. *Threshold* is usually defined as the stimulus level that evokes a positive response at least 50% of the time, and some measure of variability is used to define the range of uncertainty in the subjects' judgments. Thresholds must be defined statistically because of uncontrollable variations in the application of stimuli and in the state of the subject from moment to moment and from one set of trials to another.

The "classic" psychophysical methods incorporate procedures to control for many of these sources of variability (Engen, 1972). For example, the "method of limits" has both an ascending and descending set of stimulus intensities to balance the effects of a subject's reluctance to report sensing the stimulus during the ascending trials and tendency to continue reporting the stimulus on the descending trials. Threshold values can be markedly affected by instructions, practice, fatigue, stimulus order, the opportunity to preview stimuli, feedback on success of discrimination, and the subject's motivation and attention. These influences can never be completely eliminated, but testing procedures can be adopted that reduce them or hold them constant for the experimental conditions being compared. The systematic manipulation of these variables to reveal the size of their effect on thresholds influence is also worthwhile. There has been little work evaluating such influences on respiratory thresholds, even though methodological differences are often cited to explain discrepancies in published reports.

Traditionally it was assumed that a "true" threshold existed for each type of stimulus but that this was always obscured by the many sources of variation just mentioned. According to signal detection theory, however, there is no single, true threshold for a given stimulus. At low levels of stimulation, near threshold, the subject's uncertainty about whether a stimulus has occurred arises from the inherent instability of the sensory neural mechanisms (internal noise) on which the stimulus signal is superimposed. In addition, a stage of judgment and decision always intervenes between afferent stimulation and the subject's response. The subject might be very cautious and say "yes" only when he or she is very confident that a stimulus was presented, or on the other hand may have a tendency to say yes even when not confident that a stimulus occurred; the latter behavior would yield a lower threshold measure than the first if there were no penalty for wrong guesses. This *decision criterion* can be influenced by many nonsensory factors, including the subject's personality, emotional state, motivation, instructions, expectations, or prior experience. For instance, the consequence (reward or punishment) of making a positive or negative response has a potent effect on the subject's decisions. Consider the detection problem of a sailor on watch in wartime deciding whether to report a vague object in the sky, which might be a bird, a friendly aircraft, or an enemy aircraft. His or her decision will be different in friendly waters that at a remote station near the enemy shore.

The signal detection task for assessing decision criterion along with other factors causing *response bias* consists of many trials when a stimulus is present, interspersed randomly with trials when the stimulus is absent. The proportion of times the subject was right (said yes when there was a stimulus or no when there was not) compared to the proportion of times the subject was wrong (said yes when there was no stimulus or no when there was one) is used to obtain independent measures of the subject's ability to discriminate a sensory signal and of the decision criterion used. This method has been used either to obtain a bias free estimate of the subject's sensory threshold or to study the influence of the various situational and personal factors that can influence it. Several laboratories have recently begun to use detection tasks in the study of respiratory thresholds (Banzett et al., 1987; Bloch-Salisbury and Harver, 1994; Bonnel et al., 1985; Narbed et al., 1983).

If observer biases are so potent an influence, how is it that precise and reproducible threshold data has been obtained in numerous studies over the years using the traditional psychophysical methods? Observer bias is probably held constant, if not eliminated, through the use of highly experienced observers (often the experimenters themselves) and standardized testing procedures. Insertion of catch trials to prevent false positive responses and instructing the subject that stimuli above threshold should be clearly perceived, procedures often used to stabilize response bias, no doubt also result in higher threshold values because subjects set a higher criterion for reporting a stimulus change.

The forced-choice method, which derives from signal detection procedures, is designed to negate the effect of the subject's expectations and decision criteria, thus providing a very sensitive, bias-free measure of sensory discrimination (Green and Swets, 1966; Jones, 1956; Swets, 1959). The forced-choice method has been used to test the discrimination of tidal volume changes and the sensory effects of hypercapnia (Banzett et al., 1987, 1989). In the two-alternative forced-choice procedure, each trial consists of two successive time intervals; the stimulus is presented in only one of these, and the subject indicates which interval contains the stimulus; a response is required even if the subject believes it is only a guess. The stimulus is presented an equal number of times in the first and second intervals in random progression, and the subject's percentage of correct choices is tested against chance. Correct choices on 50% of the trials are expected by guessing, and 75% correct is usually taken as evidence for detection of the stimulus; the exact percentage for statistically significant detection depends on the number of choice trials and the confidence level required. Differences in the percentage of correct responses can also be used to test the effect of different experimental conditions on the discrimination of suprathreshold stimuli. If 20–50 trials are required to test detection at each stimulus level adequately, the number of trials and the time required to determine a threshold value can become a serious problem. This can be partly overcome with a preliminary short series of trials to narrow the range of stimuli to be used in the main experiment or by a tracking procedure in which short series of trials repeatedly step above and below the chance detection level (Dyck, 1986).

In addition to the smallest discriminable stimulus (threshold), the strongest tolerable stimulus can be measured, thus defining a person's perceptual range. The value for this upper perceptual limit is determined by the degree of discomfort produced, the subject's willingness to tolerate it, and the experimenter's reluctance to approach harmful stimulus intensities. Thresholds and tolerance levels clearly reflect different sensory and judgmental processes, so it is not surprising to find that they are often poorly correlated. Tolerance measures are especially susceptible to the influence of personality differences and motivational factors.

Psychophysical Scaling

A usable internal representation of the intensity of physical events, ordered from weak to strong, is apparently possessed by animals, children, and preliterate societies; it does not require an internalized number system. Nonnumerical representation is evidenced to muscle contractions (increased force to adjust for heaviness), hand gestures ("it was this long"), language ("small," "tiny," and "teeny-tiny"), and symbols (the musician's pianissimo, pp, to fortissimo, ff). Numerical measurement is so much a part of our popular culture, however, that people find it easy to assign numbers to rate experiences; a scale of 1–10 is commonplace (Edwards, 1979). Some psychophysical scaling methods ask the subject to report perceived intensity using numbers; others require a nonnumerical report (verbal, analog rating scale, and muscle contractions) that can then be assigned numbers. All these are "direct scales" because final numbers are closely related to the judgments that generated them, but internal cognitive events always intervene between afferent signals and reports of perceived intensity. Private experience on which the judgments are based cannot be directly observed and must be inferred from people's scaling behavior. They may choose to scale perceptions in ways not intended by the experimenter (a numerical scale does not prevent the subject from covertly transforming the numbers to verbal categories).

Ultimate validation that intensity scales truly register private sensations is not possible, but their usefulness in describing sensory responses can judged by several criteria: (1) repeatability; (2) the degree to which they are sensitive to the stimuli of interest; (3) whether the results are consistent with those of other scaling methods; (4) "face validity," or reasonableness of the what the subject is asked to report; and (5) the degree to which the subjective scaling matches the behavioral use of gradations in physical intensity (discussed by Marks, 1974; pp. 271–278, and Mahler and Harver, 1990). By these standards the most widely used scaling procedures appear to provide reasonable estimates of several respiratory sensations (Adams and Guz, 1991; Wilson and Jones, 1989). Of the several scaling methods available there is little basis for using a particular method because of its superior ability to "capture" the inner perceptions of the subject. Selecting a scaling method is more sensibly based on the convenience of its use for specific subjects and situations, the kind of statistical treatment it permits (see scale properties), the need to compare results with that of other studies using the same procedure, stability over the time period of interest, and the experience and skill a laboratory has developed with a particular method.

Types of Scales

Scales may have ordinal, interval, or ratio properties. Ordinal data imply only that the order of the points is known; for instance, we may know that if a subject rates the sensation as severe, it feels more intense than when it is rated slight; likewise we may know that a rating of 2 is greater than a rating of 1. An interval scale implies that the increase in sensation when moving from a rating of 1 to 2 is equal to that when moving from 2 to 3, for instance, the Celsius temperature scale. A ratio scale implies that 2 is twice as big as 1, for instance, the Kelvin temperature scale. (Ordinal and interval properties are inherent in ratio scales.) All mathematical operations may not be appropriate for all types of scale: for instance, averaging and parametric statistics are not designed for use with ordinal scaling. It is difficult to verify that psychophysical scales have interval or ratio properties; the production of data in numerical form does *not* imply such properties.

Verbal category scales consist of familiar words arranged in a fixed order of increasing intensity (e.g., "none," "slight," "moderate," "strong," and "strongest"), and the subject's selections are limited by the words that anchor the extremes and define the steps between them. Giving definitions of the words increases their separation from one another and increases the consistency of their use between trials and between subjects (e.g., "extreme breathlessness means the most you have ever experienced"). This method can only be assumed to register judgments of order; because there are no numbers there is little temptation to treat the data with inappropriate parametric statistics. Verbal rating scales are especially useful for experiences subjects have described verbally over their lifetimes ("I am slightly out of breath") and for sensations that cannot be discriminated in many fine steps. Such scales are easily understood, and subjects learn to use them reliably with repeated testing.

Numerical interval scales consist of numbers assigned to the extremes of perceived intensity (e.g., 0–10) and to equal intervals along the scale. The derived psychophysical functions do not have inherent ratio properties and are not necessarily linearly related to those obtained with magnitude estimation procedures. Caution is advised in the employment of parametric statistics. The fixed range prevents the subject from reporting sensations that, in the course of the experiment, appear to lie above or below the extreme numbers. This limitation is partly countered by giving the subject a preview of the intensity range and defining more clearly what the extreme numbers mean. The size of steps between the extremes limits the resolution of the scale. Some subjects may favor certain numbers and are reluctant to move away from them, thus introducing a decision bias not unlike those described for threshold measures.

Borg Scales

The addition of familiar verbal expressions to a numerical scale can increase the consistency with which subjects use the scale positions; for example, the "Borg scales," now widely used to study respiratory sensation, were originally created to provide psychophysical measures of perceived exertion during exercise (Borg, 1962, 1970, 1982a). Beginning in the early 1960s, Borg and his associates developed scales that subjects could understand and use easily and that allowed the judgments of different subjects to be compared. Previously Borg, using Steven's method of open magnitude estimation, found that judgments of exertion were related to workload by a power function (Borg, 1962). The numbers obtained had relative but not absolute meaning and could not be used for interindividual comparisons. He developed a combined verbal-numerical category scale to overcome this problem. It was based on the reasoning that if people have acquired a common language for describing the degree of their experienced exertion (e.g., fairly light somewhat hard, hard, very hard, and so on), these words, placed along a numerical scale, could also give numbers a common meaning. Added to this was the idea that the judgments of different people could be equated by positioning the categorical steps in relation to each person's "perceptual range," bounded by the smallest perceptible and maximum tolerable sensations. Despite objections that might be raised about the comparability of these range boundaries and the meaning of the category terms for different people, the various forms of these scales have found wide usage in a variety of laboratory and clinical settings and the values obtained have been found to be consistent for an individual from time to time and to allow comparisons among subjects (Borg, 1962; Marks et al., 1983). These categorical judgments of perceived exertion were highly correlated with the size of the workload and associated physiological changes, such as heart rate (Borg, 1962).

Borg also developed a category-ratio scale that had true ratio properties as well as providing an absolute measure of perceived intensity (Borg, 1982a). This was accomplished by physically spacing the verbal expressions along the numbered scale in a manner that would yield subject ratings that were related to workload load by a power function with an exponent similar to that obtained with open magnitude procedures. The validity of this type of scale rests on evidence that the power function for perceived exertion parallels important physiological changes during work (Noble et al., 1983) and on its ability to achieve ratio scaling in other sensory modalities, such as taste and sound (Borg, 1982b; Marks et al., 1983). Although now used to study of a variety of respiratory sensations (e.g., Burdon et al., 1982; Wilson and Jones, 1989), validation of either the category or category-ratio scales against known physiological sources of these sensations is still not possible.

Visual Analog Scales

In analog scaling the subject is presented with a line representing the range of experienced intensities. The extremes may be bounded by numbers (e.g., 0 and 100) or words (e.g., "not at all breathless" and "extremely breathless"), or both. The subject judges intensity by marking a point on the line (or moving a pointer), and distance along the line is taken as the measure of sensation. In theory the subject has a continuous interval scale available for judging, with resolution limited only by the visuomotor act of marking and the ability to keep in mind the meaning of scale locations from trial to trial. In practice some subjects may elect to use only certain broad regions of the scale, especially when judging sensations that cannot be finely discriminated. Occasionally segments of the line are marked, and numbers or words added to encourage subjects to use the whole scale and to help them remember previous ratings. These scales have been widely used to study respiratory sensations, such as breathlessness (Adams and Guz, 1991). Subjects find them easy to use. Visual analog scales are especially useful in studying relative changes in respiratory sensation from one condition to another, situations in which it is not necessary to make assumptions about the formal scalar meaning of the numbers obtained. They can be used rapidly by the subject, to monitor continuously the time course of changing sensations (Adams et al., 1985; Harty et al., 1993).

Magnitude Estimations

In this method the subject selects numbers to match the perceived magnitude of a range of stimulus intensities. The experimenter may attempt to define closely how the numbers are to be used by presenting one or more levels of the stimulus; alternatively, the subject may be allowed to assign numerical values to perceived intensities, with no limitation on the numbers that can be used. (In an alternative method, magnitude production, the subject adjusts the stimulus to match a number on the perceptual scale.)

Owing to the work of Stevens and later investigators, the relationship between perceived magnitude and stimulus intensity is commonly described by a function having the form

$$R = cS^n$$

where R is the perceived intensity, S is the physical stimulus, c is a constant defining the slope, and n is the exponent of the function. In practice, the exponent is often determined by plotting log R versus log S and determining the slope of the resultant straight line (log c is the y intercept of that line). The equation is not applicable, however, if the original data have a nonzero intercept. In this case an intercept term b must be added:

$$R = cS^n + b$$

If the intercept is nonzero, the log-log plot does not yield a straight line unless the intercept is subtracted before log transformation.

Because the slope c and the intercept b can vary with such factors as the subject's choice of how to use the scale, experimental conditions, and background noise and because the exponent n is thought to reflect underlying properties of neural processing (Stevens, 1970), many investigators have concentrated on n to the exclusion of other parameters. It must be realized, however, that a great deal of information is lost when exponents alone are reported. One must know all parameters of the fitted curve to know whether sensation has changed after an intervention or is different between two groups of subjects. A difference in intercept or slope, even in the absence of a change in exponent, can imply a large difference in perceived magnitude evoked by a given stimulus. Although c and b may vary among subjects because of their choices in using the scale, they are often quite stable in an individual subject under the same conditions: in some cases a population can agree on the meaning of a scale (take, for instance, the common agreement of musicians on the meaning of a tonal scale). The usefulness of absolute numbers is reviewed by Gescheider (1988), and caution has been advised in their use in measuring respiratory sensations (Harver et al., 1986).

Figure 1 shows four hypothetical data sets (A, B, C, and D) in an individual subject. In Figure 1a, R is plotted against S; in Fig. 1b, $\log R$ is plotted against $\log S$. Note that, although the exponents are all the same (n = 0.5), the sensory

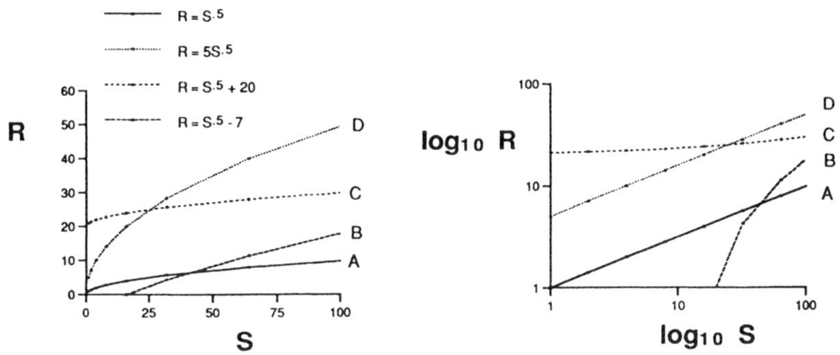

Figure 1 Hypothetical data sets in an individual subject.

responses are very different. When stimulus intensity = 65, the evoked sensations are 8 in A, 12 in B, 28 in C, and 40 in D. Notice also that in A and D, where the intercept is zero, the log-log plots are straight lines with slopes of 0.5, but B and C have curvilinear slopes. Lines A and D represent simple models of sensory response with different constants (i.e., in A, $c = 1$ and in D, $c = 5$). Line C shows a situation in which the subject reports sensation even when the experimental stimulus is turned off (i.e., $b = 20$). Line B represents a situation in which stimuli below a certain threshold are not perceived (i.e., $b = -7$).

The exponents and the shape of the sensation-stimulus plot can differ considerably among subjects; group averages often obscure the great range of individual differences (Luce and Mo, 1965; Teghtsoonian and Teghtsoonian, 1971; Teghtsoonian, 1989). The variation of exponents among subjects reflects the way they respond to the testing protocol and use the scale, as well as basic differences in their sensory neural processing (Stevens and Greenbaum, 1966). For respiratory studies, this is evident when individual data are reported (see, for example, Bakers and Tenney, 1970; Killian et al., 1981; Katz-Salamon, 1984; Stubbing et al., 1981). The exponents for a given subject, however, are usually quite consistent across experimental sessions (Hellman, 1981), giving an advantage to within-subject comparisons in studying the perceptual effect of various conditions. Lengthening the interval between testing periods reduces this consistency (Teghtsoonian, 1989). Some of the difficulties in scaling can be circumvented with cross-modality matching procedures, which do not require the use of numbers; subjects report the perceived intensity of one stimulus modality by adjusting the intensity of another (Stevens, 1959, 1975). The size of an inspiratory load, for example, can be rated by varying the strength of hand grip (Burki et al., 1978; Muza and Zechman, 1984).

The variations in testing procedure that can bias a subject's intensity scaling have been well documented for many kinds of nonrespiratory stimuli (see Gescheider, 1988; Marks, 1974; Poulton, 1968). The more prominent variations are caused by (1) the choice of an initial standard stimulus (Hellman and Zwislocki, 1961); (2) the spacing and number of stimulus levels (Teghtsoonian, 1989); and (3) order of presentation (often the judgment given on a trial is biased toward that of the immediately preceding trial) (Cross, 1973). These procedural biases may be unimportant when studying relative differences in perception between experimental conditions, when the protocol is constant and subjects are used as their own control. This does not rule out the possibility that the experimental treatment itself introduced a response bias not present under the control condition, for example, introduced a distraction that made it difficult for the subject to remember the initial standard.

IV. Psychophysics and Neural Events

Psychophysics and sensory electrophysiology provide different but complementary information about the functioning of afferent systems. The relationships between psychophysical judgments and the electrophysiological signals recorded from primary sensory afferents, central pathways, or cerebral cortex have been studied in an attempt to understand the neural processes that underlie perceptual phenomena.

A. Single Afferent Neurons

The response thresholds and power functions of single mechanoreceptive afferents have been compared to those obtained with psychophysically measured thresholds. Two important questions have been addressed. (1) Are the limits of perceptual performance set at the peripheral or at the central stages of neural processing? (2) Which receptors or primary sensory afferents contribute to the perceptual response?

Thresholds for mechanoreceptor response to vibratory stimuli in monkeys were found to correspond closely to psychophysical thresholds for vibration in both monkeys and humans (La Motte and Mountcastle, 1975; Merzenich and Harrington, 1969; Talbot et al., 1968), suggesting that, in this system, the subjective thresholds are set by the properties of peripheral neurons rather than by central mechanisms (Mountcastle, 1975). Simultaneous thresholds for single afferents and for perception have recently been obtained in response to tactile stimuli in normal alert humans using microneurographic and microstimulation techniques (Johansson and Vallbo, 1979; Vallbo, 1981; Vallbo and Johansson, 1976). For some afferents, and for some skin locations, perceptual and neural thresholds were the same, but for others the perceptual threshold was higher, showing that perception may in some cases be limited by receptor performance and in other cases by later processing stages (Vallbo, 1984). These techniques have also shown that humans can detect the firing of a single afferent neuron and that individual skin afferents can evoke specific sensations, such as pressure or tickling (Ochoa and Torebjork, 1983). Similar experiments on the relation of afferent discharge to respiratory sensory thresholds do not seem feasible at present given that the sensory neurons are less accessible for recording and discrete stimulation.

Power function exponents for peripheral nerve responses have been compared to exponents for magnitude estimations. Mountcastle and associates found a close correspondence between the intensity function of mechanoreceptor responses to tactile stimulation in monkeys and human psychophysical judgments of comparable stimuli (Mountcastle, 1967; Mountcastle and Darian-Smith, 1968). These results led to the general hypothesis that the form and slope of the psychophysical function reflect the properties of mechanoreceptive afferents and that central stages of processing are linear transformations of this input. Notwithstanding the remarkable similarities observed between neural and perceptual data, the interpretation of these results has been criticized on the grounds that the neural and perceptual measures were obtained in separate experiments (and different species), that were was great variability in the threshold and response curves of individual receptors, and that the mechanoreceptors recorded may not have been responsible for the perceptual responses (Kruger and Kenton, 1973; Uttal, 1973).

Others argue that psychophysical functions need not be determined in all cases by receptor properties because further stages of synaptic processing can easily transform the stimulus-response function (see MacKay, 1963; Stevens, 1970). Indeed, simultaneous measurements of afferent discharge and judgments of tactile intensity in humans failed to show a close agreement between the neural and psychological responses (Knibestol and Vallbo, 1980). The power exponents obtained in different individuals and different experiments varied widely for the neural recordings (0.26–1.92) and the psychophysical measures (0.36–2.09), and the exponents were not correlated. In view of these findings it is unwarranted to expect that the afferent path responsible for a specific respiratory sensation could be identified on the basis of a close match between the psychophysical power function and that of a few sampled afferent neurons.

B. Cortical Event-Related Potentials

The brain's response to sensory stimulation can be recorded from the scalp of intact human subjects as event-related potentials (ERPs), also frequently called evoked potentials. The ERPs evoked by visual, auditory, and somatosensory stimuli are well described and have been extensively studied (see Regan, 1989). Only recently have ERPs evoked by respiratory stimuli been recorded. In 1986, Davenport et al. reported that cortical potentials could be evoked by occlusion of the airway during inspiration. Since that time various laboratories have recorded ERPs following negative pressures applied at the mouth (Strobel and Daubenspeck, 1993), resistive and elastic loading (Bloch et al., 1990; Bloch-Salisbury and Harver, 1994), and electrical stimulation of intercostal nerves (Gandevia and Macefield, 1989). Respiratory ERPs are influenced by sleep (Wheatley and White, 1993), by aging (Harver et al., 1995), and by respiratory disease (Cruz et al., 1992; Harver et al., 1991; Harver and Bloch, 1992). Respiratory afferents projecting to the somatosensory cortex evoke waveforms similar to those found for somatosensory stimulation of limbs and face (Gandevia and Macefield, 1989; Davenport et al., 1986; Desmedt, 1971). The latency and amplitude of these responses can vary with the strength of the respiratory stimulus (Bloch et al., 1990; Strobel et al., 1993; Bloch-Salisbury and Harver, 1994) and the phase of the breathing cycle (Revelette and Davenport, 1990).

Apart from relationships that may exist between ERPs and psychophysical measures, respiratory ERPs have many potential applications in the study of sensory systems (Regan, 1989, reviews such applications in other modalities), for example (1) testing the integrity of sensory paths in neurological disease or during surgery; (2) providing evidence of a sensory response when a verbal report is not possible, as in infants, animals, or sleeping or sedated subjects; (3) following the functional status of the sensory paths during early development and aging; and (4) studying the effect of various neurological disorders on sensory responses. They may also be used to estimate which portions of the sensory path are affected by various interventions or clinical states: there is now considerable information about which cortical and subcortical structures give rise to the principle components of the somatosensory ERP (Allison et al., 1980; Desmedt, 1986; Goff et al., 1980). There is still doubt, however, about the precise origin of certain individual waves, and some components are thought to have several sources (Johnson, 1993; Okada et al., 1983).

Our interest here is in the relation of ERPs to psychophysical data. Can ERPs give us insight into sensory neural events not revealed by psychophysical judgments? Can certain ERP components provide a physiological index of conscious sensation? It is hoped by some that a physiological response in the form of electrical deflections can provide an objective measure of perceptual reactions without the need for psychophysical judgments. At one time Stevens saw the value of such a goal:

> If good fortune should favor us and we should find a point in the auditory system where the neural potentials keep pace with the loudness function, the happy prospect of an objective measure of the loudness exponent would appear to be opened. We could then presumably bypass the cross-modality matching procedures and their attendant variability, in favor of a signal read directly by a meter (Stevens, 1970).

In the same paragraph, however, he described the variability and noise in the electrical responses that would make such an outcome unlikely. There are several other technical reasons that a close relationship between ERPs and perception might not be found. The most important of these is the possibility that the scalp recordings of massed neural activity cannot reflect the complex patterns of neural activity that lead to or comprise perceptual judgments. The series of waveforms making up the ERP can reflect both cortical and subcortical activity, but the only neural elements that make a significant contribution to the ERP are those whose activity is highly synchronized and consistently time locked to the stimulus and that have a geometric alignment and orientation allowing their potentials to summate and be detected at the scalp (see Allison et al., 1986; Regan, 1989; Schlag, 1973). A further complication is that the spatial and temporal overlapping of the field potentials from different sources makes it difficult to determine whether an ERP waveform has a single neural origin or is a composite of several cerebral generators. These generators may even include motor pathways if the stimulus elicits a voluntary movement (Vaughan et al., 1968); cortical motor potentials have been reported during voluntary breathing movements (Lansing et al., 1973; Macefield and Gandevia, 1991). There are also procedural problems. Choices must be made about how to obtain the psychological and electrophysiological measures. The evoked potentials can vary depending on electrode sites selected, the pass band and gain of the recording system, the number of stimulus repetitions, the wave components recorded, and the features selected for measurement (amplitude, latency, and duration). Considering that different kinds of perceptual responses undoubtedly use different neural pathways, the choice of perceptual measure could determine whether a psychophysical-ERP correlation was found.

Direct comparisons of ERPs and psychophysical measures have been made for responses to visual, auditory, and somatosensory stimuli (see Regan, 1989), but to our knowledge only one such comparison has been made for responses to respiratory stimuli (Bloch-Salisbury and Harver, 1994). In some studies the ERP and perceptual judgments corresponded closely (Bloch et al., 1990; Campbell et al., 1977; Chapman et al., 1981; Ruchkin et al., 1980; Squires et al., 1975), and in others they did not (Libet et al., 1967; Regan and Spekreijse, 1986). The same was true when the power function exponents for ERP and psychophysical measures were compared (Franzen and Offenloch, 1969; Hashimoto et al., 1988; Stevens, 1970; Uttal, 1965). A close correspondence between the latency or amplitude of an ERP component and a perceptual response does not necessarily mean that the two have identical neural generators. They may simply have a common sensory input, causing the two to vary together as the stimulus intensity changes. Nevertheless, certain waveforms (e.g., long latency potentials from association cortex) are often highly correlated with perceptual measures and subject to the same behavioral influences, such as attention, motivation, expectation, and learning (Hillyard and Picton, 1987). The challenge to investigators is to devise experiments that could disprove the hypothesis that ERP and perceptual responses register the activity of different, temporally coincident, cortical systems.

Aside from the search for psychophysical-neural equivalents, how might ERP measurements be useful in understanding neural processes underlying respiratory sensation? Work with other modalities suggests that the different stages in sensory transmission and perception might be studied. The ERPs, presumed to arise from different portions of the sensory pathway, may be affected differently by the physical properties of the stimulus and by the subject's state and perceptual task. The early waves are quite sensitive to physical features of the stimulus, and later components are markedly influenced by the attentional state of the subject and cognitive aspects of the perceptual task, such as memory, recognition, and decisions (Desmedt et al., 1983; Hillyard and Picton, 1987; Pritchard, 1981). The later waves are not modality specific and are more closely related to perceptual judgments than the earlier potentials. It appears from the limited work available that these distinctions will hold for respiratory-related potentials (Strobel and Daubenspeck, 1993). This approach, which assumes a serial processing system in which each stage depends on the output of the one preceding it (Gevins, 1986; Regan, 1989), has its limitations because there are also pathways for parallel processing that bypass the serial transmission of somatosensory signals (Merzenich and Kaas, 1980).

V. Summary

Considering the known complexity of the cerebral networks responsible for perception, it is clear that no single measure can reveal how this system functions. The value of standard psychophysical methods lies in their ability to constrain the manner of stimulus presentation, control the subject's attentional state, define the perceptual task, and provide a measure of the natural output or end point of the sensory neural system. The objective measures of perception made possible by psychophysical methodology are a great improvement on anecdotal reports of symptoms and sensations. They facilitate the determination of afferent pathways available for perception and reveal effects of experimental or clinical interventions. They may even better our understanding of the language patients use to communicate respiratory symptoms. Other methods of observing sensory and perceptual functions (electrophysiological recordings, neurological lesions, brain imaging, and behavioral measures) will complement, but not supplant, psychophysical studies.

Acknowledgments

The authors thank Dr. Steven Shea, Dr. Elisabeth Bloch-Salisbury, and Dr. Neil Bartlett for helpful criticism. Supported by Grants HL46690 and HL19170 from the National Institutes of Health.

References

Adams, L., and Guz, A. (1991). Dyspnea on exertion. In: Exercise, Pulmonary Physiology and Pathology. Edited by B.J. Whipp and K. Wasserman. Dekker, New York, pp. 449–494.

Adams, L., Lane, R., Shea, S.A., Cockcroft, A., and Guz, A. (1985). Breathlessness during different forms of ventilatory stimulation: a study of mechanisms in normal subjects and respiratory patients. Clin. Sci. 69:663–672.

Aitken, R.C.B., Zealley, A.K., and Rosenthal, S.V. (1970). Some psychological and physiological considerations of breathlessness. In: Breathing: Hering Breuer Centenary Symposium. (Ciba Foundation Symposium). Edited by R. Porter. Churchill, London, pp. 253–273.

Algom, D. (1992). Psychophysical Approaches to Cognition. North Holland, Amsterdam.

Allison, T., Goff, W.R., Williamson, P.D., and Van Glider, J.C. (1980). On the neural origin of the early components of the human somatosensory potential. In: Progress in Clinical Neurophysiology, Vol. 7. Edited by J.E. Desmedt. Karger, Basel, pp. 51–68.

Allison, T., Wood, C.C., and McCarthy, G. (1986). The central nervous system. In: Psychophysiology. Edited by M.G.H. Coles, E. Donchin, and S.W. Porges. Guilford, New York, pp. 5–12.

Arieli, R. (1990). Can the rat detect hypoxia in the expired air? Respir. Physiol. 79: 243–253.

Bakers, J.H.C.M. and Tenney, S.M. (1970). The perception of some sensations associated with breathing. Respir. Physiol. 10:85–92.

Banzett, R.B., Lansing, R.W., and Brown, R. (1987). High-level quadriplegics perceive lung volume change. J. Appl. Physiol. 62:567–573.

Banzett, R.B., Lansing, R.W., Reid, M.B., Adams, L., and Brown, R. (1989). "Air hunger" arising from increased P_{CO_2} in mechanically ventilated quadriplegics. Respir. Physiol. 76:53–68.

Bartoshuk, L.M. (1977). Methodological problems in the psychophysical testing of taste and smell. In: Special Senses in Aging. Edited by S.S. Han and D.H. Coons. University of Michigan, Ann Arbor, pp. 9–20.

Bloch, E., Harver, A., and Squires, N.K. (1990). Event-related potentials elicited by resistive loads in normal subjects. Am. Rev. Respir. Dis. 141:A30B.

Bloch-Salisbury, E., and Harver, A. (1994). Effects of detection and classification of resistive and elastic loads on endogenous event-related potentials. J. Appl. Physiol. 77:1246–1255.

Bonnel, A.M., Mathiot, M.J., and Grimand, C. (1985). Inspiratory and expiratory resistive load detection in normal and asthmatic subjects: a sensory decision theory analysis. Respiration 48:12–23.

Borg, G. (1962). Physical Performance and Perceived Exertion. Gleerup, Lund, pp. 1–63.

Borg, G. (1970). Perceived exertion as an indicator of somatic stress. Scand. J. Rehab. Med. 2:92–95.

Borg, G.A.V. (1982a). Psychophysical bases of perceived exertion. Med. Sci. Sports Exerc. 14:377–381.

Borg, G.A.V. (1982b). A category scale with ratio properties for intermodal and interindividual comparisons. In: Psychophysical Judgment and the Process of Perception. Edited by H. Geissler and P. Petzold. North Holland, Amsterdam, pp. 25–34.

Boring, E.G. (1950). A History of Experimental Psychology, 2nd edition. Appleton-Century-Crofts, New York.

Bornstein, R.F., and Pittman, T.S. (1992). Perception Without Awareness. Guilford, New York.

Bridgman, P.W. (1927). The Logic of Modern Physics. Macmillan, New York.

Burdon, G.W., Juniper, E.F., Killian, K.J., Hargreave, F.E., and Campbell, E.J.M. (1982). The perception of breathlessness in asthma. Am. Rev. Respir. Dis. 126:825–828.

Burki, N.K., Davenport, P.W., Safdar, F., and Zechman, F.W. (1978). The effects of airway anesthesia on magnitude estimation of added inspiratory resistive and elastic loads. Am. Rev. Respir. Dis. 117:71–75.

Burns, B.H., and Howell, J.B.L. (1969). Disproportionately severe breathlessness in chronic bronchitis. Q. J. Med. 38:277–284.

Campbell, E.J.M., Freedman, S., Smith, P.S., and Taylor, M.E. (1961). The ability of man to detect added non-elastic loads to breathing. Clin. Sci. 20:223–231.

Campbell, F.W., Atkinson, J., Francis, M.R., and Green, D.M. (1977). Estimation of auditory thresholds using evoked potentials. In: Visual Evoked Potentials in Man: New Developments, Vol. 2. Edited by J.E. Desmedt. Karger, Basel, pp. 67–78.

Chapman, C.R., Chen, A.C.N., Colpitts, Y.M., and Martin, R.W. (1981). Sensory decision theory describes evoked potentials in pain discrimination. Psychophysiology 18: 114–120.

Cheesman, J., and Merikle, P.M. (1986). Distinguishing conscious from unconscious perceptual processes. Can. J. Psychol. 40:343–367.

Clark, W.C. (1984). Application of multidimensional scaling to problems in experimental and clinical pain. In: Pain Measurement in Man: Neurophysiological Correlates of Pain. Edited by B. Brown. Elsevier, Amsterdam, pp. 349–369.

Cross, D.V. (1973). Sequential dependencies and regression in psychophysical judgments. Percept. Psychophys. 14:547–552.

Cruz, M., Stecenko, A., and Davenport, P.W. (1992). Respiratory related evoked potentials in asthmatic children. Am. Rev. Respir. Dis. 145:A631.

Davenport, P.W., Friedman, W.A., Thompson, F.J., and Franzen, O. (1986). Respiratory related cortical potentials evoked by inspiratory occlusion in humans. J. Appl. Physiol. 69:1843–1848.

Davenport, P.W., Dalziel, D.J., Webb, B., Bellah, J.R., and Vierck, C.J. (1991). Inspiratory resistive load detection in conscious dogs. J. Appl. Physiol. 70:1284–1289.

Desmedt, J.E. (1971). Somatosensory evoked potentials in man. In: Handbook of Electroencephalography and Clinical Neurophysiology. Edited by A. Remond. Elsevier, Amsterdam, pp. 55–82.

Desmedt, J.E. (1986). Generator sources of SEP in man. In: Evoked Potentials. Edited by R.Q. Craco and I. Bodis-Wollner. A.R. Liss, New York, pp. 235–245.

Desmedt, J.E., Huy, N.T., and Bourquet, M. (1983). The cognitive P40, N60 and P100 components of somatosensory potentials and the earliest signs of sensory processing in man. Electroenceph. Clin. Neurophysiol. 56:272–283.

Dickinson, J. (1976). Proprioceptive Control of Human Movement. Princeton Books, Princeton, pp. 46–51.

Dixon, N.F. (1981). Preconscious Processing. Wiley, Chichester.
Dyck, P. (1986). Detection thresholds of cutaneous sensations in health and disease in man. In: Spinal Afferent Processing. Edited by T.L. Yaksh. Plenum, New York, pp. 345–362.
Edwards, B. (1979). "10" [motion picture]. Warner Bros., Los Angeles.
Elliott, M.W., Adams, L., Cockroft, A., MacRae, K.D., Murphy, K., and Guz, A. (1991). The language of breathlessness. Use of verbal descriptors by patients with cardiopulmonary disease. Am. Rev. Respir. Dis. 144:826–832.
Engen, T. (1972). Psychophysics. In: Experimental Psychology, Vol. 1, Sensation. Edited by J. W. Kling and L.A. Riggs. Holt-Rhinhart and Winston, New York, pp. 11–86.
Franzen, O., and Offenloch, K. (1969). Evoked response correlates of psychophysical magnitude estimates for tactile stimulation in man. Exp. Brain Res. 8:1–18.
Gandevia, S.C., and Macefield, G. (1989). Projection of low-threshold afferents from human intercostal muscles to the cerebral cortex. Respir. Physiol. 77:203–214.
Geissler, H.G. (1990). Psychophysical Explorations of Mental structures. Hogrefe and Huber, Toronto.
Geldard, F.A. (1953). The Human Senses. Wiley & Sons, New York, pp. 53–54.
Gescheider, G.A. (1988). Psychophysical scaling. Annu. Rev. Psychol. 39:169–200.
Gevins, A.S. (1986). Quantitative human neurophysiology. In: Experimental Techniques in Human Neuropsychology. Edited by H.J. Hannay. Oxford, New York, pp. 419–456.
Goff, W.R., Williamson, P.D., Van Glider, J.C., Allison, T., and Fisher, T.C. (1980). Neural origins of long latency evoked potentials recorded from the depths and from the cortical surface of the brain in man. In: Progress in Clinical Neurophysiology, Vol. 2. Edited by J.E. Desmedt. Karger, Basel, pp. 126–145.
Green, D.M., and Swets, J.A. (1966). Signal Detection Theory and Psychophysics. Wiley, New York.
Harty, H., Heywood, P., and Adams, L. (1993). A comparison between continuous and discrete measurements of breathlessness during exercise in normal subjects using a visual analog scale (VAS). Clin. Sci. 85:229–236.
Harver, A., and Bloch, E. (1992). Correlation among age, lung function, and event-related potentials to airway occlusion. Psychophysiology 29:537.
Harver, A., and Mahler, D.A. (1990). The symptom of dyspnea. In: Dyspnea. Edited by D.A. Mahler. Futura, Mount Kisko, NY, pp. 1–53.
Harver, A., Baird, J.C., and McGovern, J.F. (1988). Grouping and multidimensional organization of respiratory sensations. Percept. Psychophys. 44:285–292.
Harver, A., Bloch, E., Sampson, M., and Carter, D. (1991). Respiratory related evoked potentials in patients with obstructive sleep apnea and age-matched controls. FASEB J. 5:A735.
Harver, A., Squires, N.K., Bloch-Salisbury, E., and Katkin, E.S. (1995). Event-related potentials to airway occlusion in young and old subjects. Psychophysiology 32:121–129.
Harver, A.S., Tenney, S.M., and Baird, J.C. (1986). A cautionary note on the interpretation of the power law for respiratory effort. Am. Rev. Respir. Dis. 133:341–342.
Hashimoto, I., Yoshikawa, K., and Sasaki, M. (1988). Somatosensory evoked potential correlates of psychophysical magnitude estimations for tactile air-puff stimulation in man. Exp. Brain Res. 73:459–460.

Hellman, R.P. (1981). Stability of individual loudness functions obtained by magnitude estimation and production. Percept. Psychophys. 29:63–70.
Hellman, R.P., and Zwislocki, J.J. (1961). Some factors affecting the estimation of loudness. J. Acoust. Soc. Am. 33:687–694.
Hillyard, S.A., and Picton, T.W. (1987). Electrophysiology of cognition. In: Handbook of Physiology. Section 1. The Nervous System, Vol. V. Edited by V.B. Mountcastle and F. Plum. American Physiological Society, Bethesda, MD, pp. 519–584.
Hochberg, J. (1984). Perception. In: Handbook of Physiology. Section 1. The Nervous System. Vol. III, Sensory Processes, Part 1. Edited by J.M. Brookhart and V.B. Mountcastle. American Physiological Society, Bethesda, MD, pp. 75–101.
Howell, J.B.L. (1970). Respiratory sensation in pulmonary disease. In: Breathing: Hering-Breuer Centenary Symposium. Edited by R. Porter. Churchill, London, pp. 287–295.
Johansson, R.S., and Vallbo, A.B. (1979). Detection of tactile stimuli. Thresholds of afferent units related to psychophysical thresholds in the human hand. J. Physiol. (Lond.) 297:405–422.
Johnson, R., Jr. (1993). On the neural generators of the P300 even-related potential. Psychophysiology 30:90–97.
Jones, F.N. (1956). A forced-choice method of limits. Am. J. Psychol. 19:672–673.
Katz-Salamon, M. (1984). Assessment of ventilation and respiratory rate by healthy subjects. Acta Physiol. Scand. 120:53–60.
Katz-Salamon, M. (1988). Respiratory psychophysics: a methodological overview. In: Respiratory Psychophysiology. Edited by C. von Euler and M. Katz-Salamon. Macmillan, London, pp. 65–78.
Kelvin, W.T. Popular Lectures and Addresses, 1891–1894. In, J. Bartlett (1980), Familiar Quotations. Little, Brown and Company, Boston. p. 594.
Kihlstrom, J.F., Barnhardt, T.M., and Tataryn, D.J. (1992). Implicit perception. In: Perception Without Awareness: Cognitive, Clinical and Social Perspectives. Edited by R.F. Bornstein and T.S. Pittman. Guilford, New York, pp. 17–54.
Killian, K.J., Mahutte, C.C., and Campbell, E.J.M. (1981). Magnitude scaling of externally added loads to breathing. J. Appl. Physiol. 123:12–15.
Knibestol, M., and Vallbo, A.B. (1980). Intensity of sensation related to activity of slowly adapting mechanoreceptive units in the human hand. J. Physiol. (Lond.) 300: 251–267.
Kruger, L., and Kenton, B. (1973). Quantitative neural and psychophysical data for cutaneous mechanoreceptor function. Brain Res. 49:1–24.
LaMotte, R.H., and Mountcastle, V.B. (1975). Capacities of humans and monkeys to discriminate between vibratory stimuli of different frequency and amplitude: correlation between neural events and psychophysical measurement. J. Neurophysiol. 38:539–559.
Lansing, R., Schoepflin, C., Schoepflin, W., and Stein, P. (1973). Brain potentials associated with voluntary respiratory movements in man. Electroencephal. Clin. Neurophysiol. 35:757–758.
Libet, B., Alberts, W.W., Wright, E.W., and Feinstein, B. (1967). Responses of human somatosensory cortex to stimuli below threshold for conscious sensation. Science 158:1597–1600.

Luce, R.D., and Mo, S.S. (1965). Magnitude estimation of heaviness and loudness by individual subjects. Br. J. Stat. Psychol. 18:159–174.

Macefield, G., and Gandevia, S.C. (1991). The cortical drive to human respiratory muscles in the awake state assessed by premotor cerebral potentials. J. Physiol. (Lond.) 439:545–558.

MacKay, D.M. (1963). Psychophysics of perceived intensity: a theoretical basis of Fechner's and Steven's laws. Science 1:1–27.

Mahler, D.A., and Harver, A. (1990). Clinical measurement of dyspnea. In: Dyspnea. Edited by D.A. Mahler. Futura, Mount Kisko, NY, pp. 75–100.

Marcel, A.J. (1983). Conscious and unconscious perception: an approach to the relations between phenomenal experience and perceptual processes. Cognitive Psychol. 15: 238–300.

Marks, L.E. (1974). Sensory Processes: The New Psychophysics. Academic Press, New York.

Marks, L.E. (1986). Context and sensory processes: in search of basic laws. Cah. Psychol. Cognit. 2:121–136.

Marks, L.E., Borg, G., and Ljunggren, G. (1983). Individual differences in perceived exertion assessed by two new methods. Percept. Psychophys. 34:280–288.

Martenuik, R.G., and Ryan, M.L. (1972). Psychophysics of kinesthesis: angular movement. J. Motor Behav. 4:135–142.

Martenuik, R.G., Shields, K.W., and Campbell, S. (1972). Amplitude, position, timing and velocity as cues in reproduction of movement. Percept. Motor Skills 35:51–58.

Matthews, P.B.C. (1977). Muscle afferents and kinaesthesia. Br. Med. Bull. 33:137–142.

Melzack, R. (1975). The McGill pain questionnaire: major properties and scoring methods. Pain 1:277–299.

Melzack, R., and Torgerson, W.S. (1971). On the language of pain. Anesthesiology 34:50–60.

Merzenich, M.M., and Harrington, T. (1969). The sense of flutter-vibration evoked by stimulation of the hairy skin of primates: comparison of human sensory capacity with the responses of mechanoreceptive afferents innervating the hairy skin of monkeys. Exp. Brain Res. 9:236–260.

Merzenich, M.M., and Kaas, J.H. (1980). Principles of organization of sensory-perceptual systems. In: Progress in Psychobiology and Physiological Psychology. Vol. 9. Edited by J.M. Sprague and A.N. Epstein. Academic Press, New York, pp. 1–42.

Mountcastle, V.B. (1967). The problem of sensing and neural coding of sensory events. In: The Neurosciences. Edited by G.C. Quarton, T. Melnechuk, and F.O. Schmitt. Rockefeller University Press, New York, pp. 393–408.

Mountcastle, V.B. (1975). The view from within: pathways to the study of perception. John Hopkins Med. J. 136:109–131.

Mountcastle, V.B., and Darian-Smith, I. (1968). Neural mechanisms in somesthesia. In: Medical Physiology. Edited by V.B. Mountcastle. Mosby, Baltimore, pp. 1372–1423.

Muza, S.R., and Zechman, F.W. (1984). Scaling of added loads to breathing: magnitude estimation vs. handgrip matching. J. Appl. Physiol. 57:888–891.

Narbed, P.G., Mercer, D., Howell, J.B.L., and Spencer, E. (1983). A signal detection theory analysis of the effect of chest cage constriction upon the detection of inspiratory resistive loads. Clin. Sci. 64:417–421.

Noble, B.J., Borg, G.A.V., Jacobs, I., Ceci, R., and Kaiser, P. (1983). A category-ratio perceived exertion scale: relationship to blood and muscle lactates and heart rate. Med. Sci. Sports Exerc. 15:523–528.

Ochoa, J.L., and Torebjork H.C. (1983). Sensations evoked by intraneural microstimulation of single mechanoreceptor units innervating the human hand. J. Physiol. (Lond.) 342:633–654.

Okada, Y.C., Kauffman, L., and Williamson, S.J. (1983). The hippocampal formation as a source of slow endogenous potentials. Electroenceph. Clin. Neurophysiol. 55: 417–426.

Pierce, C.S., and Jastrow, J. (1884). On small differences in sensation. Mem. Natl. Acad. Sci. 3:75–83.

Plassman, B.L., and Lansing, R.W. (1990). Perceptual cues used to reproduce an inspired lung volume. J. Appl. Physiol. 69:1123–1130.

Poulton, E.C. (1968). The new psychophysics: six models for magnitude estimation. Psychol. Bull. 69:1–19.

Pritchard, W.S. (1981). Psychophysiology of P300. Psychol. Bull. 89:506–540.

Ratliff, L. (1976). On the psychophysiological bases of universal color terms. Proc. Am. Philos. Soc. 120:31–330.

Regan, D. (1989). Human Brain Electrophysiology. Elsevier, New York.

Regan, D., and Spekreijse, H. (1986). Evoked potentials in vision research, 1961–1985. Vision Res. 26:1461–1480.

Revelette, W.R., and Davenport, P.W. (1990). Effects of timing of inspiratory occlusion on cerebral evoked potentials in humans. J. Appl. Physiol. 68:282–288.

Revelette, W.R., Zechman, F.W., Jr., Parker, D.E., and Wiley, R.L. (1984). Effect of background loading on perception of inspiratory loads. J. Appl. Physiol. 56:404–410.

Riggs, L.R. (1987). Recollection of early laboratory experiments on vision. In: Foundations of Sensory Science. Edited by W.W. Dawson and J.M. Enoch. Springer-Verlag, Berlin, pp. 191–228.

Ruchkin, D.S., Sutton, S., Keitzman, M.G., and Silver, K. (1980). Slow wave and P300 in signal detection. Electroenceph. Clin. Neurophysiol. 50:45–47.

Schiffman, S.S., and Erickson, R.P. (1971). A theoretical review: a psychophysical model for gustatory quality. Physiol. Behav. 1:617–633.

Schlag, J. (1973). Generation of brain evoked potentials. In: Bioelectric Recording Techniques: Part A, Cellular Processes and Brain Potentials. Edited by R.F. Thompson and M.M. Patterson. Academic, New York, pp. 385–404

Sekular, R., Nash, D., and Armstrong, R. (1973). Sensitive, objective procedure for evaluating response to light touch. Neurology 23:1282–1291.

Simon, P.M., Schwartzstein, R.M., Weiss, J.W., Lahive, K., Fencl, V., Teghtsoonian, M., and Weinberger, S.E. (1989). Distinguishable sensations of breathlessness induced in normal volunteers. Am. Rev. Respir. Dis. 140:1021–1027.

Simon, P.M., Schwartzstein, R.M., Weiss, J.W., Fencl, V., Teghtsoonian, M., and Weinberger, S.E. (1990). Distinguishable types of dyspnea in patients with shortness of breath. Am. Rev. Respir. Dis. 142:1009–1014.

Squires, K.C., Squires, N.C., and Hillyard, S.A. (1975). Decision related cortical potentials during an auditory signal detection task with cued observation intervals. J. Exp. Psychol. Hum. Percept. Perform. 1:268–269.

Stebbins, W.C., Brown, C.H., and Petersen, M.R. (1984). Sensory functions in animals. In: Handbook of Physiology, Section 1. The Nervous System. Vol. III. Sensory Processes. Part 1. Edited by J.M. Brookhart and V.B. Mountcastle. American Physiological Society, Washington, D.C., pp. 123–148.
Stevens, S.S. (1956). The direct estimation of sensory magnitudes-loudness. Am. J. Psychol. 69:1–25.
Stevens, S.S. (1959). Cross-modality validation of subjective scales for loudness, vibration, and electric shock. J. Exp. Psychol. 57:201–209.
Stevens, S.S. (1961). The psychophysics of sensory function. In: Sensory Communication. Edited by W.A. Rosenblith. Wiley, New York, pp. 1–33.
Stevens, S.S., and Greenbaum, H.B. (1966). Regression effects in psychophysical judgment. Percept. Psychophys. 1:439–446.
Stevens, S.S. (1970). Neural events and the psychophysical law. Science 170:1043–1050.
Stevens, S.S. (1975). Psychophysics. Wiley, New York.
Strobel, R.J., and Daubenspeck, J.A. (1993). Early and late respiratory-related potentials evoked by pressure pulse stimuli in humans. J. Appl. Physiol. 74:1484–1491.
Stubbing, D.G., Killian, K.J., and Campbell, E.J.M. (1981). The quantification of respiratory sensations by normal subjects. Respir. Physiol. 44:251–260.
Swets, J. (1959). Indices of signal detectability obtained with various psychophysical procedures. J. Acoust. Soc. Am. 31:511–513.
Talbot, W.H., Darian-Smith, I., Kornhuber, H.H., and Mountcastle, V.B. (1968). The sense of flutter vibration: comparison of the human capacity with response patterns of mechanoreceptive afferents from the monkey hand. J. Neurophysiol. 31:301–334.
Tanner, W.P., Jr., and Swets, J.A. (1954). A decision-making theory of visual detection. Psychol. Rev. 61:401–409.
Taylor, J.L., and McCloskey, D.I. (1990). Triggering of preprogrammed movements as reactions to masked stimuli. J. Neurophysiol. 63:439–446.
Teghtsoonian, R. (1989). The study of individuals in psychophysical measurement. In: Psychophysics in Action. Edited by G. Ljunggren and S. Dornic. Springer-Verlag, Berlin, pp. 95–102.
Teghtsoonian, M., and Teghtsoonian, R. (1971). How repeatable are Steven's power law exponents for individual subjects? Percept. Psychophys. 10:147–149.
Teuber, H.L. (1960). Perception. In: Handbook of Physiology. Section 1. Neurophysiology. Vol. III. Edited by J. Field, H.W. Magoun and V.E. Hall. American Physiological Society, Washington, D.C., pp. 1595–1668.
Uttal, W.R. (1965). Do compound evoked potentials reflect psychological codes? Psychol. Bull. 64:377–392.
Uttal, W.R. (1973). The Psychophysiology of Sensory Coding. Harper and Row, New York.
Vallbo, A.B. (1981). Sensations evoked from the glabrous skin of the human hand by electrical stimulation of unitary mechanoreceptive afferents. Brain Res. 215:359–363.
Vallbo, A.B. (1984). Tactile sensations related to activity in primary afferents with special reference to detection problems. In: Somatosensory Mechanisms. Edited by C. von Euler, O. Franzen, U. Lindblom, and D. Ottoson. Plenum, New York, pp. 163–172.
Vallbo, A.B., and Johansson, R. (1976). Skin mechanoreceptors in the human hand: neural and psychophysical thresholds. In: Sensory Functions of the Skin of Primates. Edited by Y. Zotterman. Pergamon Press, Oxford, pp. 29–54.

Van Essen, D.C., and Maunsell, J.H.R. (1983). Hierarchical organization and functional streams in the visual cortex. Trends Neurosci. 9:370–375.

Vaughan, H.G., Costa, L.D., and Ritter, W. (1968). Topography of the human motor potential. Electroenceph. Clin. Neurophysiol. 25:1–10.

Weiskrantz, L. (1986). Blindsight: A Case Study and Implications. Oxford University Press, Oxford.

Wheatley, J.R., and White, D.P. (1993). Influence of NREM sleep on respiratory related cortical evoked potentials in normal humans. J. Appl. Physiol. 74:1803–1810.

Wilson, R.C., and Jones, P.W. (1989). A comparison of the visual analog scale and modified Borg scale for measurement of dyspnea during exercise. Clin. Sci. 76:277–282.

Zechman, F.W., Jr., and Wiley, R.L. (1986). Afferent inputs to breathing: respiratory sensation. In: Handbook of Physiology. Section 3. The Respiratory System. Vol. II. Control of Breathing, Part 1. Edited by Cherniack, N.S., and Widdicombe, J.G. American Physiological Society, Bethesda, MD, pp. 449–474.

4

Perception of Respiratory Mechanical Events

PAUL W. DAVENPORT

University of Florida
Gainesville, Florida

W. ROBERT REVELETTE

University of Kentucky
Lexington, Kentucky

I. Introduction

Ventilation of the lung is a mechanical process produced by pumping forces generated by the respiratory muscles. The pump generates the driving force for air to flow and increase the lung volume. The movement of air into the lung is opposed by the mechanical properties of the respiratory system, which act as a load on the pumping action of the respiratory muscles. The resistance and compliance of the respiratory system combine to produce a mechanical impedance to the expansion of the thorax. Acute changes in mechanical load can result from intrinsic mechanical changes in the respiratory system or extrinsic mechanical loads. An increase in mechanical load requires an increase in the driving force of the pump for maintenance of ventilation. Increases in mechanical loads of sufficient magnitude, intrinsic and extrinsic, elicit the sensation of dyspnea.

The perception of respiratory mechanical events is dependent on two processes. The first is the detection of the change in breathing pattern. The threshold for detection of changes in impedance can be quantified in the laboratory. When a ventilatory mechanical parameter has changed to sufficient magnitude, the subject attends to the stimulus and detection results. The magnitude that elicits detection of 50% of the stimulus presentations is defined as the *detection threshold.* It is difficult for the subject to differentiate changes in resistance from changes in compliance at the detection threshold. The second perceptual process, differentiation of the load, improves with increasing magnitudes of stimulation. As the magnitude of the stimulus increases, the subject is able to provide an estimate of the magnitude of the stimulus. In addition, the type of stimulus, such as resistive or elastic loads, is discriminated with increasing accuracy as the stimulus magnitude increases. Thus, the ability of a subject to evaluate a change in respiratory mechanics is a temporal process dependent on the initial detection of a change and then an assessment of the type and magnitude of the change. The adjustment of breathing pattern in response to the change in mechanics is appropriate to the stimulus.

II. Detection of Respiratory Mechanical Loads

External mechanical loads have been used as an effective tool to study the sensory processes involved with the perception of mechanical events related to breathing. Campbell et al. (1961) studied the ability of human subjects to detect graded elastic loads (1.4–4.9 cm H_2O/L) applied to inspiration. They plotted the percentage of the loads detected against the load magnitude and defined the threshold for detection as the load magnitude detected 50% of the time, 2.47 cm H_2O/L. Subsequently, Zechman and Davenport (1978) used elastic loads ranging from 0.48 to 5.27 cm H_2O/L to determine the detection threshold. The subjects were allowed only one inspiration against the load. The mean detection threshold was 1.86 cm H_2O/L, with a range of 0.7–2.0 cm H_2O/L.

The detection of resistive loads has been studied much more extensively. Bennet et al. (1962) found the detection threshold to be 0.59 cm H_2O/L/s, with a range of 0.40–0.98 cm H_2O/L/s. They noted that this represented a 25% increase above the mean intrinsic resistance for the subject. Wiley and Zechman (1966) studied the relationship between the background resistance and the detection threshold. They found considerable variability in the resistive load detection threshold, but this variability was reduced when the detection threshold was expressed as the ratio of the subject's background resistance. The background resistance included the subject's intrinsic resistance and the minimal resistance of the apparatus. The mean resistive load detection threshold was 0.6 cm H_2O/L/s. The ratio of the resistance at detection to the total background resistance was 0.25–0.30. This ratio remained constant when the background resistance was increased with the addition of a continuous extrinsic resistive load and for a patient with an elevated intrinsic background resistance. Thus, subjects with an elevated background resistance require a greater magnitude of added resistance for detection to occur.

III. Magnitude Estimation of Loads

Subjects have been exposed to suprathreshold loads and asked to provide an estimate of the load magnitude (Burki et al., 1983; Gamberale et al., 1978; Gottfried et al., 1978; Killian et al., 1981; Tack et al., 1981, 1982; Wolkove et al., 1981). The method of estimation has ranged from numerical scales to cross-modality matching. The result of these studies has shown that increasing load magnitude is associated with an increasing perceptual estimate of the load. There is a linear relationship between the load magnitude and the perceptual estimate of the load using a log-log transformation. The slope of the line is a measure of the sensitivity of the subject to the stimulus.

Magnitude estimation studies are performed by allowing the subjects to inspire against the load and then report the magnitude of the load. Each load magnitude is presented several times in random order with or without a cue to warn the subject of an upcoming load presentation. Inspiration against suprathreshold mechanical loads results in a reduction of airflow for a resistive load (Zechman et al., 1957) and volume for an elastic load (Zechman and Davenport, 1978). When subjects were required to maintain the airflow for resistive loads at a target control value, there was an increase in the estimated magnitude of the load (Killian et al., 1982). When the airflow target was increased, the magnitude estimation of the load increased further. Conversely, when inspiration is interrupted with a load for only a portion of the inspiration, there is a reduction in the perceived magnitude of the load (Knafelc and Davenport, 1991). These results suggest that the perceived magnitude of a load is in part proportional to the duration it is maintained; that is, perception of mechanical loads is a function of the magnitude and duration of the stimulus. This implies that spatial and temporal processes are involved in the perception of suprathreshold mechanical loads.

Ventilation against an increased load increases the work of breathing (Zechman et al., 1957). The steady-state ventilatory pattern may be altered to minimize the work of breathing (Otis et al., 1950; Mead, 1960). The application of graded extrinsic loads is detected with an elevated absolute threshold that is a function of the ratio of the background to added load (Weber-Fechner relationship). Magnitude estimation of added extrinsic resistive loads while breathing with an elevated background produces a shift in the log-log relationship resulting from an increased threshold for detection and decreased perceived estimate for the same magnitude of the load (Revelette et al., 1984). This suggests that the central nervous system can suppress increases in sensory input when that information is applied continuously. Thus, subjects are desensitized with a background load and the added load must be elevated above the background "noise" level for detection and magnitude estimation to occur.

IV. Perception of Mechanical Load Pattern

The generation of the inspiratory driving pressure creates the pressure gradient for air to flow into the lung. The resistive component of impedance opposes airflow (Milic-Emili and Zin, 1986). The airflow pattern has a low flow at the onset of inspiration, and the pressure change related to resistance is small. Increasing flow rate augments the resistive component of Ppl pattern to a peak when airflow is maximal at approximately midinspiration. There is then a reduction in the resistive component of Ppl as airflow returns to zero at the end of the inspiration. The Ppl profile related to compliance is dependent on the expansion of the lung and thorax and is linked to volume. This elastic component gradually increases as the Ppl becomes more negative over the entire inspiration, to reach a maximum at the end of inspiration. The net pressure profile related to the mechanical load for an inspiration is function of the total impedance to inspiration, a combination of the resistive and elastic patterns. There is a gradual change in intrapleural pressure that reaches a peak before the end of inspiration and a gradual decline, as airflow ceases, to the Ppl for the elastic component at end inspiration.

The application of extrinsic mechanical loads produces changes in the profile of volume, airflow, and pressure. A large resistive load opposes the movement of air and results in a reduction in airflow (Zechman et al., 1957). Ppl becomes more negative, and the transdiaphragmatic pressure (Pdi) is augmented (Zechman et al., 1985). The pattern of these mechanical changes is directly related to the airflow, and the magnitude of the change is dependent on the load magnitude. Resistive load magnitudes near the threshold of detection (Zechman and Davenport, 1978) produce very small changes in airflow (from control) but are associated with a more negative Pm and augmented Pdi (Zechman et al., 1985). The Pdi becomes augmented above control progressively earlier in the inspiration as the load magnitude increases (Fig. 1). This is also associated with a progressive decrease in the detection latency.

Extrinsic elastic loads are produced by having the subject inspire from a closed rigid container. These loads oppose the inflation of the lung and contraction of the inspiratory muscles by the generation of a negative pressure in the load chamber during inspiration. To produce a given tidal volume, a greater driving pressure is required to maintain lung inflation (Milic-Emili and Zin, 1986). This results in an increased negative pressure measured at the mouth (Pm), a more negative Ppl, and an augmented Pdi (Zechman et al., 1985). It has been shown that elastic load magnitudes near the detection threshold produce little change in the

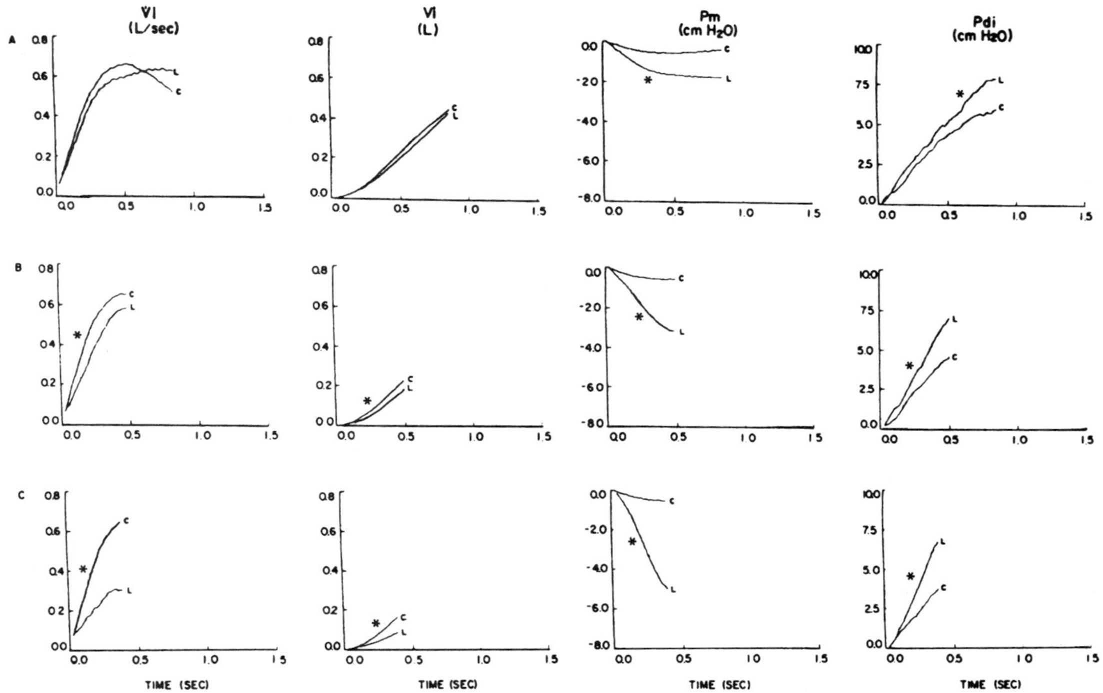

Figure 1 Group mean patterns of inspiratory flow ($\dot{V}_I$), inspired volume (V_I), mouth pressure (Pm), and transdiaphragmatic pressure (Pdi) for added inspiratory resistive loads. Plotted as a function of time are mean instantaneous values of each variable sampled every 10 ms during loaded breaths (L) and corresponding unloaded breaths (C) from onset of inspiration up to Tdet for three resistive loads: 1.8 (A), 4.5 (B), and 22.9 cm H_2O/L/s. *First point at which control and loaded breath patterns significantly ($p < 0.05$) deviate. (From Zechman et al., 1985.)

inspired volume (Zechman and Davenport, 1978). There is a more negative Pm, and the Pdi is augmented late in the inspiratory cycle (Zechman et al., 1985). Increasing magnitudes of elastic loads are associated with reduction in the inspired volume and a progressively greater negative Pm and augmented Pdi (Fig. 2). These mechanical changes are associated with a decreased detection latency.

Inspiratory mechanical loads oppose the pumping action of the respiratory muscles regardless of the type of load. When loads are applied, increased force generated by the respiratory muscles is necessary to maintain the inspiratory driving pressure (Milic-Emili and Zin, 1986). This is reflected in associated changes in the related pressures: Pdi, Ppl, and Pm (Zechman et al., 1985). If the opposition (load) to the inspiratory pump exceeds 25–30% of the background load, then the threshold is reached and detection results. This suggests that any measure of a change in driving pressure related to the application of a load correlates with the detection and magnitude estimation of that load. The mechanics of the system are changing such that the ability of the respiratory muscles to produce pumping forces is compromised.

The perceptual system mediating the sensation of mechanical loads must receive an information pattern that is load dependent. The airflow-related information should increase rapidly early in the breath, reach a maximum at peak airflow, and dissipate late in the breath. Information related to the tidal volume profile should increase slowly as the inspiration proceeds. There should be a progressive increase in volume-related information throughout the inspiration to a maximum at end inspiration. With increased mechanical loads, the information pattern should reflect the load-specific mechanical changes.

The mechanical changes associated with ventilation of the lung are transduced by respiratory mechanoreceptors. The conducting airways have afferents with activity patterns that are related to the airflow, airway distension, and lung volume (Sant' Ambrogio, 1982). The respiratory muscles have mechanoreceptors that transduce the changes in muscle length and force (Corda et al., 1965a; Critchlow and von Euler, 1963; Holt et al., 1991). The activity of these mechanoreceptors is a function of their adequate stimulus. The pattern of afferent activity, threshold and discharge frequency, is linked to the pattern of their mechanical stimulus (Corda et al., 1965b; Davenport et al., 1981). The application of mechanical loads changes the pattern of the mechanical forces related to ventilation in a load-specific manner, and there will be an associated change in the afferent activity of those mechanoreceptors. It is therefore reasonable to conclude that the detection, localization, discrimination, magnitude estimation, and behavioral compensation are a function of the change in mechanoreceptor activity patterns resulting from the application of a mechanical load. The mechanical parameters associated with increased load change the pattern of mechanoreceptor activity, resulting in a load-dependent information pattern provided to the central nervous system. Using a collage of afferent activity from the respiratory tract and respira-

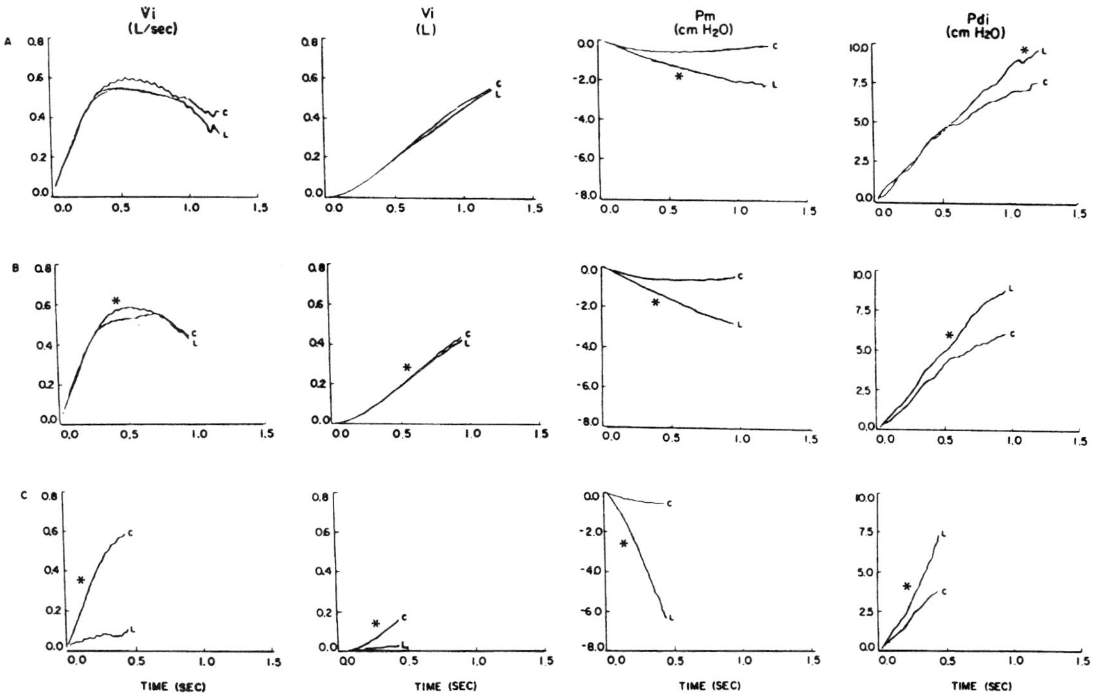

Figure 2 Group mean patterns of inspiratory flow ($\dot{V}_I$), inspired volume (V_I), mouth pressure (Pm), and transdiaphragmatic pressure (Pdi) for added inspiratory elastic loads. Plotted as a function of time are mean instantaneous values of each variable sampled every 10 ms during loaded breaths (L) and corresponding unloaded breaths (C) from onset of inspiration up to Tdet for three elastic loads: 3.5 (A) and 5.2 (B) cm H_2O/L and airway occlusion (C). *First point at which control and loaded breath patterns significantly ($p < 0.05$) deviate. (From Zechman et al., 1985.)

tory muscles, the cortex can then sense that there is a load-related change, locate the source of the change, and determine the type of change that is occurring.

Patterning of information is therefore an important parameter that provides the transduction of the respiratory mechanical changes into a sensory code that is used by the higher brain centers during respiratory perception. The latency of detection (Tdet), the time required for the subject to signal the perception of a load, is dependent on the magnitude and type of load (Zechman and Davenport, 1978). The detection latency for both resistive and elastic loads decreases with increasing load magnitude (Fig. 3). The resistive load information pattern is maximal early in the breath at peak flow, and detection occurs early in inspiration if the load-related information exceeds the threshold. Volume-related elastic loads have an information pattern that gradually increases to a maximum at the end of

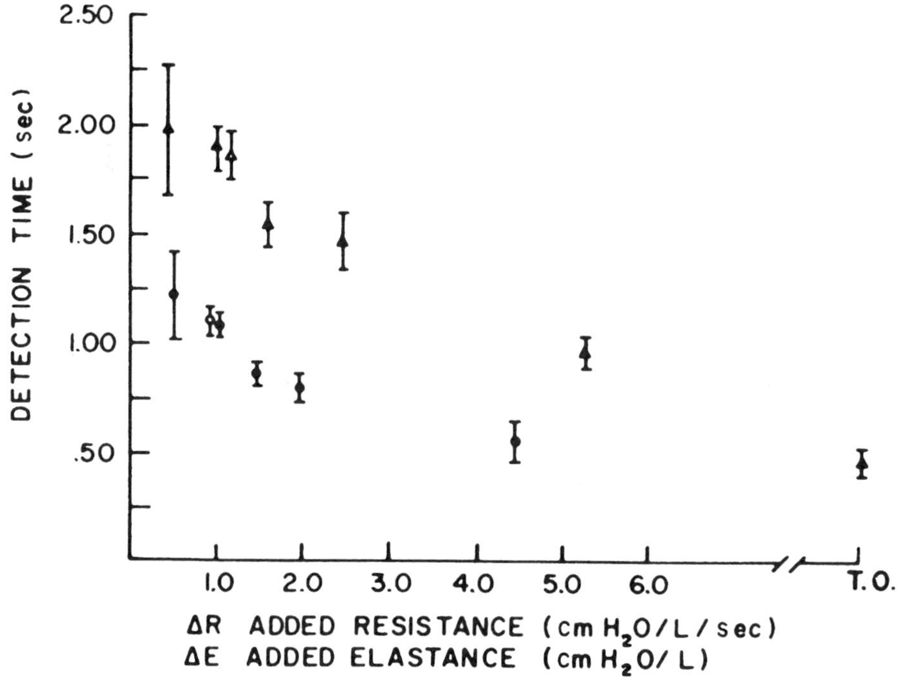

Figure 3 Effect of graded resistive and elastic loads on detection time. The closed circles represent Tdet for R loads and the closed triangles represent the Tdet for E loads. The Tdet values associated with threshold R and E loads (ΔR_{50} and ΔE_{50}) are represented by the open circles and triangles, respectively. Values plotted are group mean ± standard error of the mean. (From Zechman and Davenport, 1978.)

inspiration. If this load information exceeds the threshold, then detection occurs late in inspiration. This suggests that the detection of a mechanical load is related to the mechanical effect of the load on breathing pattern and thereby mechanical load-specific effects on the afferent activity pattern.

The pattern of information is also important after the load exceeds threshold. The subject then has information directly related to the pattern of the load available for use in discrimination of the type of load. The differences between resistive and elastic loads on the pattern of breathing allow the subject to discriminate these types of loads. Resistive and elastic loads at threshold or greater than threshold have been presented and the subject asked to discriminate between the type of load (Zechman et al., 1981; Campbell et al., 1963). If the load is very close to threshold, it is very difficult for a subject to discriminate correctly between the two types of loads. The near threshold loads were discriminated at the level of chance. One of the reasons for this poor discrimination is the low magnitude and short duration of information patterning available for discrimination. The information must exceed threshold for sufficient lengths of time for the subject to perceive the pattern produced by the load. If the subject is given an easily detected suprathreshold load, however, then the subject can discriminate the type of load with a greater degree of accuracy (75–90%). The greater the level of the load, the greater the ability of the subject to discriminate the type the load.

The relationship between load information pattern and the subject's perception of the load is further shown in Fig. 4 (Zechman et al., 1981). The subjects were presented near threshold and suprathreshold resistive and elastic loads. They signaled the detection of the load by squeezing a hand grip and matched the perceived pattern of the load with hand grip pattern. The subjects were asked to discriminate between the types of load. The near threshold loads were poorly discriminated, yet there was a significant difference in the detection latency: resistive load Tdet was shorter than elastic load Tdet. This result suggests that the load magnitude was sufficient to exceed the threshold for detection but insufficient for discrimination. The subjects sensed the presence of the load, but the load-specific information available for discrimination was inadequate. Larger, suprathreshold resistive and elastic loads were detected earlier in the breath, and the significant difference remained between their respective detection latencies. However, the discrimination of these larger magnitude loads was greatly improved. The hand grip pattern for resistive loads had an early onset, reached a peak near midinspiration, and decreased late in inspiration. The hand grip pattern matched the airflow pattern for the time that the airflow was sufficient to produce information above the detection threshold. The onset of hand grip represents the time at which the load information reached threshold, and the duration indicates the time the load information exceeded threshold. The onset of hand grip response for the suprathreshold elastic load occurred later in the breath and increased throughout the breath in a pattern similar to the inspired volume. Again, the onset represents

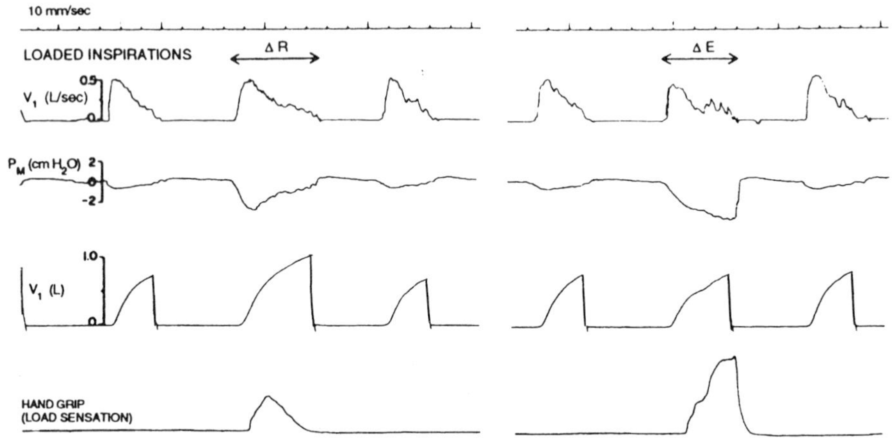

Figure 4 Temporal patterns of load sensation expressed by hand grip tension in response to added resistive (ΔR) and elastic (ΔE) loads. ΔR = 4.5 cm H_2O/L/s. ΔE = 4.8 cm H_2O/L, $\dot{V}_I$ = inspiratory airflow, Pm = mouth pressure, and V_I, inspiratory volume. (From Zechman et al., 1981.)

the point at which the load exceeded threshold and the duration represents the time the load was above threshold.

These results are consistent with a subsequent study of the correlation of the detection of resistive and elastic loads and Pdi (Zechman et al., 1985). Both types of loads produced an augmentation of Pdi. This augmentation occurred progressively earlier in the inspiration with increasing load magnitude. The Tdet was correlated with the progressively earlier deviation of the loaded Pdi from the control pattern. The significant differences in the Tdet were a function of load type, resistive load Tdet shorter than elastic load Tdet. These results suggest that the threshold for detection is related to the increased mechanical load to the pump exceeding a sensory threshold that is a ratio of the background load. When the threshold is exceeded, detection follows and information on the type and magnitude of the load becomes available in a mechanical pattern-specific manner as long as the load stimulus remains above threshold.

Animal studies of the mechanisms mediating respiratory sensations are limited. An animal model of resistive load detection was developed in dogs with a tracheal stoma (Davenport et al., 1991). The dogs were behaviorally conditioned to signal the detection of occlusions and inspiratory resistive loads. The dogs easily detected the loads and signaled their detection by lifting their front paws from a lever. The resistive load detection threshold and Weber fraction were found to be similar to these values in humans. The application of the loads through the tracheal stoma of the dogs excluded afferent systems in the mouth, nose, pharynx, larynx, and upper trachea from mediating this sensation. The remaining afferents would be lung vagal and respiratory muscle mechanoreceptors. The breathing pattern, as measured by tidal volume (VT, inspiratory and expiratory time (TI and TE), frequency, minute ventilation, and expired P_{CO_2}, was not altered by near threshold, detected loads. This would make it unlikely that vagal afferents or chemoreceptors mediated this load detection. Respiratory muscle afferents in the pump have been hypothesized to be mediating this sensation and may be operant in this animal study.

It is impossible to conclude, however, that the perception of respiratory load is caused solely by a change in afferent activity. An inspiratory mechanical load is perceived only if the subject breathes. The perception of inspiratory loads is part of an active mechanical pumping event. Inspiration requires the motor act of driving the respiratory pump, which generates the forces to produce ventilation. Motor drive provides the activation of the respiratory muscles that produce the pumping forces that generate the driving forces for inspiratory airflow and volume. Changes in the respiratory muscle afferent activity related to respiratory muscle mechanics produced by the motor drive to the muscles is expected. This suggests that inspiratory effort is directly related to the pattern of afferent activity and the perception of the load. Both resistive and elastic loads act on the pump, and the perception of the load is result of the central processing of information related to the motor drive to the pump and the associated patterning of the load-related mechanical changes producing characteristic changes in afferent activity patterns. Subjects who have participated in discrimination experiments report that a suprathreshold load was an elastic load because it continued to increase in magnitude and was present late in the breath. Subjects were aware of a resistive load because they sensed it early in the inspiration.

V. Respiratory System–Related Evoked Potentials

The transduction of mechanical events related to breathing produces a change in the sensory activity going to the cerebral cortex. Afferents from various regions of the respiratory system project specifically to the somatosensory region of the cerebral cortex. Although somatosensory cortical activation by vagal afferents in the human are unknown, stimulation of vagal and superior laryngeal afferents elicits neural activity in this region of the cortex of cats (Aubert and Guilhen, 1971; Aubert, 1970; Aubert and Legros, 1970). Electrical and mechanical stimulation of the diaphragm elicits an evoked potential in the dorsal spinal cord (Revelette et al., 1990). Diaphragmatic afferents also activate neurons in the VPL nucleus of the thalamus (Fig. 5). These thalamic neurons increase their activity in response to either electrical or mechanical stimulation of diaphragmatic afferents.

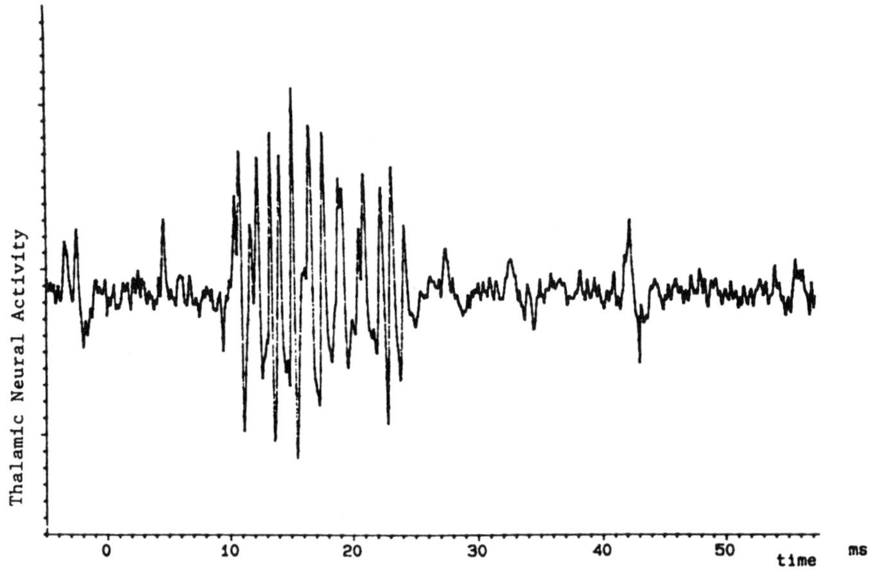

Figure 5 Thalamic neural activity elicited by electrical stimulation of the phrenic nerve. The recording site was marked and found by histological analysis to be in the ventroposterior lateral (VPL) nucleus of the thalamus.

Mechanical and electrical stimulation of intercostal afferents activates a separate population of neurons in the VPL nucleus of the thalamus. These thalamic regions have anatomical connections with the somatosensory region of the cerebral cortex (Sallach et al., 1991). Electrical stimulation of phrenic and intercostal muscle afferents activates neurons in the somatosensory region of the cat cerebral cortex (Davenport et al., 1985). Specific mechanical stimulation of intercostal mechanoreceptors elicits a short-latency activation of cat somatosensory cortical neurons (Davenport et al., 1993). Electrical stimulation of intercostal muscles in humans also elicits a cortical evoked potential in the somatosensory region, suggesting that this pathway is present in humans (Gandevia and Macefield, 1989). This intercostal and phrenic afferent projection via the thalamus is similar to other muscle proprioceptive systems (Anderson et al., 1966; Landgren and Silfvenius, 1969; Oscarsson and Rosen, 1963; Phillips et al., 1971). Thus, the neural substrate exists for mechanoreceptors in the pump muscles to provide transduction of pump mechanics and projection of this activity to the somatosensory region of the cerebral cortex via a dorsal column-lemniscal pathway that is relayed by the VPL region of the thalamus. This neural pathway may be part of the sensory limb for perception of mechanical loads.

The presence of a somatosensory cortical pathway in experimental animals suggests that one should be able to record some measure of this change in sensory processing in humans. Evoked potentials have been used in other sensory systems to record the cortical neural activity elicited by a synchronous stimulation of a population of afferents that project to a specific colony of cerebral cortical neurons (Kakigi and Shibasaki, 1984; Larsson and Prevec, 1970; Pratt and Starr, 1981; Pratt et al., 1979; Starr et al., 1981; Allison et al., 1989a, b; Huttunen and Homberg, 1991; McCloskey et al., 1983; Wood et al., 1988). This afferent activation causes simultaneous depolarization of a cortical column of neurons, creating a dipole recorded with electrodes placed in close proximity to that dipole (Desmedt et al., 1987; Deiber et al., 1986). A dipole in the somatosensory cortex elicited by cutaneous and muscle afferent stimulation is routinely recorded in human subjects using scalp electrodes (Hämäläinen et al., 1990; Kakigi and Shibasaki, 1984).

The activation of cortical neurons by mechanical loads has been studied using the evoked potential technique modified to meet the unique requirements for respiratory load stimulation (Davenport et al., 1986). A mechanical load (inspiratory occlusion) was applied while simultaneously recording over the somatosensory region of the cortex in the adult human. Inspiratory occlusion should produce a maximal activation of the load-related afferents. This load was presented at the onset of an inspiration. Electroencephalographic (EEG) activity was recorded from scalp electrodes placed over the frontal (Fz) and somatosensory (Cz and C3) regions of the cerebral cortex. Bipolar recordings were obtained with a cephalic reference Cz. The EEG activity was recorded for 800 ms after the onset of the occlusion. The inspiratory occlusion pressure at the onset of the inspiratory effort was used to synchronize the occlusions and trigger the signal averager. In addition, the inspiration preceding each occlusion was averaged as the control. A specific occlusion-related evoked potential (RREP) was recorded; however, the evoked potential was absent in unoccluded averages (Fig. 6). This EEG pattern was recorded from the electrodes, Cz–C3, over the left somatosensory region. The evoked potential was similar to somatosensory evoked potentials reported for the hand and leg. Four voltage peaks were consistently observed. The first peak, P1, was a positive voltage produced by the dipole generated when a cerebral cortical column was depolarized by the arrival of activity from a population of afferents that were activated by the occlusion stimulus. This first peak signals the arrival of the afferent information at the somatosensory cortex. No evoked potential was observed in the frontal region using a cephalic reference. When a control trial using averages of unoccluded breaths was performed, this RREP was not observed.

It was subsequently found that the RREP could be recorded bilaterally from the somatosensory region of the cortex with a cephalic reference, Cz–C3 and Cz–C4 (Revelette and Davenport, 1990). It could be elicited by presentation of occlusion at that beginning of the breath and by an occlusion interruption of the

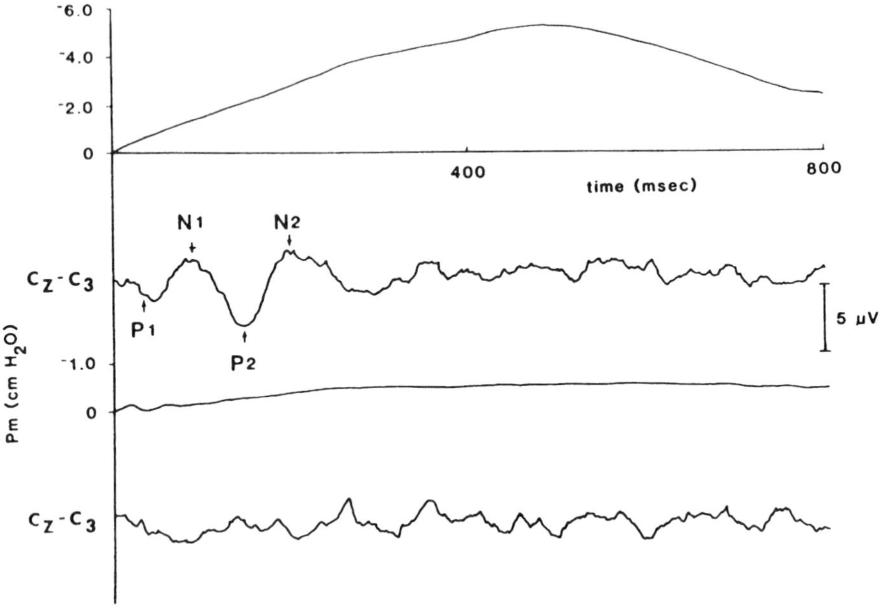

Figure 6 Averaged control and occluded breath responses. Top two traces, mouth pressure (Pm), and Cz–C3 evoked potential average with inspiratory occlusion. Bottom two traces, average control, unoccluded Pm, and Cz–C3 activity. Identifiable peaks for evoked potential related to inspiratory occlusion are indicated. No comparable peaks were discernible in the control recording. (From Davenport et al., 1985.)

breath at approximately midinspiration. Interruption of inspiration produced a larger amplitude RREP with a shorter latency than the onset occlusion. The RREP was observed with as few as 32 midinspiratory occlusions. The interrupted breath methodology is easier to use and has been the preferred method for eliciting the RREP in subsequent studies.

The peak latencies varied between subjects. The P1 latency was correlated with the P0.1, that is, decreased P1 latency with increased P0.1 (Davenport et al., 1986). This suggested that the stimulus threshold was exceeded sooner, with larger driving pressures resulting in a shorter time required for the onset of the sensory signal. The P1 latency was shorter in some subjects because of a decrease in the transduction time required for generating the sensory signal to the cortex.

This observation suggests that the generation of the P1 peak is in part related to the breathing pattern. The initiation of cortical activity is a function of the activation of the afferent system mediating the response. With occlusion, there is a respiratory drive-dependent ramp increase in the stimulus. Increases in respiratory drive increase the rate of change in the stimulus during an occlusion. This results in a decrease in the time required for the stimulus to exceed threshold and a corresponding decrease in the P1 latency. The initial observation of a relationship between P0.1 and P1 latency was made between subjects. If the rate of change in stimulus results in a decrease in the time required to exceed threshold, then an increase in respiratory drive within a subject should decrease the P1 latency. The relationship between inspiratory drive and P1 latency was investigated by comparing the RREP with steady-state hypercapnia and normocapnia (Davenport et al., 1992a). The RREP was initially observed in normocapneic subjects. These subjects were then exposed to steady-state hypercapnia, which caused a fourfold increase in the occlusion pressure elicited with onset and interrupted inspiratory occlusions. The amplitude of the P1 potential in other sensory systems is directly related to the stimulus magnitude (Franzén and Offenloch, 1969). If the mouth pressure was the source of the afferent information, then the increases in negative Pm during hypercapnia should have produced an increased amplitude for the P1 potential. However, the amplitude was not significantly different between normocapneic and hypercapnic conditions. The only parameter of the evoked potential that changed was a small but significant decrease in the P1 latency, correlated with the increase in P0.1. The decrease in latency suggests there is increase in the rate of stimulation, bringing the afferents to threshold quicker. The rate of stimulation is increased between the greater respiratory drive to the pump is increasing the rate of occlusion-related mechanoreceptor stimulation. The latency of the evoked potential is related to the time required to bring the afferents to threshold and the transmission properties of the neural pathway. The pathway properties were unlikely to change in these subjects, and hence the decrease in latency is the result of a decreased time required to bring the afferents to threshold. The lack of change in amplitude further suggests that negative mouth pressure is not the source of the afferent information mediating the RREP elicited by inspiratory occlusion.

However, an important issue arises of nonrespiratory artifacts contaminating the RREP. Possible contamination or even generation of the RREP could result as an artifact of signal-averaging electrocardiographic (ECG) activity from scalp electrodes. In addition, the inspiratory occlusion method produces auditory signals that may produce an auditory evoked potential artifact, further contaminating the RREP. The inspiratory interrupted occlusion-elicited RREP was recorded from Cz–C3 and Cz–C4 (Davenport and Hill, unpublished results). C3 and C4 were also referenced to an electrode placed over the lower cervical spine and on the lower leg. The RREP recorded with the cephalic Cz reference was unaffected by ECG activity. However, the use of noncephalic references resulted in large voltage peaks in the RREP average produced by ECG transients. This was particularly true with the leg reference. The RREP was also recorded in a deaf subject in the same study. The RREP was present in the deaf subject and was similar to that in subjects with no hearing deficit. The RREP was then recorded without using headphones for auditory masking in both occlusion and control trials. The averaged control evoked potential was electrically subtracted from the occlusion-elicited RREP. This removed the averaged activity that may be related to auditory cues and motion of the breathing apparatus. The RREP was again present and similar to that in previous reports. The absence of auditory contamination is further evidenced by the original report of the RREP (Davenport et al., 1986), in which the occlusion was produced by silently placing a stopper in the inspiratory inlet of the breathing circuit. These results demonstrate that the RREP recorded from the Cz–C3 and Cz–C4 electrode pairs is not contaminated by ECG, is not an auditory evoked potential, is not an artifact of mechanical motion of the breathing circuit, and is of cephalic origin.

The RREP has been primarily recorded with a cephalic reference Cz. The scalp distribution of the RREP remained unknown. A series of experiments were performed in children aged 10–13 to determine the scalp topographical distribution of the RREP (Davenport et al., 1992b). EEG activity was recorded from 17 electrode sites, referenced to the joined earlobes. Cz–C3 and Cz–C4 were recorded simultaneously. Inspiratory interrupted occlusions were the stimulus. The RREP was observed in the Cz–C3 and Cz–C4 recordings in all the children tested. With the joined earlobe reference, the early P1 peak predominated in the postcentral electrodes (C3, C4, P3, and P4). This suggests a sensory cortical source intermediate, rostral-caudal, between the C and P locations (the C′ site). The P1 was not observed in the midline electrodes (Fz, Cz, or Pz). A negative peak, N_f, was found in the precentral electrodes (F3, F4, F7, F8, and, to a lesser extent, C3 and C4). The N_f peak occurred approximately 13 ms after P1 and was probably generated from a different cortical source than the P1 peak. The source of this N_f peak may be associated with the motor cortex. This negativity is not observed with the Cz, the cephalic reference. The results of this study demonstrate that the early components of the RREP are of cephalic origin and the signal-to-noise ratio is greatly improved with the Cz reference. There are potentially two load-related generator sites, in the somatosensory cortex and possibly in the motor cortex.

The RREP provides a measure of neural activity related to the sensation of mechanical loads. In other somatosensory systems, there is a correlation between the amplitude of the peak analogous to P1 elicited by tactile stimulation and the magnitude of the stimulus (Franzén and Offenloch). This suggests that the amplitude of the P1 peak should be correlated with the magnitude of the inspiratory load. The correlation of the RREP with the perception of resistive loads and the associated changes in mechanics in adults was studied (Knafelc, 1992). The RREP was recorded (Cz–C3 and Cz–C4) with three graded resistive loads of 2, 9, and 21 cm $H_2O/L/s$. The loading protocol was designed to remove order effects. Four trials were used to provide 80 presentations of each load (and no load) for averaging. The RREP was obtained by averaging the presentations for each load magnitude separately. The averaged control, no-load presentations were subtracted from each averaged load RREP. The subjects also provided a magnitude estimation of the load. The log of the P1 peak amplitude linearly correlated to the log of the magnitude estimation of the loads (Fig. 7) and log of the resistive load magnitude (Fig. 8). The correlation of the P1 amplitude with the perception and mechanical changes associated with load perception supports the idea of the RREP as a neural measure of the cortical activity related to respiratory load sensation.

Asthmatic children who attend the asthma clinic at the University of Florida have been tested for the presence of mid-inspiratory occlusion-elicited RREP (Cruz et al., 1992). These patients had moderate to severe asthma. The RREP was observed bilaterally and was absent on unoccluded breaths. In the same study, children with a history of life-threatening asthma were also subjects for the recording of inspiratory occlusion elicited RREP. The P1 peak was absent in four of the nine children with life-threatening asthma tested. A somatosensory evoked potential elicited by median nerve stimulation was present in all these patients,

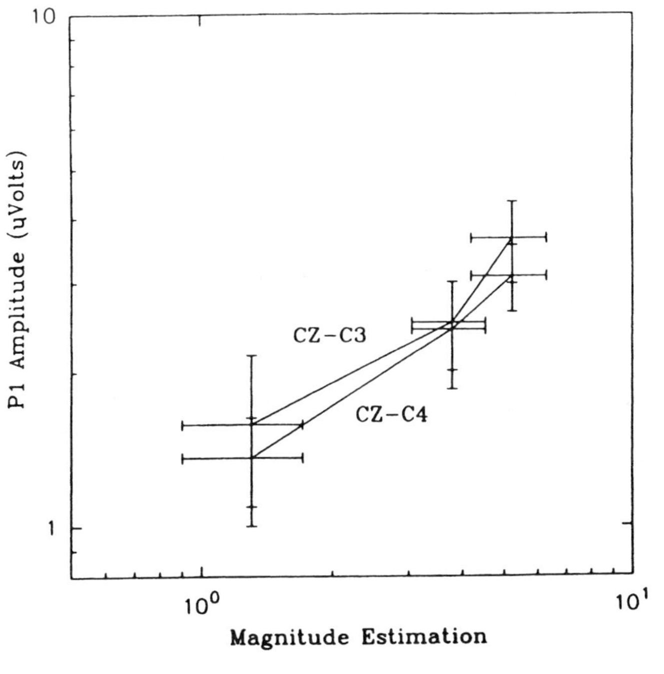

Figure 7 Relationship (log-log) between resistive load magnitude estimation and the P1 amplitude of the RREP. There was no significant difference between the electrode pairs.

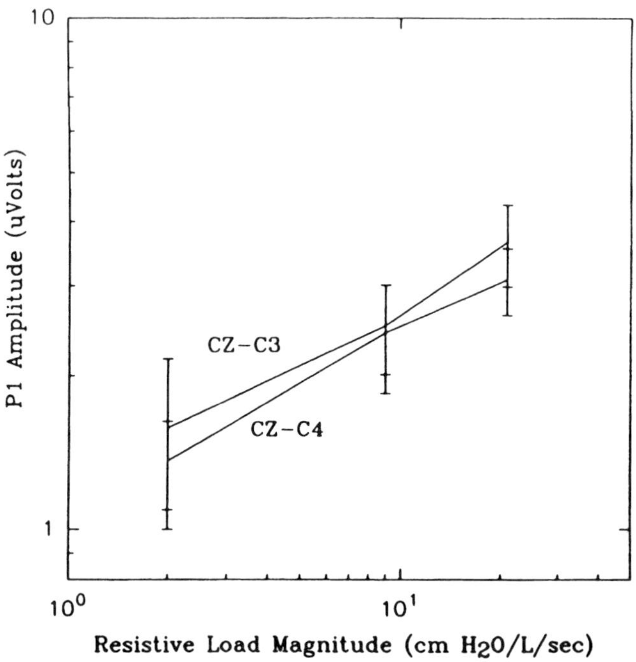

Figure 8 Relationship (log-log) between the resistive load magnitude and the amplitude of the P1 peak of the RREP. The P1 peak amplitude increased with increasing load magnitude. There was no significant difference between electrode pairs.

however. The RREP was present bilaterally in patients without life-threatening asthma. The RREP was found bilaterally in all nonasthmatic children. This suggests that this region of the somatosensory cortex is not activated by inspiratory occlusion in this subpopulation of asthmatic patients. Kikuchi et al. (1994) found a reduced perceptual sensitivity in similar adult asthmatic patients using magnitude estimation of resistive loads. Future studies combining neural and perceptual measures in these asthmatic patients are necessary to determine whether some patients are at risk of a life-threatening asthmatic attack because of a failure in the afferent transduction and/or sensory processing of respiratory load information.

The RREP is thus a bilaterally represented measure of neural activity elicited by inspiratory mechanical loads in adults and children. Inspiratory occlusions and graded suprathreshold resistive loads elicit the RREP. The P1 peak of the RREP, however, is absent in a subpopulation of asthmatic patients with life-threatening asthma. The afferents mediating the RREP remain unknown. Respiratory muscle afferents have transduction properties and cortical projection pathways consistent with their hypothesized role in respiratory load sensation. If this respiratory-related cortical activity is similar to evoked potentials for other sensory systems, then the early P1 potential represents the arrival of the sensory signal in the somatosensory region of the cerebral cortex, similar to the primary evoked potential found with cortical surface recordings in the cat.

VI. Summary

Mechanical loads increase the load to the pump, resulting in a dyspneic sensation. The correlation of the RREP with the ventilatory response to a respiratory load suggests that conscious humans use cerebral cortical sensory and motor systems as one response mechanism to respiratory loads. Perception is most likely the result of a combination of sensory processes, interacting with motor processes, leading to the sensation the subject reports. Mechanical loads act on the respiratory system and change the patterning of mechanoreceptor information. The change in pump information patterning correlates with the perceptual events related to load sensation.

The detection of the presence of resistive or elastic loads can occur without a major change in the patterning of flow or volume. However, flow- and volume-related mechanoreceptors may be participating in the perceptual process. Flow and volume afferents provide information to the central nervous system signaling the maintenance of volume or flow. However, pump afferents during a loaded breath provide information indicating altered pump performance. The net result is an increase in acuity and localization of the specific afferent change. Essential information is provided to the central nervous system, allowing the system to discriminate the presence, type, and magnitude of the mechanical load to breathing. This sensory information can then be used to develop a behavioral breathing strategy to compensate for the added load.

References

Allison, T., McCarthy, G., Wood, C.C., Williamson, P.D., and Spencer, D.D. (1989a). Human cortical potentials evoked by stimulation of the median nerve. II. Cytoarchitectonic areas generating long-latency activity. J. Neurophysiol. 62:711–722.

Allison, T., McCarthy, G., Wood, C.C., Darcey, T.M., Spencer, D.D., and Williamson, P.D. (1989b). Human cortical potentials evoked by stimulation of the median nerve. I. Cytoarchitectonic areas generating short-latency activity. J. Neurophysiol. 62: 694–710.

Anderson, S.A., Landgren, S., and Wolsk, D. (1966). The thalamic relay and cortical projection of group I muscle afferents from the forelimb of the cat. J. Physiol. (Lond.) 183:576–591.

Aubert, M. (1970). Topographie des projections de la sensibilite viscerale sur l'ecorce cerebrale du chat. II. Etude des projectoins corticales du vague cervical chez le chat anesthesie au chloralose. Arch. Ital. Biol. 108:447–461.

Aubert, M., and Guilhen, C. (1971). Topographie des projections de la sensibilite visverale sur l'ecorce cerebrale du chat. III. Etude des projections corticales du nerf larynge superieur. Arch. Ital. Biol. 109:236–252.

Aubert, M., and Legros, J. (1970). Topographie des projectoins de la sensibilite viscerale sur l'ecorce cerebrale du chat I. Etude des projections corticales du vague cervical chez le chat anesthesie. Arch. Ital. Biol. 109:423–446.

Bennet, E.D., Jayson, M.I.V., Rubenstein, D., and Campbell, E.J.M. (1962). The ability of man to detect non-elastic loads to breathing. Clin. Sci. 23:155–162.

Burki, N.K., Davenport, P.W., Safdar, F., and Zechman, F.W. (1983). The effect of airway anesthesia on magnitude estimation of added inspiratory resistive and elastic loads. Am. Rev. Respir. Dis. 127:2–4.

Campbell, E.J.M., Freedman, S., Smith, P.S., and Taylor, M.E. (1961). The ability of man to detect added elastic loads to breathing. Clin. Sci. 20:223–231.

Campbell, E.J.M., Bennet, E.D., and Rubenstein, D. (1963). The ability to distinguish between added elastic and resistive loads to breathing. Clin. Sci. 24:201–207.

Corda, M., von Euler, C., and Lennerstrand, G. (1965a). Proprioceptive innervation of the diaphragm. J. Physiol. (Lond.) 178:161–177.

Corda, M., Eklund, G., and von Euler, C. (1965b). External intercostal and phrenic α motor responses to changes in respiratory load. Acta Physiol. Scand. 63:391–400.

Critchlow, V., and von Euler, C. (1963). Intercostal muscle spindle activity and its γ-motor control. J. Physiol. (Lond.) 168:820–847.

Cruz, M., Stecenko, A., and Davenport, P.W. (1992). Respiratory related evoked potentials in asthmatic children. Am. Rev. Respir. Dis. 145(4):A631.

Davenport, P.W., Frazier, D.T., and Zechman, F.W. (1981). The effect of the resistive loading of inspiration and expiration on pulmonary stretch receptor discharge. Respir. Physiol. 43(3):299–314.

Davenport, P.W., Thompson, F.J., Reep, R.L., and Freed, A.N. (1985). Projection of the phrenic nerve afferents to the cat sensorimotor cortex. Brain Res. 328:150–153.

Davenport, P.W., Friedman, W.A., Thompson, F.J., and Franzén, O. (1986). Respiratory related cortical evoked potentials in humans. J. Appl. Physiol. 60:1843–1848.

Davenport, P.W., Dalziel, D.J., Webb, B., Bellah, J.R., and Vierck, Jr., C.J. (1991). Inspiratory resistive load detection in conscious dogs. J. Appl. Physiol. 70(3):1284–1289.

Davenport, P.W., Holt, G.A., and Hill, P.M. (1992a). The effect of increased inspiratory drive on the sensory activation of the cerebral cortex by inspiratory occlusion. In: Respiratory Control: Central and Peripheral Mechanisms. Edited by D.F. Speck, M.S. Dekin, W.R. Revelette, and D.T. Frazier. University Press of Kentucky, pp. 216–221.

Davenport, P.W., Colrain, I., and Hill, P. McN. (1992b). Scalp topography of the short latency components of the respiratory related evoked potential in children. Australasian Psychophysiology Conference (abstracts).

Davenport, P.W., Shannon, R., Mercak, A., Reep, R.L., and Lindsey, B.G. (1993). Cerebral cortical evoked potentials elicited by cat intercostal muscle mechanoreceptors. J. Appl. Physiol. 74(2):799–804.

Deiber, M.P., Giard, M.H., and Mauguiere, F. (1986). Separate generators with distinct orientations for N20 and P22 somatosensory evoked potentials to finger stimulation? Electroenceph. Clin. Neurophysiol. 65:321–334.

Desmedt, J.E., Nguyen, T.H., and Bourguet, M. (1987). Bit-mapped color imaging of human evoked potentials with reference to the N20, P22, P27 and N30 somatosensory responses. Electroenceph. Clin. Neurophysiol. 68:1–19.

Franzén, O., and Offenloch, K. (1969). Evoked response correlates of psychophysical magnitude estimates for tactile stimulation in man. Exp. Brain Res. 8:1–18.

Gamberale, F., Holmér, I., Kindblom, A.-S., and Nordström, A. (1978). Magnitude perception of added inspiratory resistance during steady-state exercise. Ergonomics 21: 531–538.

Gandevia, S.C., and Macefield, G. (1989). Projection of low-threshold afferents from human intercostal muscles to the cerebral cortex. Respir. Physiol. 77:203–214.

Gottfried, S.B., Altose, M.D., Kelsen, S.G., Fogarty, C.M., and Cherniack, N.S. (1978). The perception of changes in airflow resistance in normal subjects and patients with chronic airways obstruction. Chest 73:286–288.

Hämäläinen, H., Kekoni, J., Sams, M., Reinikainen, K., and Näätänen, R. (1990). Human somatosensory evoked potentials to mechanical pulses and vibration: contributions of SI and SII somatosensory cortices to P50 and P100 components. Electroenceph. Clin. Neurophysiol. 75:13–21.

Holt, G.A., Dalziel, D.J., and Davenport, P.W. (1991). The transduction properties of diaphragmatic mechanoreceptors. Neurosci. Lett. 122:117–121.

Huttunen, J., and Homberg, V. (1991). Modification of cortical somatosensory evoked potentials during tactile exploration and simple active and passive movements. Electroenceph. Clin. Neurophysiol. 81:216–223.

Kakigi, R., and Shibasaki, H. (1984). Scalp topography of mechanically and Velectrically evoked somatosensory potentials in man. Electroenceph. Clin. Neurophysiol. 59: 44–56.

Kikuchi, Y., Okabe, S., Tamura, G., Hida, W., Homma, M., Shirato, K., and Takishima, T. (1994). Chemosensitivity and perception of dyspnea in patients with a history of near-fatal asthma. N. Engl. J. Med. 330(19):1329–1334.

Killian, K.J., Mahutte, C.K., and Campbell, E.J.M. (1981). Magnitude scaling of externally added loads to breathing. Am. Rev. Respir. Dis. 123:12–15.

Killian, K.J., Bucens, D.D., and Campbell, E.J.M. (1982). Effect of breathing patterns on the perceived magnitude of added loads to breathing. J. Appl. Physiol. 52:578–584.

Knafelc, M.E. (1992). Effect of ventilatory loads on respiratory mechanics and dyspnea. Doctoral Dissertation, University of Florida.

Knafelc, M.E., and Davenport, P.W. (1991). Magnitude estimation of resistive loads presented at the onset of inspiration and mid-inspiration. FASEB J. 5:A1480.

Landgren, S., and Silfvenius, H. (1969). Projection to cerebral cortex of group I muscle afferents from the cat's hindlimb. J. Physiol. (Lond.) 200:353–372.

Larsson, L.-E., and Prevec, T.S. (1970). Somato-sensory response to mechanical stimulation as recorded in the human EEG. Electroenceph. Clin. Neurophysiol. 28:162–172.

McCloskey, D.I., Cross, M.J., Honner, R., and Potter, E.K. (1983). Sensory effects of pulling or vibrating exposed tendons in man. Brain 106:21–37.
Mead, J. (1960). Control of respiratory frequency. J. Appl. Physiol. 15:325–336.
Milic-Emili, J., and Zin, W.A. (1986). Breathing responses to imposed mechanical loads. In: Handbook of Physiology, The Respiratory System: Control of Breathing, Vol. II. Edited by N.S. Cherniak and J.G. Widdicombe. American Physiological Society, Washington, D.C., pp. 751–769.
Oscarsson, O., and Rosen, I. (1963). Projection to cerebral cortex of large muscle spindle afferents in forelimb nerves of the cat. J. Physiol. (Lond.) 169:924–945.
Otis, A.B., Fenn, W.O., and Rahn, H. (1950). Mechanics of breathing in man. J. Appl. Physiol. 2:592–607.
Phillips, C.G., Powell, T.P.S., and Wisendanger, M. (1971). Projection from low-threshold muscle afferents of hand and forearm area 3a of baboon's cortex. J. Physiol. (Lond.) 217:419–446.
Pratt, H., and Starr, A. (1981). Mechanically and electrically evoked somatosensory potentials in humans: scalp and neck distributions of short latency components. Electroenceph. Clin. Neurophysiol. 51:138–147.
Pratt, H., Amlie, R.N., and Starr, A. (1979). Short latency mechanically evoked somatosensory potentials in humans. Electroenceph. Clin. Neurophysiol. 47:524–531.
Revelette, W.R., and Davenport, P.W. (1990). Effects of timing of inspiratory occlusion on cerebral evoked potentials in humans. J. Appl. Physiol. 68(1):282–288.
Revelette, W.R., Zechman, F.W., Parker, D.E., and Wiley, R.L. (1984). Effect of background loading on perception of inspiratory loads. J. Appl. Physiol. 56(2):404–410.
Revelette, W.R., Taylor, R.F., Davenport, P.W., Reynolds, S.M., and Frazier, D.T. (1990). Effect of diaphragmatic muscle spindle activation on inspiratory drive. Modulation of Respiratory Pattern: Peripheral and Central Mechanisms International Conference.
Sallach, J., Davenport, P.W., and Reep, R.L. (1994). Thalamocortical projections activated by phrenic nerve afferents in the cat. Neurosci. Lett. 180:114–118.
Sant'Ambrogio, G. (1982). Information arising from the tracheobronchial tree of mammals. Physiol. Rev. 46(2):531–569.
Starr, A., McKeon, B., Skuse, N., and Burke, D. (1981). Cerebral potentials evoked by muscle stretch in man. Brain 104:149–166.
Tack, M., Altose, M.D., and Cherniack, N.S. (1981). Effect of aging on respiratory sensations produced by elastic loads. J. Appl. Physiol. 50(4):844–850.
Tack, M., Altose, M.D., and Cherniack, N.S. (1982). Effect of aging on the perception of resistive ventilatory loads. Am. Rev. Respir. Dis. 126:463–467.
Wiley, R.L., and Zechman, F.W. (1966). Perception of added airflow resistance in humans. Respir. Physiol. 2:73–87.
Wolkove, N., Altose, M.D., Kelsen, S.G., Kondapalli, P.G., and Cherniack, N.S. (1981). Perception of changes in breathing in normal human subjects. J. Appl. Physiol. 50: 78–83.
Wood, C.C., Spencer, D.D., Allison, T., McCarthy, G., Williamson, P.D., and Goff, W.R. (1988). Localization of human sensorimotor cortex during surgery by cortical surface recording of somatosensory evoked potentials. J. Neurosurg. 68:99–111.

Zechman, F.W., and Davenport, P.W. (1978). Temporal differences in detection of resistive and elastic loads to breathing. Respir. Physiol. 34:267–277.
Zechman, F.W., Hall, F.G., and Hull, W.E. (1957). Effects of graded resistance to tracheal airflow in man. J. Appl. Physiol. 10:356–362.
Zechman, F.W., Wiley, R.L., and Davenport, P.W. (1981). Ability of healthy men to discriminate between added inspiratory resistive and elastic loads. Respir. Physiol. 45:111–120.
Zechman, F.W., Muza, S.R., Davenport, P.W., Wiley, R.L., and Shelton, R. (1985). Relationship of transdiaphragmatic pressure and latencies for detecting added inspiratory loads. J. Appl. Physiol. 58:236–243.

5

Qualities of Respiratory Sensation

RICHARD M. SCHWARTZSTEIN

Harvard Medical School
and Beth Israel Hospital
Boston, Massachusetts

LYNDA M. CRISTIANO

Harvard Medical School
and Brigham and Women's Hospital
Boston, Massachusetts

I. Introduction: The Importance of Language

Imagine for a moment a world without language. There are no words, no letters, and no symbols. Would there be ideas and thoughts, and if so, how would they be expressed? Language is largely the product of our need to give form and shape to our ideas and to communicate these ideas to others. Thus, language is determined by the thoughts we hold and wish to transit to others.

Language is not merely the product of ideas, however, but also has a role molding those ideas. Buller (1966) outlines nicely the dilemma one might face, for example, in trying to describe a cow the first time you see one without having a word for cow. This might well prove to be a challenging if not somewhat daunting task. If describing an external object or experience, one that is easily visible to others, were difficult without appropriate language, imagine the assignment of trying to communicate to others an internal sensation or experience. To make things even a little more interesting, let us imagine that you are describing this internal sensation to someone who has never experienced it. Here is one of the major hurdles in the study of dyspnea.

In describing the study of pain, Reading (1989) wrote, "Man's unique verbal abilities open a window to private experience and only through such experience is pain defined." Dyspnea, like pain, is an internal, private experience (Comroe, 1956). However, although most of us at one time or another have experienced aching, burning, or sharp pains, it is not clear whether those of us without cardiopulmonary disease have truly experienced the respiratory sensations associated with asthma, congestive heart failure, or emphysema. Therefore, if Campbell and Howell (1963) are correct and "we can only describe sensations to others who have experienced them," then physicians and physiologists may be at a distinct disadvantage in studying dyspnea other than that associated with exercise.

The act of breathing is unique among physiological functions in that there is an automatic aspect to it and, yet, we have voluntary control over the muscles critical to performing the function. As Richards (1953) stated, "Breathing is truly a strange phenomenon of life, caught midway between the conscious and unconscious, and peculiarly sensitive to both." In nature, dyspnea usually occurs when ventilation is being stimulated, when the "automatic" control of breathing is turned up as with exercise, asthma, pulmonary embolism, or respiratory infection. Yet, studies of dyspnea often have focused on the sensations produced when subjects perform "voluntary" breathing tasks, such as breathing to achieve certain pressure or volume targets. It is not always clear how the data from such studies bear upon dyspnea associated with pathological conditions.

When studying dyspnea, are the investigators and subjects always discussing the same sensation? From one study to another, are investigators measuring the same thing? Is dyspnea a single sensation, or like pain, does it refer "not to a specific sensation which can vary only in intensity, but to an endless variety of qualities that are categorized under a single linguistic label (Melzack and Torgerson, 1971)?

Definitions of dyspnea have tended to focus on the sensations of "increased respiratory effort" (Meakins, 1934), "difficulty in breathing" (Campbell and Cuz, 1981), or "labored breathing" (Burki, 1987; Comroe, 1966a). Wasserman and Casaburi (1988) define dyspnea as the "sensation of feeling breathless or experiencing air hunger" and emphasize the role of increased ventilation in the origins of the sensation. Most acknowledge that there is an element of "distress" (Wright and Branscomb, 1954) or that it is an "unpleasant" (Burki, 1987) or "uncomfortable" (Comroe, 1966a) sensation rather than merely an awareness of increased ventilation. Using an analogy with pain, one would not say that "burning" is only an awareness of "heat," nor would one claim that to say that something is "warm" implies that there is "discomfort."

Campbell and Guz (1981) make the distinction between dyspnea as a symptom rather than a sensation. They argue that "we must not think that the symptom of breathlessness is just a bad dose of the normal sensation." Similarly,

Burki (1980) distinguishes physiological breathlessness from pathological breathlessness to denote whether the sensation occurs in healthy subjects or results from a cardiopulmonary disorder. We agree that the "context" or circumstances in which a sensation becomes apparent may impact the affective component of the sensation, but we believe that the quality of the sensation is independent of the context in which it arises. For example, if the sensation is unexpected it may be associated with more anxiety and discomfort than if it is expected for a given activity. However, the quality of the sensation should be the same. Therefore, it may be possible for normal subjects and patients with lung disease to experience similar sensations.

Much of the apparent confusion and conflict in the literature on breathing discomfort arises because of an attempt to channel a variety of respiratory sensations into a single concept of dyspnea or shortness of breath (Comroe, 1956; Tobin, 1990). However, if we view dyspnea, like pain, as a term that subsumes many sensations and then attempt to describe and define the language that qualifies each of these sensations, we gain a much clearer understanding of this often very distressing problem. For the purposes of this discussion, we use the term "dyspnea" as a generic term for breathing discomfort and consider it synonymous with the term "breathlessness."

II. The Language of Pain

Scientists often take pride in being able to quantify the natural world in which we live. They observe, measure, apply statistical tests, and, in some cases, try to reduce a complex system to a series of mathematical expressions. These efforts have greatly increased the understanding of our world, but they do not always give us a complete picture. This is particularly true with respect to the study of pain and dyspnea. To describe these sensations "solely in terms of intensity is like specifying the visual world only in terms of light flux without regard to pattern, color, texture and many other dimensions of visual experience" (Melzack, 1975).

Attempts to find physiological measures of pain that are more objective than verbal responses have largely been unsuccessful (Gracely, 1989). Changes in the autonomic nervous system are often associated with painful stimuli but tend to habituate quickly and may be nonspecific responses to stressful situations. Similarly, cortical evoked potentials may not associate closely with perceived pain (Gracely, 1989). Pain likely represents many different experiences, and there is not a distinct separate nerve for every kind of pain (Melzack and Torgerson, 1971). Often it is difficult to specify and quantify the pain stimulus as well as the pain response. In addition, any measuring tool must be able to account for the affective component of the painful experience as well as the sensory-discriminative qualities.

Pain researchers have attempted to deal with the problem of measuring uncomfortable sensations by focusing on the language of pain. This work also influenced many of the early studies on the qualities of respiratory perceptions, and a review of the major investigations in this area will help us to understand how to approach dyspnea.

A. Development of Pain Questionnaires

Approximately 70 years ago, Titchener (1920) described four distinctive qualitatively different categories of pain: prick, clear pain, quick pain, and ache. Dallenbach (1939) amplified on this concept by developing a list of 44 words describing pain qualities. This list was divided further into five categories that defined different attributes of the painful experience: temporal aspects (palpitating and throbbing), spatial aspects, integration with pressure (heavy and pressing), qualitative attributes (dull and sharp), and the affective component (savage and ugly).

Melzack and Torgerson (1971) refined this approach by adding 60 words to Dallenbach's list and regrouping them into only three categories: sensory qualities (temporal, spatial, pressure, and thermal), affective qualities (tension and fear), and evaluative qualities (the overall subjective intensity of the experience). In addition, they found that some words connoted an intensity of pain. For example, although the words *stabbing* and *pricking* may describe similar qualities of sensation, the word *stabbing* connotes a more intense pain. When subjects with different socioeconomic, educational, and linguistic backgrounds were asked to order the words within a grouping based on intensity, there was a high degree of agreement about the ordering (Melzack and Torgerson, 1971).

Melzack (1975) took the next step in the development of his pain questionnaire by presenting his list of descriptors to 297 patients with different pain syndromes. Interestingly, the patients were highly selective in the words they chose to describe the pain and were frequently quite grateful to be provided finally with the right word, in their minds, to describe their pain. It was as if the patients previously had not been able to communicate adequately about their pain because the appropriate language was not available to them. This inability to communicate, undoubtedly worsened by the fact that the doctors, friends, and relatives with whom they had spoken had not experienced the pain, likely led to considerable frustration.

As in this previous work (Melzack and Torgerson, 1971), Melzack again found that the descriptors contained within the words themselves implied intensities (Melzack, 1975). He suggested that an assessment of the intensity of the pain based upon the intensity implied by the descriptors chosen to qualify the pain may be more reliable than a single numerical value. The number may be more susceptible to the "vagaries of the moment" than the qualifying word (Melzack, 1975). Finally, Melzack proposed that the questionnaire would be useful to detect differences among methods to relieve pain by providing information about the relative effects of an intervention on the sensory, affective, and evaluative dimensions of the pain.

B. Application of the Pain Questionnaire

In the first application of the McGill pain questionnaire, Dubuisson and Melzack (1976) administered the questionnaire to 95 patients suffering from one of eight pain syndromes (menstrual pain, arthritic pain, labor, degenerative joint disease, toothache, metastatic carcinoma, phantom limb pain, and posttherapeutic neuralgia). The goal of the study was to determine whether the words chosen from the questionnaire by each patient would discriminate the different pain syndromes. Each type of pain appeared to be characterized by a discrete or distinctive grouping of verbal descriptors (Table 1). Furthermore, 77% of all the patients in the study resembled other patients of their diagnostic category based upon the qualifying terms they selected to describe the pain.

Subsequently, the McGill pain questionnaire has been used to discriminate different pathologic entities that at first glance may appear to have common pain qualities. Hunter and Philips (1981) administered the questionnaire to 65 patients with chronic headaches. Based on the quality of the pain, one could retrospectively distinguish between tension headaches (tight) and migraine headaches (sharp, binding, and nauseating). In addition, the authors looked at the relationship between mood and personality and the subjective experience of pain. The intensity of pain and the affective component of pain were associated with the general mood state of the patient, but no measures correlated with personality type. These results suggested that tension and migraine headaches were discrete entities rather than a continuum varying primarily in intensity and that the questionnaire might be a useful diagnostic tool in this setting.

In a related study, Grushka and Sessle (1984) applied the McGill pain questionnaire in an effort to distinguish between two causes of toothache: reversible inflammation and a necrotic pulp. The questionnaire was administered to 102 patients with toothache and correctly classified 73% of the patients. The patients with a necrotic pulp tended to select words that ranked higher in intensity than patients with reversible inflammation.

Melzack et al. (1986) utilized the McGill pain questionnaire to discriminate patients with trigeminal neuralgia from those with "atypical facial pain." Of these patients 90% were correctly classified based on the qualifiers chosen. The two syndromes were discriminated primarily on the basis of the affective components of the pain.

Table 1 Descriptions Characteristic of Clinical Pain Syndromes[a]

Menstrual pain ($N = 25$)	Arthritic pain ($N = 16$)	Labor pain ($N = 11$)	Disk disease pain ($N = 10$)	Toothache ($N = 10$)	Cancer pain ($N = 8$)	Phantom limb pain ($N = 8$)	Postherpetic pain ($N = 6$)
Sensory							
Cramping Aching	Gnawing Aching	Pounding Shooting Stabbing Sharp Cramping Aching	Throbbing Shooting Stabbing Sharp Cramping Aching Heavy Tender	Throbbing Boring Sharp	Shooting Sharp Gnawing Burning Heavy	Throbbing Stabbing Sharp Cramping Burning Aching	Sharp Pulling Aching Tender
Affective							
Tiring Sickening	Exhausting	Tiring Exhausting Fearful	Tiring Exhausting	Sickening	Exhausting	Tiring Exhausting Cruel	Exhausting
Evaluative	Annoying	Intense	Unbearable	Annoying	Unbearable		
Temporal: constant	Constant Rhythmic	Rhythmic	Constant Rhythmic	Constant Rhythmic	Constant Rhythmic	Constant Rhythmic	Constant Rhythmic

[a]A total of 95 patients suffering from one of eight clinical pain syndromes offered these responses to characterize the quality of the pain when presented with the McGill pain questionnaire. Note that each pain syndrome is identified by a unique set of descriptors. For example, even though arthritic pain and postherpetic pain have similar temporal and affective qualities, arthritic pain has a "gnawing" aspect not present in postherpetic pain. Conversely, postherpetic pain has a "sharp" and "pulling" quality not described by patients with arthritic pain.

Source: Modified from Dubuisson and Melzack (1976).

III. The Language of Breathlessness

A. Problems in the Study of Breathlessness

In the study of pain, investigators are often able to localize specific neural end organs and pathways responsible for transmitting the consequences of a noxious stimulus to the central nervous system. In the study of breathlessness, on the other hand, it is much less clear that there are "dyspnea receptors." Afferent information arises from multiple locations in the respiratory system during breathing and is conveyed centrally (Plum, 1966). The information is integrated centrally, perhaps along with a corollary discharge from the motor cortex (see section on sense of effort and Chap. 9), and the individual responds. The sensations of breathlessness should be viewed as arising from an organ system rather than from specific receptors.

If the absence of a dyspnea receptor does not make the study of breathlessness difficult enough, one is also faced with the problem that it is often impossible to define the stimulus that produces the sensation. Brightness, loudness, heat, and pressure can be easily measured and quantified, and the size of the stimulus can be correlated with a consequent rating for pain. What is the stimulus for a patient with chronic obstructive lung disease who complains of shortness of breath walking up a flight of stairs? Is it a change in arterial blood gases? Is it the resistive or elastic load on the system? Is it tension in the muscles? Is it the work of going up a flight of stairs? What about the patient with asthma or pulmonary embolism? What role does airways inflammation or pulmonary hypertension play in the sensations of dyspnea? Some of these factors can be measured with relative ease; others require invasive techniques or are difficult to determine in the intact organism. In patients it is often particularly difficult to isolate a specific stimulus and correlate this with a resulting level of dyspnea. Furthermore, as suggested by Comroe (1966a), this approach may be entirely wrong: it may lead to the asking the wrong questions. Rather than measure everything that can be measured physiologically about the respiratory system and then correlate these data with the patient's dyspnea, one must look at the sensations themselves and the subject's reaction to the sensations (Comroe, 1966a).

Finally, as noted earlier, the study of breathlessness is complicated by the duality of respiratory control, that is, our breathing is under both reflex and volitional control. It is not always clear how we can apply the knowledge gained from studies employing volitional, task-oriented breathing to further our understanding of dyspnea arising from reflex changes in ventilation.

Given these problems, how should one approach the study of breathlessness? This volume is testament to the fact that there are many approaches that will yield useful information about the origins of dyspnea and the factors that modulate respiratory sensations. Nevertheless, it is our bias that if one is truly to understand the "experience" of dyspnea given the complexity of factors impacting the sensations of respiratory discomfort, one must listen to what the patient or experimental subject tells us. We must use the language of dyspnea as a tool to understand the physiology of the sensations.

B. Early Thoughts on the Qualities of Breathlessness

Observers of the descriptions of dyspnea offered by patients and normal subjects alike repeatedly note that there is more than one kind of breathlessness. Richards (1953) contrasted the dyspnea of the mountain climber, a powerful muscular effort, from that of the asthmatic (gasping) and from that of the patient with a tracheal tumor (suffocating). Underlying these sensations, he believed, were three factors: breathing capacity, breathing effort, and respiratory drive. He described these categories of dyspnea as "restricted breathing," "labored breathing," and "increased or hyperpneic breathing."

The notion of an "urge to breathe" was presented by Wright and Branscomb (1954). They believed that there were two characteristic types of dyspnea. In one instance, the act of taking a deep breath relieved the urge to breathe. In the second instance, the deep breath did not relieve the uncomfortable urge to breathe and the circumstances ultimately led to a sense of smothering if pushed to a high intensity.

Comroe, in summing up the prevailing views on dyspnea in the mid-1960s (1966b) listed six grades or types of sensations. Some of these pertained to specific activities (deep breathing associated with exercise and the sensation associated with breath hold), some appeared to characterize sensations associated with impediments to breathing (harder to get one's breath and hindered breathing), and one recalled the concept of Wright and Branscomb (1954) of a need for a deep inspiration or a sensation of suffocating. The final sensation was an awareness that there is an increased ventilation.

Because most individuals spend the greater part of their lives without giving much thought to their breathing, merely becoming aware of one's breathing has been thought by some to be a major feature of dyspnea. Stuart-Harris (1966) described three types of "awareness of breathing": awareness of an increase in ventilation, of difficulty breathing, and of a need to breathe. It is not obvious, however, that an awareness of an increase in ventilation implies discomfort, which sets it apart from his other two categories.

An awareness of increased ventilation was also key to two of the four "elemental sensations" that, according to Campbell and Guz (1981), "singly or in combination underlie breathlessness." Tightness, excessive ventilation, excessive frequency of breathing, and difficulty in the act of breathing comprised the four elemental sensations. Tightness was distinguished from the other sensations because it is a sensation present even when the subject does not breathe. A sense of "irritation" usually residing in the anterior chest was thought to be closely allied to the sense of tightness. The awareness of excessive ventilation, to the extent that it was manifest as an increase in tidal volume, was thought to be a weak stimulus to perception; an increased respiratory rate, especially if it were interrupted by speech, was thought to be a potent source of breathlessness. Hypoxia and hypercapnia were thought to produce breathlessness to the extent that they stimulated an increase in ventilation and respiratory rate. Finally, the sensation of "difficulty in the act of breathing" was thought to be related to the concept of "inappropriateness" (Campbell and Howell, 1963). The individual becomes aware of difficulty breathing when the displacement of the respiratory system, expressed as either airflow or volume change, is less than the displacement expected. (This concept is discussed in greater detail in the section on the "sense of effort.")

C. Direct Studies of the Language of Breathlessness

In their attempts to understand the natural and physical world, scientists usually begin by observing, measuring, and quantifying the phenomena that surround them. The study of dyspnea, to the extent that individuals have focused on quantifying the intensity of breathlessness and have then tried to correlate that intensity with various physiological variables, has generally been characterized by this same approach. Comroe (1956) critiqued the attempts to determine the nature of dyspnea by trying to correlate the intensity of dyspnea with something that we can measure. As with pain (Gracely, 1989), there are no physiological measures of dyspnea that are more objective than the verbal responses provided by individuals experiencing the sensations of breathlessness. There have now been three major studies that have borrowed from the techniques of pain research to try to elaborate the language of dyspnea.

Using normal subjects, Simon et al. (1989) induced breathlessness by asking the subjects to perform a series of eight respiratory tasks. The stimuli by which dyspnea was induced, included breath holding, CO_2 inhalation, inhalation of CO_2 with ventilation voluntarily targeted below the level dictated by chemical drive, breathing with a resistive load, breathing with an elastic load, voluntary elevation of functional residual capacity, voluntary limitation of tidal volume, and exercise. After completing each task, subjects selected phrases that best described their respiratory sensations during the application of the stimulus. These phrases were selected from a list of qualifying phrases (Table 2) that had been compiled from patient interviews and pilot studies in normal subjects. A cluster analysis was used to determine whether there were natural classes or categories of respiratory sensations that would be reflected in groupings of descriptors.

Subjects were quite certain that they experienced qualitatively different sensations when performing the various tasks. Nine groups or clusters of phrases emerged (Table 3). Furthermore, the stimuli that were used to induce breathless-

Table 2 Descriptors

1.	My breath does not go in all the way.
2.	My breathing requires effort.
3.	I feel that I am smothering.
4.	I feel a hunger for more air.
5.	My breathing is heavy.
6.	I cannot take a deep breath.
7.	I feel out of breath.
8.	My chest feels tight.
9.	My breathing requires more work.
10.	I feel that I am suffocating.
11.	I feel that my breath stops.
12.	I am gasping for breath.
13.	My chest is constricted.
14.	I feel that my breathing is rapid.
15.	My breathing is shallow.
16.	I feel that I am breathing more.
17.	I cannot get enough air.
18.	My breath does not go out all the way.
19.	My breathing requires more concentration.

Source: From Simon et al. (1989).

Table 3 Clusters

Cluster name	Descriptor	Descriptive phrase
1. Rapid	14	I feel that my breathing is rapid.
2. Exhalation	18	My breath does not go out all the way.
3. Concentration	19	My breathing requires more concentration.
4. Shallow	1	My breath does not go in all the way.
	6	I cannot take a deep breath.
	15	My breathing is shallow
5. Work	2	My breathing requires effort.
	9	My breathing requires more work.
6. Suffocating	3	I feel that I am smothering.
	8	My chest feels tight.
	10	I feel that I am suffocating.
	11	I feel that my breath stops.
	13	My chest is constricted.
7. Hunger	4	I feel a hunger for more air.
	17	I cannot get enough air.
8. Heavy	5	My breathing is heavy.
	16	I feel that I am breathing more.
9. Gasping	7	I feel out of breath.
	12	I am gasping for breath.

Source: From Simon et al. (1989).

ness were characterized by different combinations of clusters (Table 4). These data suggest that there are multiple distinct sensations of dyspnea and raise the question of whether there are different physiological mechanisms underlying these sensations. Earlier, Kontos and coworkers (1963), using nonstandard phrases and different numbers and types of stimuli, observed that subjects used different phrases to describe their respiratory sensations when performing similar ventilatory tasks. However, their study was not designed to examine systematically the language of dyspnea, used stimuli that were all associated with an increase in neuromuscular output of the respiratory system, and elicited qualifying phrases that interestingly fell primarily within the clusters "suffocating" and "hunger" as described by Simon et al. (1989).

There have been two studies of patients with cardiopulmonary disease that have utilized respiratory questionnaires to examine the quality of the sensations of dyspnea. Simon and colleagues (1990) examined 53 patients representing six different pathophysiological states, including pulmonary vascular diseases, neuromuscular and chest wall disease, congestive heart failure, asthma, interstitial lung disease, chronic obstructive pulmonary disease, and pregnancy. As in their previous study (Simon et al., 1989), a subject selected the phrases from a list of 19 qualifiers that best applied to his or her "uncomfortable awareness of breathing."

Table 4 Clusters Associated with Particular Stimuli[a]

		Stimuli							
Cluster	Descriptors	BrHo	CO_2	DTV	Res	Elas	FRC	V_T	Exercise
1. Rapid	14		X				X	X	X
2. Exhalation	18						X		
3. Concentration	19			X				X	
4. Shallow	1, 6, 15							X	
5. Work	2, 9		X		X				
6. Suffocating	3, 8, 10, 11, 13								
7. Hunger	4, 17	X		X	X	X			
8. Heavy	5, 16								X
9. Gasping	7, 12								

[a]Clusters, groups of phrases that tended to be used together by subjects when describing their respiratory sensations, characterized the respiratory sensations associated with eight respiratory stimuli. Each respiratory stimulus is associated with a distinct cluster or group of clusters.

Respiratory stimuli: BrHo = breath holding; CO_2 = hypercapnia; DTV = suppressed ventilation during hypercapnia; Res = external resistive load; Elas = external elastic load; FRC = increased end-tidal lung volume; V_T = voluntary limitation of tidal volume.

Source: From Simon et al. (1989).

Table 5 Revised Clusters Associated with Particular Conditions[a]

Clusters	Descriptors	Vasc	Neuro	CHF	Preg	Inters	Asthma	COPD
1. In	1	X	X					
2. Deep	6				X		X	
3. Stops	11							
4. Gasping	12		X			X		X
5. Rapid	14	X		X				
6. More	16							
7. Exhalation	18						X	
8. Concentration	19						X	
9. Suffocating	3, 10			X				
10. Hunger	4, 7, 17			X	X			X
11. Heavy	2, 5		X	X			X	X
12. Effort	2, 7, 9		X		X	X		X
13. Tight	8, 13						X	
14. Shallow	9, 15		X			X		

[a]Vasc = pulmonary vascular disease; Neuro = neuromuscular and chest wall disease; Preg = pregnancy; Inters = interstitial lung disease.
Source: From Simon et al. (1990).

Again, a cluster analysis was used to search for similarities among descriptors chosen. A series of 14 clusters emerged (Table 5), and after further refinement of the analysis, the particular pathophysiological conditions were characterized by 8 different clusters. From these data one can conclude that patients with breathlessness resulting from a variety of pathophysiologic conditions experience qualitatively different sensations.

The analysis performed by Simon and coworkers (1990) demonstrated several other features of the respiratory sensations underlying dyspnea: multiplicity, uniqueness, and sharing. All the pathophysiological conditions were characterized by more than one cluster, suggesting that breathlessness is a composite of more than one sensation. Second, each condition was characterized by a unique set of clusters, indicating that the breathlessness in each condition is a different composite of sensations. Third, some clusters were shared by more than one condition, suggesting that dyspnea in these conditions may be mediated by similar pathways or receptors.

Drawing upon the experience of Simon et al. (1989, 1990), Elliot and colleagues (1991) developed an expanded questionnaire of phrases used to characterize respiratory sensations. They presented this questionnaire to 208 patients with cardiopulmonary disease and asked each subject to respond "yes" or "no" to each of the items to describe the feeling they experience when their breathing "troubles them" during walking, running, or climbing stairs. First they established the validity of the questionnaire by inserting a number of repeated phrases. Of the 208 patients, 169 were considered reliable in their responses. A cluster analysis was then applied, and 12 groupings of phrases emerged (Table 6). These data confirm the findings of Simon et al. (1990) that the dyspnea experienced by patients with different pathophysiological maladies is characterized by different clusters and again suggest that there are multiple separate and distinct sensations subsumed by the concept of breathlessness.

The three studies cited (Simon et al., 1989, 1990; Elliott et al., 1991) utilized questionnaires derived from the experiences of English-speaking subjects and patients in the United States and Great Britain. It is unclear at this point whether these questionnaires can simply be translated into other languages and used with patients in different countries or whether similar results will be obtained if they are administered to patients for whom English is not the native language. In addition to the linguistic problems inherent in translating the somewhat colloquial terms found in questionnaires, cultural influences may lead to the use of very different language when describing unpleasant respiratory sensations.

Attempts are being made to employ dyspnea questionnaires in France and Portugal. Preliminary results from France suggest that there are significant cultural impediments to this approach (C. Peiffer, personal communication). French patients appear uncertain about the meaning of the idiomatically translated phrases and reluctant to discriminate among different sensations. As the migration of individuals around the world increases, the need to clarify cultural influences on the language of dyspnea will grow in importance.

IV. Language of Common Respiratory Sensations

Focusing largely on the chest wall as the source of respiratory sensations, Killian and Campbell (1985) described three types of proprioceptive sensations—displacement, force, and effort—that they believed were the underpinnings of dyspnea. There are many other sources of information throughout the respiratory system, however, including the upper airway, pulmonary receptors, and chemoreceptors. It is likely that information from these sites also contributes to the sensations of breathlessness. We examine in more detail three of the most common sensations of dyspnea, air hunger, effort, and chest tightness, which reflect the contribution of several of these sites in producing breathlessness.

A. The Sense of Air Hunger

The "urge to breathe" may be one of the strongest impulses we experience. Dyspnea, it has been stated, occurs when the act of breathing does not satisfy the urge to breathe (Wright and Branscomb, 1954). The urge to breathe or need to

Table 6 Descriptors of Breathing Trouble and Their Groupings Resulting from Cluster Analysis

Grouping	*Y*	*N*
Cluster 1		
1. I feel out of breath.	137	15
2. I feel short of breath.	146	13
3. I feel puffed.	131	16
4. I feel breathless.	136	16
5. I am aware of my breathing.	141	9
6. I feel a need to breathe.	102	25
7. My breathing takes too much effort.	96	41
8. It is difficult to breathe.	110	37
9. I can't get enough air into my chest.	110	31
10. My breathing is not sufficient.	96	23
11. My breath does not go in enough.	85	34
12. I feel I cannot breathe deeply enough.	101	29
13. I feel I cannot breathe enough.	99	32
14. I want to take in more air.	119	29
15. I feel a need to take a deeper breath.	119	26
16. My breathing feels uncomfortable.	97	33
17. My breathing is too shallow.	79	43
18. I do not feel satisfied by my breathing.	90	28
Cluster 2		
19. I feel I am fighting for breath.	91	54
20. I feel desperate for breath.	71	58
21. I feel I am grasping for breath.	101	50
22. I feel a hunger for more air.	88	50
Cluster 3		
23. I feel wheezy.	84	67
Cluster 4		
24. My breathing feels tiring.	77	52
25. My chest feels tired.	63	69
26. My breathing feels unpleasant.	62	65
Cluster 5		
27. My chest feels tight.	85	54
Cluster 6		
28. My chest aches.	56	88
Cluster 7		
29. I feel I am suffocating.	49	87
30. I feel I am smothering.	43	92
31. I feel that my breath stops.	29	113
Cluster 8		
32. I feel that I am breathing bad air.	11	129
33. I feel that air does not taste right.	8	128

Table 6 Continued

Grouping	*Y*	*N*
Cluster 8 (continued)		
34. My breathing is too deep.	10	108
35. I feel a raw sensation in my chest.	30	108
36. I feel a raw sensation deep in my throat.	30	121
Cluster 9		
37. I cannot breathe fast enough.	50	72
38. I cannot breathe in fast enough.	56	62
39. I feel I can't control my breathing.	61	63
40. My breath does not go out enough.	38	74
41. I cannot breathe out fast enough.	31	78
42. My breathing is too heavy.	42	73
Cluster 10		
43. My breathing is too fast.	59	59
Cluster 11		
44. I feel winded in my chest.	38	72
Cluster 12		
45. I feel I want to sigh.	50	86

Source: Modified from Elliott et al. (1991).

breathe appears to require an enhanced "respiratory drive" or increase in neural output to the ventilatory muscles. Kontos et al. (1963) studied 11 normal subjects who were given carbon dioxide to breathe, made to exercise, or given a respiratory stimulant. They all developed breathing discomfort characterized by such phrases as "could not get enough air," "could not breathe fast or deep enough," and "suffocating." The intensity of these sensations was relieved by breathing with larger tidal volumes.

In the absence of an intact respiratory controller, of an automatic or reflex drive to breathe, these sensations do not arise. Plum (1966) described patients with lesions of the brain stem who did not have an "automatic" control of ventilation but did have intact voluntary respiratory movements. These subjects reportedly did not experience breathlessness. Similarly, subjects with congenital central hypoventilation syndrome, who maintain relatively normal ventilation while awake but require mechanical ventilation when asleep to prevent apneic respiratory failure, develop neither an increase in ventilation nor a sense of an urge to breathe when exposed to CO_2 or made to exercise (Shea, personal communication). These findings suggest that this type of breathlessness can occur only if the stimulus retains the ability to excite the medullary center (Plum, 1966).

The phrases "need to breathe," "urge to breathe," and "cannot get enough air" fit most closely with the cluster "air hunger" (Simon et al., 1990). Four experimental stimuli, exercise, hypoxia, hypercapnia, and suppressed ventilation, have been employed to study the sensation of air hunger.

Exercise

Adams and Guz (1991) have detailed the debate about whether the term "dyspnea" should be applied to the sensations experienced by normal subjects when exercising. As stated earlier, we contend that the concept of whether a sensation is appropriate or expected (or inappropriate or unexpected) for a particular condition may impact the affective component of the sensation. However, we do not believe it alters the basic phrases used to qualify or describe the sensation.

Lane et al. (1987a) describe 18 subjects who exercised and described their associated respiratory sensation as "an uncomfortable need to breathe." Interestingly, this sensation was not altered by the addition of resistive loads to the breathing circuit during exercise. The subjects were able to distinguish the increased difficulty breathing associated with the resistors from the need to breathe arising from the exercise. Simon and colleagues (1989) found that exercise was characterized by the sensations of "rapid" and "heavy" breathing. It is possible that the intensity of exercise in this study was not sufficient to produce a sensation of air hunger.

Hypoxia

Until recently, hypoxia and hypercapnia were believed to be perceived only to the extent that they resulted in an increase in respiratory frequency and total ventilation (Campbell and Guz, 1981). A more recent study of normal subjects made hypoxic during exercise (Chronos et al., 1988), however, dispels this notion. Subjects performed steady-state exercise with varying levels of inspired oxygen and were asked to rate "the uncomfortable need to breathe." Breathing a gas mixture containing 15% oxygen, subjects noted that changes in breathlessness occurred more quickly than changes in ventilation. This contrasted with the trials in which subjects breathed 100% oxygen and breathlessness tracked with changes in ventilation. These data suggest that hypoxia may contribute to dyspnea independently of ventilation and lead to air hunger.

Hypercapnia

A number of studies have shown that hypercapnia causes breathing discomfort and that restriction of ventilation during hypercapnia increases the intensity of the discomfort (Remmers et al., 1968; Chonan et al., 1987; Schwartzstein et al., 1989). These results are consistent with the concept that information from the chest wall is important in modulating the dyspnea associated with hypercapnia (Campbell and Howell, 1963; Killian and Campbell, 1985; Schwartzstein et al.,

1989, 1990). Investigations into the quality of breathlessness associated with hypercapnia have largely utilized experimental models that attempt to minimize the information arising from the chest wall to establish whether hypercapnia independently gives rise to breathlessness.

Patients with complete high cervical spinal cord injuries who are maintained chronically on mechanical ventilators develop breathing discomfort characterized as air hunger in association with hypercapnia (Banzett et al., 1989). Despite the absence of chest wall afferent information, these patients developed progressive air hunger with acute incremental changes in end-tidal P_{CO_2} produced by changing the inspired concentration of carbon dioxide.

Manning and colleagues (1992) also demonstrated that patients with high cervical spinal cord injury develop air hunger or an urge to breathe in association with hypercapnia. Furthermore, the same sensation was produced when end-tidal P_{CO_2} was held constant but tidal volume was decreased. This suggests that pulmonary receptors rather than muscle and chest wall receptors are the source of information that "satisfies" the urge to breathe (Wright and Branscomb, 1954).

An alternative approach to dissociating the breathlessness of hypercapnia from ventilation was provided by Demediuk et al. (1992). Normal subjects maintained a constant level of ventilation by following a visual display and periodically rated their effort to breathe and their sense of an unpleasant urge to breathe. Carbon dioxide was added surreptitiously to the inspired gas. Subjects were able to rate the two sensations independently. At a constant level of ventilation, the urge to breathe increased with elevations in end-tidal P_{CO_2} while the sense of effort to breathe decreased (Fig. 1). Thus, the urge to breathe characterizes the breathlessness of hypercapnia and is distinct from the sense of effort. One cannot help but wonder whether these differences in language imply differences in the physiological mechanisms producing the sensations.

Suppressed or Restricted Ventilation

At some point in their lives most individuals have attempted to hold their breath either as a game or to swim underwater. It is clear that during a breath hold an uncomfortable sensation develops that ultimately forces the individual to take a breath. The potential sources of the unpleasant sensation, including chest wall muscles (Noble et al., 1971; Campbell et al., 1967; Whitelaw et al., 1981), pulmonary afferents (Guz et al., 1966), and blood gas derangements (Fowler, 1954), have received considerable attention, but the quality of the sensation has generally not been studied in a systematic way. Guz et al. (1966) found that normal subjects described an unpleasant sensation from the chest that developed almost immediately after initiating the breath hold, worsened with the duration of the breath hold, and ultimately forced the subject to take a breath. The chest sensation was relieved almost immediately with the first breath.

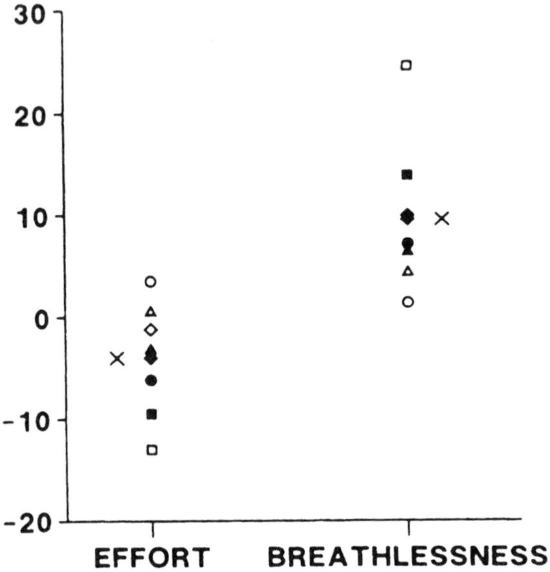

Figure 1 Mean change in effort and breathlessness ratings of normal subjects maintaining a constant level of hyperpnea when carbon dioxide was added to the inspired gas in quantities sufficient to induce mild hypercapnia. Under conditions of mild hypercapnia, the sense of "effort" associated with maintaining the targeted ventilation was reduced but the sense of "breathlessness" or "unpleasant urge to breathe" increased. (Modified from Demediuk et al., 1992.)

Banzett and colleagues (1990) paralyzed normal subjects with a neuromuscular blocker and found that they developed a sensation of air hunger even in the absence of active muscle contraction. They commented further that the sensation was similar to that of a standard breath hold. This suggests that the sensation of air hunger associated with a breath hold does not depend on the willful suppression of breathing.

An alternative model for studying the breathlessness associated with restricted or suppressed ventilation requires subjects either to restrict tidal volume voluntarily (Simon et al., 1989) or to limit chest wall excursion by mechanical means (Wright and Branscomb, 1954). The subjects who voluntarily restrict tidal volume at rest describe their respiratory sensations as rapid and shallow breathing (Simon et al., 1989), and subjects with a mechanical impediment to deep breathing (binding of the chest and abdomen with tape) who are stimulated to breathe with exercise describe a sensation of air hunger (Wright and Branscomb, 1954).

B. Sense of Effort

The majority of patients with chronic pulmonary problems and dyspnea, including patients with chronic obstructive pulmonary disease (COPD), asthma, interstitial lung disease, and kyphoscoliosis, have an increased work of breathing as a result of the resistive and elastic loads that are prominent features of the pathophysiology of their underlying diseases. This has led to considerable research on load compensation (Axen and Haas, 1982; Burdon et al., 1983; Axen et al., 1983), load perception (Campbell et al., 1980; Revelette and Wiley, 1987; Killian et al., 1982), and the mechanisms underlying load perception (Noble et al., 1972; Whitelaw et al., 1976; DiMarco et al., 1982; Gottfried et al., 1984). It has also led to an emphasis on the sense of effort as the specific sensation most closely related to dyspnea (Killian and Campbell, 1985).

There is considerable evidence that the sense of effort plays a role in breathlessness in many disease states and experimental conditions (see Chap. 9), but one must be cautious about equating the grading of effort with dyspnea in all situations (Wasserman and Casaburi, 1988). If one requires the definition of dyspnea to include a quality of discomfort, there are clearly circumstances in which one can experience an increased effort to breathe without experiencing discomfort and thus without provoking dyspnea. Using an analogy with limb muscles, one can lift a weight and describe the effort involved in performing the task yet not experience pain. Similarly, one can breathe against a resistive load and describe the effort involved in performing the task yet not experience dyspnea.

The Sense of Effort and the Concept of "Inappropriateness"

In the early 1960s, Campbell and Howell (1963) grappled with the relationship between dyspnea and loaded breathing and proposed the concept commonly referred to as length-tension inappropriateness. At its core, this concept encompasses the idea of a comparison between two kinds of information, central and peripheral. As neural impulses leave the cerebral cortex ultimately to stimulate the muscles of ventilation, a "corollary discharge" (Sperry, 1950) is sent to the sensory cortex and is perceived as "effort" (Killian and Campbell, 1985; Gandevia, 1988). If there is a load on the respiratory system, then the ventilatory muscles do not contract to the same degree, nor do the lungs inflate to the same degree as they would for the same neural stimulation in the unloaded state. Thus, the introduction of a load "alters the relationship between the demand for, and the effort of, breathing" (Campbell and Howell, 1963). They suggested that "this imbalance" was "ultimately responsible for the unpleasant sensation" (1963). The notion of an imbalance between efferent neural impulses from the central nervous system and the afferent information returning from the respiratory system has been generalized to include the contribution from upper airway and pulmonary receptors as well as chest wall receptors (Plum, 1966; Schwartzstein et al., 1990). This imbalance has been termed efferent reafferent dissociation and is thought to impact the intensity of breathlessness rather than produce an independent sensory experience (Schwartzstein, 1990).

Campbell (1966) subsequently stated that "hindered hyperpnea" is not a cause for respiratory disease. Rather, in the circumstance of increased ventilation without a mechanical load, the individual merely recognizes that breathing is increased. This is likely to be true for a subject performing isocapnic hyperpnea in a laboratory, but it might be hard to convince an athlete who is gasping for air at the end of a hard race that he or she is not experiencing distress. The effort of breathing may not be perceived as excessive, but is there air hunger? Problems arise if we try to explain all dyspnea by a single mechanism or do not listen carefully to the description of the respiratory discomfort.

The Case for the Sense of Effort

Studies of the relationship between the sense of effort and dyspnea have often utilized normal subjects breathing with externally applied resistive and elastic loads (Killian et al., 1981, 1984). In one study, subjects varied the tidal volume and inspiratory flow rate while breathing on a load and then estimated the magnitude of the load (Killian et al., 1981). The perceived magnitude of the load depended not only on its elastance or resistance but on the "effort" of the loaded breath. Although the psychophysical technique of magnitude estimation is a well-established technique for studying sensations (see Chap. 4), it is unclear in this context whether this technique reveals much about uncomfortable respiratory sensations. Again, using the analogy to pain, one can shine lights of varying power into the eye of a subject and ask him to estimate the magnitude of the "brightness" without learning much about painful optical stimuli.

In a related study, Killian and coworkers (1984) instructed normal subjects to breathe with added external elastic loads at functional residual capacity and at increased lung volume. The subjects rated the magnitude of effort, tension, and breathlessness. All three ratings correlated with increases in mouth pressure, although effort tracked better with breathlessness than tension. Based on these data, the authors concluded that breathlessness and effort were psychophysically the same and that tension was perceived by a different sensory mechanism. Unfortunately, the specific instructions given to the subjects with respect to the sensations being rated were not delineated. It was noted that subjects, when not specifically instructed to rate effort or tension, preferentially rated effort. Effort is a familiar concept to the average person. It is possible that the subjects were equating breathlessness and effort as they performed the designated respiratory tasks.

In a group of patients with a variety of pulmonary problems, the magnitude of breathlessness associated with exercise was significantly related to the peak inspiratory pressure expressed as a fraction of the maximal inspiratory pressure (Leblanc et al., 1986). If one assumes that the peak inspiratory pressure is a measure of respiratory effort, then effort and breathlessness are related. No information was provided in this study about the quality of the sensations experienced by the subjects.

The qualitative sensory cluster "effort" comprised of the phrases "my breathing requires effort" and "my breathing is heavy" has been associated, along with other descriptors, with the dyspnea of neuromuscular disease, pregnancy, interstitial disease, and COPD (Simon et al., 1990). A sensory cluster including the phrases "my breathing takes too much effort" and "it is difficult to breathe" was frequently chosen to describe the sensation of "breathing trouble" in the other major study to date of the qualities of breathlessness in patients (Elliott et al., 1991). Thus, a sense of increased respiratory effort or work of breathing is clearly a component of the dyspnea of many patients with cardiopulmonary disease.

The Case Against the Sense of Effort

In addition to the formal studies cited earlier of the language of dyspnea in patients (Simon et al., 1990; Elliott et al., 1991), there are also a number of experimental models of dyspnea that suggest that the sense of effort alone cannot be equated with dyspnea. Adams and Guz have performed several studies in which total ventilation and/or the pattern of breathing was controlled; that is, effort was controlled and other respiratory stimuli were altered (Adams et al., 1985, 1986; Chronos et al., 1988; Lane et al., 1987b). For the same level of ventilation, isocapnic hyperpnea resulted in less breathlessness than exercise (Lane et al., 1987b) and less breathlessness than hypoxic or hypercapnic hyperpnea (Adams et al., 1985). Furthermore, for matched levels of ventilation hypercapnia and hypoxia resulted in greater breathing discomfort than exercise (Adams et al., 1985). In at least one of these studies (Adams et al., 1985), subjects rated "an uncomfortable need to breathe." Thus, the sense of effort may stay the same but the sense of air hunger may change.

This notion that two qualities of breathlessness may vary independently was also demonstrated by Demediuk and coworkers (1992). Normal subjects were asked to maintain a constant level of ventilation while end-tidal P_{CO_2} was altered by adding carbon dioxide to the inspired gas. The sensation of "urge to breathe" increased with hypercapnia while the sense of "effort" decreased. In a related study, Manning et al. (1991) found that in-phase chest wall vibration reduced the sense of effort associated with hypercapnia and an external resistive load in normal subjects. This occurred with no change in ventilation. The reduced sense of effort may have been a result of increased stimulation of chest wall receptors and diminished efferent-reafferent dissociation.

C. The Sense of Chest Tightness

Asthma is a common disease affecting approximately 10% of the population. The pathophysiology of asthma is characterized by airways inflammation, airways obstruction, and hyperinflation. Attempts to understand the dyspnea associated with asthma have focused largely on the role of airways resistance and the perception of increased resistance to flow. Only in more recent years have there been studies that directly addressed the language of breathlessness associated with asthma, and these have demonstrated that the sensations of "chest tightness" and "chest constriction" are typical of the breathlessness of asthma.

"In" Versus "Out"

When describing the severity of illness in patients with obstructive lung disease, it is common practice to make spirometric measures of expiratory airflow, such as forced vital capacity and forced expiratory volume in one second (FEV_1). Consequently, we commonly think of the obstruction and the associated respiratory discomfort as an expiratory event. Is that how patients perceive the problem?

Patients with chronic bronchitis have described their breathlessness as a sensation of difficulty getting air in and out of the chest, particularly out of the chest (Burns and Howell, 1969). Asthmatics, on the other hand, typically state that inspiration is more difficult than expiration (Chapman and Rebuck, 1983; Schwartzstein et al., 1992). Normal subjects when breathing on external resistive loads also tend to scale the inspiratory load greater than the expiratory load, perhaps because exhalation is largely a passive activity during quiet breathing (Chapman and Rebuck, 1983).

Asthma, Dyspnea, and Load Perception

Although asthma is a disease characterized by increased airways resistance, many studies comparing the sensations associated with bronchoconstriction with those accompanying external resistive loads suggest that there must be something else that plays an important role in the breathlessness of asthma. Kelsen et al. (1981) studied 11 patients with asthma who were asked to compare the sensation of "the effort involved in breathing" during methacholine-induced bronchospasm with that of external resistive loads. The effort associated with bronchoconstriction was greater than with the external loads for all levels of resistance. Similarly, Schwartzstein and coworkers (1991) found that the intensity of breathlessness was greater for a given level of airways resistance with bronchoconstriction than with external resistive loads. In addition they elicited two different sensations associated with bronchoconstriction. At mild degrees of bronchoconstriction, subjects primarily noted a sensation of "chest tightness or constriction"; at more severe levels of bronchospasm, the sense of "effort" as well as the sense of "chest tightness" were present (Fig. 2). Previously, Burki (1984) alluded to the sense of chest tightness in a study of the ability of subjects with asthma to estimate the size of externally applied respiratory resistive loads. The subjects estimated the size of the external loads both before and after a bronchodilator was given. Although the perception of the external loads did not differ between the asthmatic and normal subjects, the individuals with asthma noted a decrease in chest tightness after administration of the bronchodilator. As noted in the discussion of the sense of effort, the technique of magnitude estimation as applied to external loads may have little to do with the symptom of dyspnea.

The intensity of breathlessness in asthma appears to increase as the FEV_1 decreases. This has been shown whether the bronchoconstriction is induced with histamine (Burdon et al., 1982; Turcotte et al., 1990; Schwartzstein et al., 1992), exercise (Turcotte et al., 1990), antigen challenge (Turcotte et al., 1990), or methacholine (Schwartzstein et al., 1991). However, there may be a considerable variation in the severity of breathlessness for any particular degree of airflow obstruction (Burdon et al., 1982).

The intensity of dyspnea for a given degree of airflow obstruction does not

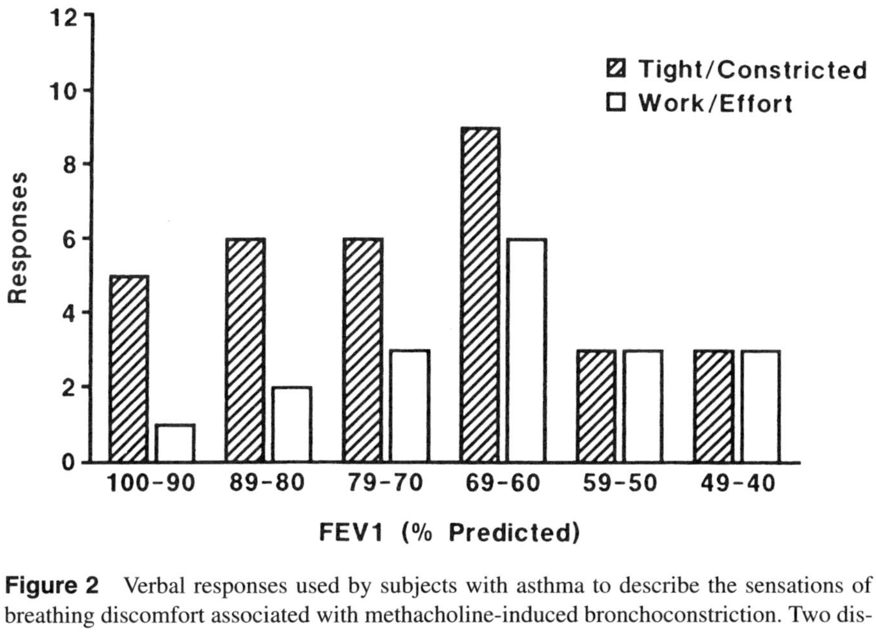

Figure 2 Verbal responses used by subjects with asthma to describe the sensations of breathing discomfort associated with methacholine-induced bronchoconstriction. Two distinct sensations emerged. At mild degrees of airways obstruction, "chest tightness or constriction" was the primary sensation. At more intense levels of bronchoconstriction, the sense of "effort" and "tightness" were used to characterize the breathing discomfort.

appear to be dependent upon the stimulus to bronchoconstriction (Turcotte et al., 1990; Schwartzstein et al., 1992), but the quality of the sensation may vary. Although subjects with bronchoconstriction induced by methacholine or histamine typically describe their discomfort associated with mild degrees of airflow obstruction as chest tightness (Schwartzstein et al., 1991, 1992), the breathlessness accompanying mild bronchospasm following inhalation of leukotrienes is also characterized by a sensation of air hunger (Fig. 3) (Schwartzstein et al., 1992). This suggests that pulmonary receptors variably stimulated by different mediators of airways inflammation play a role in the breathlessness of asthma.

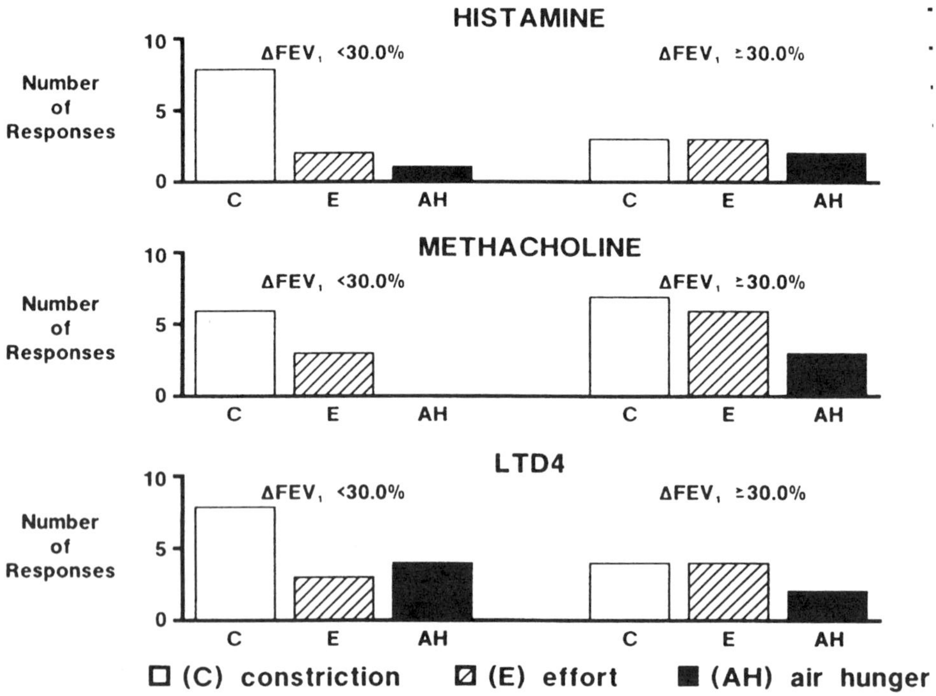

Figure 3 Verbal responses used by subjects with asthma to describe the sensations of breathing discomfort associated with bronchoconstriction induced by inhaled methacholine, histamine, and leukotrienes (LTD_4). At mild degrees of airways obstruction (change in $FEV_1 < 30\%$), the sense of "chest constriction" (C) was the most prominent sensation. The sensation of "air hunger" (AH), however, was associated with LTD_4 more often than with histamine or methacholine ($p < 0.05$). At more intense levels of bronchoconstriction all three sensations, C, effort (E), and AH, characterized the breathing discomfort.

Questionnaire Studies in Asthma

In the two major dyspnea studies utilizing questionnaires to ascertain the language of dyspnea in patients with asthma (Simon et al, 1990; Elliott, 1991), individuals with asthma described their breathlessness as a chest tightness or chest constriction as well as a sensation of increased effort or work of breathing. In addition, some subjects indicated that "their breath does not go out all the way" (Simon et al., 1990).

The source of the sensation of chest tightness remains in dispute. Permutt et al. (1991) acknowledge that the breathlessness of an acute asthma attack cannot be reproduced by breathing with an external resistive load. They believe that what is missing from experimental models that rely on external resistive loads is the hyperinflation associated with an asthma attack. Permutt argues that the sensation of chest tightness arises from the necessity to breathe at high lung volumes, and he describes one subject who, when placed on an apparatus that resulted in an elevation in functional residual capacity (FRC) of 2 L, developed chest tightness. However, studies of subjects in whom bronchoconstriction is induced with methacholine demonstrate that chest tightness develops with changes in FRC of less than 1 L (Schwartzstein et al., 1991, 1992). Studies of bronchoconstriction in patients following heart-lung transplants (Banner et al., 1988) have shown that individuals can develop chest tightness with denervated lungs, although the trachea remains a possible source of afferent information in these individuals.

V. Summary

As a general rule, we are not aware of information coming from each of our sensory organs on a moment-to-moment basis. Rather, we receive data from receptors throughout our body and integrate the information in the central nervous system to give us a "big picture" appreciation of our environment (Buller, 1966). The symptom of uncomfortable breathing, dyspnea, is in fact comprised of many sensations that likely are the result of the integration of afferent information from the chest wall, lungs, upper airways, chemoreceptors, and the corollary discharge associated with efferent impulses from the motor cortex. If we are to understand fully the sources of this information and the ways in which it is transformed into a respiratory symptom, we must pay heed to what our patients and subjects tell us. To describe dyspnea solely in terms of intensity "is like specifying the visual world only in terms of light flux without regard to pattern, color, texture and many other dimensions of visual experience" (Melzack, 1975). The qualities of dyspnea, the language employed by individuals to describe their breathing discomfort, are important keys to our understanding of an often debilitating symptom.

Acknowledgment

Supported by Pulmonary SCOR Grant HL19170-16 from the National Heart, Lung, and Blood Institute.

References

Adams, L., and Guz, A. (1991). Dyspnea on exertion. In: Exercise: Pulmonary Physiology and Pathology. Edited by B.J. Whipp and K. Wasserman. Dekker, New York, pp. 449–494.

Adams, L., Lane, R., Shea, S.A., Cockcroft, A., and Guz, A. (1985). Breathlessness during different forms of ventilatory stimulation: a study of mechanisms in normal subjects and respiratory patients. Clin. Sci. 69:663–672.

Adams, L., Chronos, N., Lane, R., and Guz, A. (1986). The measurement of breathlessness induced in normal subjects: individual differences. Clin. Sci. 70:131–140.

Altose, M., Cherniak, N., and Fishman, A.P. (1985). Respiratory sensations and dyspnea. J. Appl. Physiol. 58:1051–1054.

Axen, K., and Haas, S.S. (1982). Effect of thoracic deafferentation on load-compensating mechanisms in humans. J. Appl. Physiol. 52:757–767.

Axen, K., Haas, S.S., Haas, F., Gaudino, D., and Haas, A. (1983). Ventilatory adjustments during sustained mechanical loading in conscious humans. J. Appl. Physiol. 55: 1211–1218.

Banner, N.R., Heaton, R., Hollingshead, L., Guz, A., and Yacoub, M.H. (1988). Bronchial reactivity to methacholine after combined heart-lung transplantation. Thorax 43: 955–959.

Banzett, R.B., Lansing, R.W., Reid, M.B., Adams, L., and Brown, R. (1989). "Air hunger" arising from increased P_{CO_2} in mechanically ventilated quadriplegics. Respir. Physiol. 76:53–68.

Banzett, R.B., Lansing, R.W., Brown, R., Topulos, G.P., Yager, D., Steele, S.M., Londono, B., Loring, S.H., Reid, M.B., Adams, L., and Nations, C.S. (1990). "Air hunger" from increased P_{CO_2} persists after complete neuromuscular block in humans. Respir. Physiol. 81:1–18.

Bromm, B., and Scharien, E. (1981). Response plasticity of pain evoked reactions in man. Physiol. Behav. 28:109–116.

Buller, A.J. (1966). The muscle spindle and the control of movement. In: Breathlessness. Edited by J.B.L. Howell and E.J.M. Campbell. Blackwell Scientific, London, pp. 11–17.

Burdon, J.G.W., Juniper, E.F., Killian, K.J., Hargreave, F.E., and Campbell, E.J.M. (1982). The perception of breathlessness in asthma. Am. Rev. Respir. Dis. 126:825–828.

Burdon, J.G.W., Killian, K.J., Stubbing, D.G., and Campbell, E.J.M. (1983). Effect of background loads on the perception of added loads to breathing. J. Appl. Physiol. 54:1222–1228.

Burki, N.K. (1980). Dyspnea. In: Clinics in Chest Medicine. Edited by M.H. Williams. W.B. Saunders, Philadelphia, pp. 47–55.

Burki, N.K. (1984). Effects of bronchodilation on magnitude estimation of added resistive loads in asthmatic subjects. Am. Rev. Respir. Dis. 129:225–229.
Burki, N.K. (1987). Dyspnea. Lung 165:269–277.
Burns, B.H., and Howell, J.B.L. (1969). Disproportionately severe breathlessness in chronic bronchitis. Q. J. Med. 38:277–294.
Campbell, E.J.M. (1966). The relationship of the sensation of breathlessness to the act of breathing. In: Breathlessness. Edited by J.B.L. Howell and E.J.M. Campbell. Blackwell Scientific, London, pp. 55–64.
Campbell, E.J.M., and Guz, A. (1981). Breathlessness. In: Regulation of Breathing, Part II. Edited by T.F. Hornbein. Dekker, New York, pp. 1181–1195.
Campbell, E.J.M., and Howell, J.B.L. (1963). The sensation of breathlessness. Br. Med. Bull. 19:36–40.
Campbell, E.J.M., Freedman, S., Clark, T.J.H., Robson, J.G., and Norman, J. (1967). The effect of muscular paralysis induced by tubocurarine on the duration and sensation of breath-holding. Clin. Sci. 32:425–432.
Campbell, E.J.M., Gandevia, S.C., Killian, K.J., Mahutte, C.K., and Rigg, J.R.A. (1980). Changes in the perception of inspiratory resistive loads during partial curarization. J. Physiol. (Lond.) 309:93–100.
Chapman, K.R., and Rebuck, A.S. (1983). Inspiratory and expiratory resistive loading as a model of dyspnea in asthma. Respiration 44:425–432.
Chonan, T., Mulholland, M.B., Cherniack, N.S., and Altose, M.D. (1987). Effects of voluntary constraining of thoracic displacement during hypercapnia. J. Appl. Physiol. 63:1822–1828.
Chronos, N., Adams, L., and Guz, A. (1988). Effect of hyperoxia and hypoxia on exercise-induced breathlessness in normal subjects. Clin. Sci. 74:531–537.
Comroe, J.H. (1956). Dyspnea. Mod. Concepts Cardiovasc. Dis. 25:347–349.
Comroe, J.H. (1966a). Some theories of the mechanism of dyspnea. In: Breathlessness. Edited by J.B.L. Howell and E.J.M. Campbell. Blackwell Scientific, London, pp. 1–7.
Comroe, J. (1966b). Summing up. In: Breathlessness. Edited by J.B.L. Howell and E.J.M. Campbell. Blackwell Scientific, London, pp. 233–238.
Dallenbach, K.M. (1939). Somesthesis. In: Introduction to Psychology. Edited by E.G. Boring, H.S. Langfield, and H.P. Weld. Wiley and Sons, New York, pp. 608–625.
Demediuk, B.H., Manning, H., Lilli, J., Fencl, V., Weinberger, S.E., Weiss, J.W., and Schwartzstein, R.M. (1992). Dissociation between dyspnea and respiratory effort. Am. Rev. Respir. Dis. 146:1222–1225.
DiMarco, A.F., Wolfson, D.A., Gottfried, S.B., and Altose, M.D. (1982). Sensation of inspired volume in normal subjects and quadriplegic patients. J. Appl. Physiol. 53:1481–1486.
Dubuisson, D., and Melzack, R. (1976). Classification of clinical pain descriptions by multiple group discriminate analysis. Exp. Neurol. 51:480–487.
Elliott, M.W., Adams, L., Cockcroft, A., MacRae, K.D., Murphy, K., and Guz, A. (1991). The language of breathlessness: use by patients of verbal descriptors. Am. Rev. Respir. Dis. 144:826–832.
Ernst, M., Lee, M.H.M., Dworkin, B., and Zaretsky, H.H. (1986). Pain perception decrement produced through repeated stimulation. Pain 26:221–231.

Fowler, W.S. (1954). Breaking point of breath-holding. J. Appl. Physiol. 6:539–545.

Gandevia, S.C. (1988). Neural mechanisms underlying the sensation of breathlessness: kinesthetic parallels between respiratory and limb muscles. Aust. N.Z. J. Med. 18:83–91.

Gottfried, S.B., Leech, I., DiMarco, A.F., Zaccardelli, W., and Altose, M.D. (1984). Sensation of respiratory force following low cervical spinal cord transection. J. Appl. Physiol. 57:989–994.

Gracely, R.H. (1989). Methods of testing pain mechanisms in normal man. In: Textbook of Pain, 2nd ed. Edited by R. Melzack and P.D. Wall. Churchill Livingstone, New York, pp. 257–268.

Grushka, M., and Sessle, B.J. (1984). Applicability of the McGill pain questionnaire to the differentiation of "toothache" pain. Pain 19:49–57.

Guz, A., Noble, M.I.M., Trenchard, D., Cochrane, H.L., and Makey, A.R. (1964). Studies on the vagus nerves in man: their role in respiratory and circulatory control. Clin. Sci. 27:293–304.

Guz, A., Noble, M.I.M., Widdicombe, J.G., Trenchard, D., Mushin, W.W., and Makey, A.R. (1966). The role of vagal and glossopharyngeal afferent nerves in respiratory sensation, control of breathing and arterial pressure regulation in conscious man. Clin. Sci. 30:161–170.

Hudgel, D.W., Cooperson, D.M., and Kinsman, R.A. (1982). Recognition of added resistive loads in asthma. Am. Rev. Respir. Dis. 126:12–125.

Hunter, M., and Philips, C. (1981). The experience of headache—an assessment of the qualities of tension headache pain. Pain 10:209–219.

Kelson, S.G., Prestel, T.F., Cherniack, N.S., Chester, E.H., and Deal, E.C. (1981). Comparison of the respiratory responses to external resistive loading and bronchoconstriction. J. Clin. Invest. 67:1761–1768.

Killian, K.J., and Campbell, E.J.M. (1985). Dyspnea. In: The Thorax, Part B. Edited by C. Roussos and P.T. Macklem. Dekker, New York, pp. 787–828.

Killian, K.J., Mahutte, C.K., and Campbell, E.J.M. (1981). Magnitude scaling of externally added loads to breathing. Am. Rev. Respir. Dis. 123:12–15.

Killian, K.J., Bucens, D.D., and Campbell, E.J.M. (1982). Effect of breathing patterns on the perceived magnitude of added loads to breathing. J. Appl. Physiol. 52:578–584.

Killian, K.J., Gandevia, S.C., Summers, E., and Campbell, E.J.M. (1984). Effect of increased lung volume on perception of breathlessness, effort and tension. J. Appl. Physiol. 57:686–691.

Kontos, H.A., Shapiro, W., and Patterson, J.L. (1963). Observations on dyspnea induced by combination of respiratory stimuli. Am. J. Med. 37:374–385.

Lane, R., Adams, L., and Guz, A. (1987a). Is low-level respiratory resistive loading during exercise perceived as breathlessness? Clin. Sci. 73:627–634.

Lane, R., Cockcroft, A., and Guz, A. (1987b). Voluntary isocapnic hyperventilation and breathlessness during exercise in normal subjects. Clin. Sci. 73:519–523.

Leblanc, P., Bowie, D.M., Summers, E., Jones, N.L., and Killian, K.J. (1986). Breathlessness and exercise in patients with cardiorespiratory disease. Am. Rev. Respir. Dis. 133:21–25.

Manning, H.L., Basner, R., Ringler, J., Rand, C., Fencl, V., Weinberger, S.E., Weiss, J.W., and Schwartzstein, R.M. (1991). Effect of chest wall vibration on breathlessness in normal subjects. J. Appl. Physiol. 71:175–181.

Manning, H.L., Shea, S.A., Schwartzstein, R.M., Lansing, R.W., Brown, R., and Banzett, R.B. (1992). Reduced tidal volume increases "air hunger" at fixed P_{CO_2} in ventilated quadriplegics. Respir. Physiol. 90:19–30.

Meakins, J.M. (1934). Dyspnea. JAMA 103:1442–1445.

Melzack, R. (1975). The McGill pain questionnaire: major properties and scoring methods. Pain 1:277–299.

Melzack, R., and Wall, P.D. (1965). Pain mechanisms: a new theory. Science 150:971–979.

Melzack, R., and Torgerson, W.S. (1971). On the language of pain. Anesthesiology 34:50–59.

Melzack, R., Terrence, C., Fromm, G., and Amsel, R. (1986). Trigeminal neuralgia and atypical facial pain: use of the McGill pain questionnaire for discrimination and diagnosis. Pain 27:297–302.

Noble, M.I.M., Eisele, J.H., Frankel, H.L., Else, W., and Guz, A. (1971). The role of the diaphragm in the sensation of holding the breath. Clin. Sci. 41:275–283.

Noble, M.I.M., Frankel, H.L., Else, W., and Guz, A. (1972). The sensation produced by threshold resistive loads to breathing. Eur. J. Clin. Invest. 2:72–77.

O'Neill, P.A., Stark, R.D., Allen, S.C., and Stretton, T.B. (1986). The relationship between breathlessness and ventilation during steady-state exercise. Bull. Eur. Physiopathol. Respir. 22:247–250.

Permutt, S., Fessler, H.E., Brower, R.G., and Kosnik, E. (1991). Breathlessness in acute asthma. Breathlessness, 1991 Campbell Symposium.

Petit, J.M. (1966). Dyspnoea in bronchial asthma. In: Breathlessness. Edited by J.B.L. Howell and E.J.M. Campbell. Blackwell Scientific, London, pp. 178–185.

Plum, F. (1966). Breathlessness in neurological disease: the effects of neurological disease on the act of breathing. In: Breathlessness. Edited by J.B.L. Howell and E.J.M. Campbell. Blackwell Scientific, London, pp. 203–222.

Reading, A.E. (1989). Testing pain mechanisms in persons in pain. In: Textbook of Pain, 2nd ed. Edited by R. Melzack and P.D. Wall. Churchill Livingstone, New York, pp. 269–280.

Remmers, J.E., Brooks, J.G., and Tenney, S.M. (1968). Effect of controlled ventilation on the tolerable limit of hypercapnia. Respir. Physiol. 4:78–90.

Revelette, W.R., and Wiley, R.L. (1987). Plasticity of the mechanism subserving inspiratory load perception. J. Appl. Physiol. 62:1901–1906.

Richards, D.W. (1953). The nature of cardiac and of pulmonary dyspnea. Circulation 7: 15–29.

Schwartzstein, R.M., Simon, P.M., Weiss, J.W., Fencl, V., and Weinberger, S.E. (1989). Breathlessness induced by dissociation between ventilation and chemical drive. Am. Rev. Respir. Dis. 139:1231–1237.

Schwartzstein, R.M., Manning, H.L., Weiss, M.W., and Weinberger, S.E. (1990). Dyspnea: a sensory experience. Lung 168:185–199.

Schwartzstein, R., Lilly, J., Israel, E., Basner, R., Sparrow, D., Weinberger, S., and Weiss, J.W. (1991). Breathlessness of asthma differs from that of external resistive loads. Am. Rev. Respir. Dis. 142:A596.

Schwartzstein, R., Carpenter, E., Brughera, A., Sparrow, D., O'Donnell, C., and Banzett, R.

(1992). Quality of breathlessness during bronchoconstriction with different inhalation agents. Am. Rev. Respir. Dis. 145:A630.

Simon, P.M., Schwartzstein, R.M., Weiss, J.W., LaHive, K., Fencl, V., Teghtsoonian, M., and Weinberger, S.E. (1989). Distinguishable sensations of breathlessness induced in normal volunteers. Am. Rev. Respir. Dis. 140:1021–1027.

Simon, P.M., Schwartzstein, R.M., Weiss, J.W., Fencl, V., Teghtsoonian, M., and Weinberger, S.E. (1990). Distinguishable types of dyspnea in patients with shortness of breath. Am. Rev. Respir. Dis. 142:1009–1014.

Sperry, R.W. (1950). Neural basis of the spontaneous optokinetic response produced by visual neural inversion. J. Comp. Physiol. Psychol. 45:482–489.

Stubbing, D.G., Killian, K.J., and Campbell, E.J.M. (1981). The quantification of respiratory sensations by normal subjects. Respir. Physiol. 44:251–260.

Titchener, E.B. (1920). Notes from the psychology laboratory of Cornell University. Am. J. Psychol. 31:212.

Tobin, M.J. (1990). Dyspnea. Arch. Intern. Med. 150:1604–1613.

Turcotte, H., Corbeil, F., and Boulet, L.-P. (1990). Perception of breathlessness during bronchoconstriction induced by antigen, exercise, and histamine challenges. Thorax 45:914–918.

Wasserman, K., and Casaburi, R. (1988). Dyspnea: physiological and pathophysiological mechanisms. Annu. Rev. Med. 39:503–15.

Weisenberg, M. (1989). Cognitive aspects of pain. In: Textbook of Pain, 2nd ed. Edited by R. Melzack and P.D. Wall. Churchill Livingstone, New York, pp. 231–241.

Whitelaw, W.A., Derenne, J.-P., Couture, J., and Milic-Emili, J. (1976). Adaptation of anesthetized men to breathing through an inspiratory resistor. J. Appl. Physiol. 41:285–291.

Whitelaw, W.A., McBride, B., Amar, J., and Corbet, K. (1981). Respiratory neuromuscular output during breath holding. J. Appl. Physiol. 50:435–443.

Wright, G.W., and Branscomb, B.V. (1954). The origin of the sensations of dyspnea. Tr. Am. Clin. Climatol. Assoc. 1966:116–125.

6

Respiratory Sensations Arising from Pulmonary and Chemoreceptor Afferents

Air Hunger and Lung Volume

ROBERT B. BANZETT

Harvard School of Public Health
and Harvard Medical School
Boston, Massachusetts

ROBERT W. LANSING

University of Arizona
Tucson, Arizona

I. Introduction

There are many afferent sources that, potentially, can provide information about breathing. Physiologists have tended to concentrate on respiratory sensations arising from somatic afferents. This tendency to discount the importance of visceral afferents probably arose from several pieces of experimental evidence, discussed here, that suggested that information arising from pulmonary receptors and chemoreceptors is not consciously perceived. More recent experiments suggest that the information from visceral afferents can indeed be perceived. This evidence does not necessarily negate the importance of somatic afferents: for instance, tendon organs and spindles in the respiratory muscles are probably essential in the detection of resistive and elastic loads, and smaller fiber afferents from respiratory muscles may be important in signaling the discomfort of fatigue. Although we now know that visceral receptors can give rise to respiratory sensations, our knowledge is in a formative state. A great deal remains to be learned about the central nervous pathways involved, about the interactions between stimuli, about the nature of subjective descriptions evoked by various stimuli, and about the affective component of respiratory discomfort. One aim of this chapter is to stimulate thought and experimentation in this area; hence, we have not been hesitant to set forth hypotheses that may provoke challenge. Although much of the study in respiratory sensation has been driven by the need to understand the symptoms of cardiorespiratory disease, we concentrate here on the range of sensation that can be elicited by laboratory interventions in subjects without cardiopulmonary disease. Understanding the range of sensations that can be elicited in normal subjects will form the underpinning of any understanding of pathophysiology; clinical perspectives are discussed elsewhere in this volume (Chaps. 10, 11, 12, 15, 16).

In the present chapter we discuss the evidence that information from peripheral and central arterial chemoreceptors and from pulmonary stretch receptors reaches consciousness, and we discuss the nature of the sensations evoked by these receptors. Those receptors known to subserve cardiorespiratory reflex control are adequate to explain all described phenomena of respiratory sensation if their output ascends to the levels of conscious perception. Figure 1 depicts the pathways by which respiratory sensations could reach consciousness; the pathways from sensory receptors to the automatic respiratory centers in the medulla are accepted by most physiologists; projections to conscious perception in the forebrain are less well defined.

The study of sensations arising from internal organs is complicated by two factors. (1) In general, individuals have not developed adequate language to describe unambiguously sensations arising from within, especially when the sensations are somewhat unfamiliar. A great deal of the confusion extant in this field has probably arisen from the lack of attention paid to the words used in

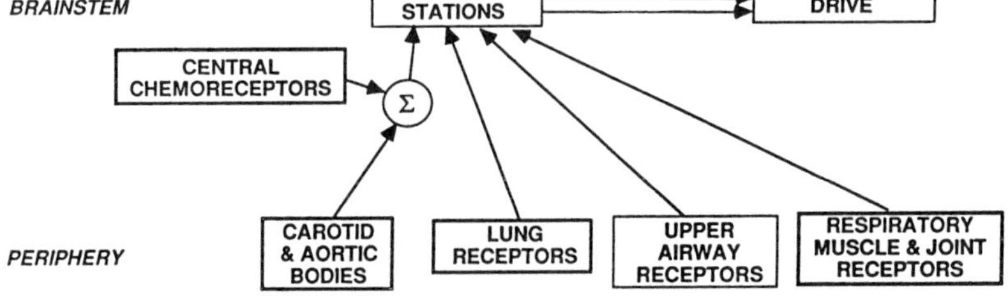

Figure 1 Possible pathways for respiratory sensations. Description in text.

communicating with subjects, the words used by subjects in describing their sensations, and the uneven reporting of such communication in published work. To a certain extent, this problem can be remedied by careful attention to developing better language with which to question subjects, as has been done in the field of pain perception (see Chaps. 3 and 5). Several studies of the language of respiratory sensation have recently been published (Simon et al., 1989, 1990; Elliott et al., 1991). We have attempted here to report descriptive language exactly when we believe it may importantly influence conclusions. (2) As in many other sensory systems, perceived sensations may result from a mixture of signals from different afferent receptors, as when the stimuli of "touch" and "cold" combine to form the apparently different sensation of "wet." In respiratory sensation it is difficult to control independently many of the variables of potential interest; for instance, gas exchange and ventilation are closely linked, both by the physical phenomena of gas exchange and by the neural phenomena of respiratory control. In the awake human, it is a difficult problem to stop ventilation without raising arterial P_{CO_2} (carbon dioxide pressure) or to raise arterial P_{CO_2} without causing automatic respiratory muscle contraction. Often, the best that can be done is to take advantage of clinical cases in whom afferent pathways are destroyed (e.g., spinal injury) or structures are altered (e.g., tracheostomy).

II. The Sense of Lung Volume: Pulmonary Stretch Receptors

It appears that all mammals have pulmonary stretch receptors whose large myelinated afferents run in the vagus nerve, as first described by Adrian (1933). Humans are no exception (Langrehr, 1964; Guz and Trenchard, 1971). Similar afferents have also been described in the pulmonary sympathetic nerves, which enter the central nervous system via the cervical cord (Kostreva et al., 1975). Slowly adapting pulmonary stretch receptors (SAPSRs) provide exquisite transduction of lung volume to action potential firing and have long been known to evoke respiratory reflexes via the medullary respiratory centers (Breuer and Hering, 1868; Head, 1889). SAPSRs are located throughout the trachea, bronchi, and lungs, being found in greater numbers in central airways. Those in central airways are in the submucosal layer; less is known about the location of those in peripheral airways, although they are more accessible to drugs given via the pulmonary circulation than those given via the bronchial circulation, suggesting that they lie quite deep in the lung. Most SAPSRs fire throughout the respiratory cycle, having some activity even at end expiration. Rapidly adapting pulmonary stretch receptors are located in the more central airways and respond to the rate of lung inflation, especially when tidal volume is large; they tend to be silent during expiration. Pronounced deflation of the lungs also stimulates these receptors; they do not adapt rapidly to deflation stimulus. The two other types of pulmonary receptors that have been described are innervated by small nonmylenated fibers, called C fibers (reviewed by Coleridge and Coleridge, 1984). Airway C fibers are located in the conducting airways and respond to a number of irritating substances. Pulmonary C fibers are located in the periphery, near the gas exchange area, and respond to pulmonary vascular congestion and to very large inflations of the lung. The stimulus-response characteristics of both categories of small fibers make it unlikely that they provide sensory feedback during normal breathing, but they may give rise to sensations experienced during the inhalation of irritant substances and inflammatory mediators or during pulmonary vascular congestion or embolism.

Pulmonary stretch receptors are only one of the several sources of afferent information that could contribute to perceptions of lung volume (see Fig. 1). In the normal intact subject, volume excursions of the lungs are inseparable from those of the chest wall (taken here to include all components of the body wall that expand with inspiration, i.e., principally rib cage, diaphragm, and abdomen). Chest wall muscles are provided with receptors like those of other skeletal muscles: the diaphragmatic, intercostal, and abdominal muscles contain muscle spindles and Golgi tendon organs; in addition, the rib cage is equipped with joint receptors. Stimulation of intercostal nerves can give rise to cortical evoked potentials (Gandevia and Macefield, 1989), although this is not sufficient to conclude that they are perceived (see Chap. 3). Although this has never been formally tested, these somatic receptors alone are presumably quite capable of detecting volume change and are likely to provide this information to conscious perception, as do other musculoskeletal receptors. Chest wall receptors are not ideally suited to volume reporting, however, for several reasons: (1) the chest wall has at least three degrees of freedom for volume change (Mead et al., 1985), making it problematical to sum volume information properly; and (2) the output of chest wall proprioceptors is affected by variables other than volume—muscle spindles are influenced by variations in γ efferent discharge, and tendon organs are influenced by changes in elastance and resistance and have essentially no response to passive inflation. In addition, other receptors may supply information relating to tidal volume in some circumstances, including upper airway flow (temperature) receptors (Sant'Ambrogio et al., 1988), thoracic and abdominal cutaneous receptors, hearing, and vision. For instance, one can gauge the size of a breath by the loudness and duration of breath sounds. It is therefore difficult to determine which receptors supply lung volume information to the forebrain under natural circumstances in the normal subject.

Despite wide variations in experimental technique, almost all studies in normal subjects have shown that subjects are able to detect changes in tidal volume as small as 50–150 ml, that is, 10–30% of a normal breath or 1–3% of vital capacity (Gliner et al., 1981; Wolkove et al., 1981; DiMarco et al., 1982; Katz-Salamon, 1984; Banzett et al., 1987). (Language does not seem to be a problem here: the average person understands quite well what is meant by "a larger breath.") Various techniques have been used to assess volume perception: some of the studies just mentioned examined the ability of subjects to reproduce standard tidal volumes using the magnitude of errors in reproduction as a measure of perceptual ability (Gliner et al., 1981; Wolkove et al., 1981; DiMarco et al., 1982; Folinsbee et al., 1982); other studies required subjects to detect changes in tidal volume imposed by the experimenter or to scale the size of breaths imposed by the experimenter (Bakers and Tenney, 1970; West et al., 1975; Katz-Salamon, 1984; Banzett et al., 1987). Some of these studies found that the minimum detectable volume change was constant, regardless of the baseline tidal volume (Wolkove et al., 1981); others found that the minimum detectable volume change increased with increasing tidal volume, that is, in accord with "Weber's law," with scaling exponents slightly more than unity (Gliner et al., 1981; DiMarco et al., 1982; Folinsbee et al., 1982; Katz-Salamon, 1984). One study, however, showed very different results: in this study experimenters altered tidal volume slowly and surreptitiously and found that subjects failed to report a change until tidal volume was more than doubled (West et al., 1975). The essence of this study was repeated, however, and the results were not borne out (Katz-Salamon, 1984). Perhaps the higher detection threshold found by West et al. was a function of a higher decision criterion adopted by their subjects (see Chap. 3). Interestingly, wind instrument players seem to be better able to gauge lung volume (Smith et al., 1990). Volume perception seems unimpaired in chronic obstructive pulmonary disease (Gottfried et al., 1985).

Much less is known about the ability of subjects to perceive absolute lung volume. Implicit in the perception of absolute volume are the abilities to sense volume relative to some fixed reference (resting functional residual capacity, FRC, total lung capacity, or residual volume, for instance) and to remember this volume for some time. When subjects attempt to reproduce a standard volume change, it is difficult to determine whether they achieve this by repeating the change in volume or by finding an absolute volume. Salamon et al. (1976) observed that subjects had great difficulty in returning to FRC after a large inspiration or expiration. Folinsbee et al. (1982) found that subjects were less precise in reproducing an absolute volume (from different starting volumes) than in reproducing a volume change. In the first case, the starting volume was changed from the end-expiratory level to residual volume, and thus recoil assistance to the movement may have contributed to the error of reproduction. Plassman and Lansing (1990), on the other hand, found that subjects could accurately reproduce an absolute volume even when the size and rate of volume change were varied. There is some evidence that pulmonary stretch receptors, as well as their central reflex pathways, adapt to continued stimulation over the course of minutes (Stanley et al., 1975; Grippi et al., 1985). This would diminish the ability of subjects to track long-term changes in mean lung volume.

A. Role of Pulmonary Receptors in Volume Perception

There is evidence in animal studies that vagal afferents project to the forebrain (Kazakov, 1966; O'Brien et al., 1971). Although there is no direct information on this point in the human, the animal studies raise the possibility that information from vagal afferents could be perceived as respiratory sensations including lung volume changes. Clinical observations suggest that patients are able to perceive pain and irritation in the lungs, however, other observations led to the conclusion that the output of pulmonary stretch receptors cannot be perceived as volume change. Two subjects underwent local anesthetic block of the vagus nerve (Guz et al., 1966a); these subjects, both respiratory physiologists, reported noticing no alteration in their perception of resting breathing, although formal tests of volume detection were not done. (Inspiratory load perception was tested and found to be normal during vagal block.) We note that ample alternative pathways for volume perception, such as chest wall and upper airway afferents, were available to these subjects, so that this dramatic experiment could not provide strong evidence that vagal receptors are not perceived.

Subjects with complete lesions of the spinal cord sensory tracts above the second cervical segment have no sensory innervation of the chest wall (functional anatomy reviewed by Banzett et al., 1987). The vagus, which provides the principal innervation of the lung, is usually undamaged in spinal injury cases. These high-level quadriplegic patients are dependent on mechanical ventilators or phrenic nerve pacers and are almost invariably tracheostomized. High-level quadriplegic subjects, then, provide an ideal opportunity to determine whether respiratory sensations can originate in visceral afferents. Brief reports of the inability of two high-level quadriplegics (Guz, 1970; Prys-Roberts, 1970; Newsom-Davis, 1979) to detect changes in their ventilator settings provided the suggestion that the traffic from pulmonary volume receptors is not perceptible. Although the rationale of these experiments was adequate to test the hypothesis under consideration, the determinations of perception were apparently informal, because no methodology was reported.

Formal psychophysical studies performed in our laboratory on five well-characterized C1–2 quadriplegic subjects determined that they could detect alterations in ventilator-delivered tidal volume. The subjects were given pairs of ventilator-delivered breaths, one having the same volume as their normal breaths, the other having a larger or smaller volume. The subjects were asked to report which breath was altered in a forced-choice study design (see Chap. 3). Quadriplegic subjects could detect changes about as well as normal subjects, and both groups localized the sensation to within the chest. Because these subjects had no chest wall afferent information and their upper airways were excluded from volume and pressure changes, it seems highly probable that they used pulmonary vagal afferents in making judgments of tidal volume.

It would be useful to confirm this conclusion by interrupting the vagal afferent pathway from the lungs, in which case the ability to perceive volume should be abolished in these subjects. Unfortunately, this is not easily accomplished in humans. Aerosolized local anesthetic has been used to block airway epithelial afferents (e.g., Cross et al., 1976; Sullivan and Yu, 1983; Easton et al., 1985; Winning et al., 1985), but the degree to which pulmonary afferents are blocked is problematical. Many pulmonary afferents lie deep in the lung in areas perfused by the pulmonary circulation (Armstrong and Luck, 1974; Sant'Ambrogio and Sant'Ambrogio, 1982). Even if central airway receptors are shown to be anesthetized by abolition of the cough reflex, pulmonary stretch receptors may escape anesthesia because the aerosol has not penetrated to the periphery of the lung or because the drug has been carried away more rapidly by the rich blood flow. The Hering-Breuer inflation reflex, useful in testing pulmonary receptor activity in animals, is weak or absent in conscious humans. Because of these technical problems, failure of aerosol anesthetic to abolish volume perception in quadriplegics would have little meaning. If, on the other hand, perception were abolished, the result would be useful. We have shown a large dose of aerosolized 20% lidocaine solution to abolish volume sensation in one quadriplegic subject on two occasions (Lansing et al., 1988). The same dose failed to block perception on another occasion in this subject and in another, similar patient on another occasion. More studies of this type would be useful.

B. Relative Roles of Pulmonary Receptors and Chest Wall Receptors in Volume Perception

What is the normal role of pulmonary receptors in relation to the alternative pathways for volume perception: chest wall receptors, motor command, and upper airway receptors? The experiments in quadriplegics can tell us only that a vagal afferent pathway exists and that vagal afferents alone can provide volume perception as sensitive as that found in the intact subject. It is possible that any one of several other pathways can provide similarly sensitive perception and that people normally attend to only one pathway if all are present. The volume perception capabilities of the alternative pathways have never been tested in isolation, but indirect tests show that they can influence volume perception.

Under usual circumstances, tidal volume is related closely to the drop in pleural pressure produced by inspiratory muscles. The force generated by inspiratory muscles is related to the activation of the muscles. Because muscle activation originates in the central nervous system, it is reasonable to surmise that one may have an awareness of the outgoing command. It is postulated that such a copy of motor command, or "corollary discharge," is important in limb kinesthesia. In theory, one might also predict tidal volume from the amount of central motor command sent to inspiratory muscles. The amount of central command necessary to produce a given inspiratory muscle pressure has been experimentally increased by weakening the muscles by fatigue or partial neuromuscular block and by imposing an external load, and it has been decreased by respiratory muscle training. Subjects having weaker muscles or breathing against a larger load tended to overestimate volume slightly compared with the control condition, but the effect was not strong (Gandevia et al., 1981; Wolkove et al., 1981; Redline et al., 1991).

Interventions thought to alter chest wall afferent activity also affect volume perception. The inspiratory muscle pressure needed to reproduce a given tidal volume has been altered by the addition of inspiratory loads to the test breath alone, and actively taken breaths have been compared with ventilator-delivered breaths (Stubbing et al., 1981; Wolkove et al., 1981; DiMarco et al., 1982; Sullivan et al., 1991). (These interventions also change the relationship between motor command and tidal volume.) Some of these experiments show that tidal volumes are overestimated when inspiratory muscles must contract more strongly, but the ability to detect volume changes was generally not much affected by these interventions. Dimarco et al., for instance, found that when subjects switched from active breathing to passive inflation, the exponent for tidal volume estimation changed insignificantly (from 1.24 to 1.32). Wolkove et al. found that errors in volume estimation in the midrange of lung volumes was increased from 100 to 200 ml. In all reports, however, volume judgments remained more closely proportional to the actual tidal volume than to the tidal pressure swings, suggesting that volume receptors (whether pulmonary or somatic) are more important in volume judgments than are muscle tension receptors or central command. Volume judgments are also slightly altered by vibration of the chest wall, thought to stimulate intercostal muscle spindles (Stubbing et al., 1981). Vibration of the rib cage is likely to be transmitted to the lung, altering gas exchange (Bitterman et al., 1983) and stimulating pulmonary receptors, making conclusions about the afferent pathway difficult.

Upper airway receptors sensitive to cooling by airflow could also provide cues to tidal volume changes; however, the existing evidence suggests that they do not have an important role. Anesthesia of the upper airway mucosa with aerosolized lidocaine does not impair the ability to perceive changes in tidal volume (DiMarco et al., 1982), and tidal volumes are not perceived differently when the subject breathes through the mouth as opposed to the nose (Fox et al., 1986).

In all it appears that volume (or displacement) receptors dominate the perception of volume and that they are capable of reasonably fine discrimination.

Although one cannot determine causality on a teleological basis, it appears that pulmonary receptors are ideally situated to provide volume information. If chest wall receptors played a major role in volume perception, one might expect changes in the expansion pattern (e.g., diaphragm inspiration versus rib cage inspiration) to cause errors in volume estimation. Upper airway cool receptors are likewise subject to error: their discharge depends not only on flow, but also on the temperature and humidity of inspired gas; thus, inspired volumes would feel smaller on hot, humid days (anecdotal observations lend credence to this proposal; people often complain of not getting enough air on hot humid days).

III. Other Pulmonary Sensations

Several other sensations can arise from the lung, such as pain and the tickle or scratch that precedes cough. Subjects can even localize the position of a foreign object to the left or right lung (Morton et al., 1950), although anecdotal reports suggest that some sensations from the distal bronchi are referred to the substernal region. Pulmonary congestion, reinflation of collapsed lung, and inhalation of particles and irritating gases produce sensation that apparently arises in the lung; some of these sensations have also been reported by high-level quadriplegics (Fillenz and Widdicombe, 1972). Capsaicin, a C fiber stimulant, inhaled as aerosol (Fuller et al., 1985) or introduced to the pulmonary artery (Winning et al., 1986), produces a raw, burning sensation within the chest, accompanied by cough; the effect following injection was blocked by inhaled local anesthetic. This stimulation of pulmonary C fibers did not produce breathlessness, however. Lobeline, another C fiber stimulant, produces cough and a burning sensation or illusion of fume inhalation localized to the upper chest or throat (Bevan and Murray, 1963; Jain et al., 1972). These data suggest that C fiber afferents may be important in the genesis of the cough and discomfort arising from pulmonary vascular congestion or unpleasant sensations evoked by the inspiration of irritant substances.

Another sensation that may arise from the lungs is the sense of "tightness" felt by asthmatics. Asthma increases the work done by respiratory muscles, and it has often been suggested that this workload is the primary cause of dyspnea in patients whose blood gases are normal (e.g., Marshall et al., 1954; Campbell and Howell, 1963; Burki, 1980; Chapman and Rebuck, 1983; Killian et al., 1984). A great deal has been learned about the perceptual response to loads (reviewed by Zechman and Wiley, 1986), but it has not been possible to explain adequately symptoms of asthma on this basis. Because the lung itself is altered in asthma, it seems reasonable to propose the hypothesis that pulmonary afferents themselves are altered by the disease. There is some evidence that asthma sensation is diminished by aerosolized local anesthetic or block of the vagus nerve, suggesting that it arises in pulmonary afferents (Petit and Delhez, 1970; Eisele and Jain, 1971;

Guz, 1977). On the other hand, lung transplant recipients, who presumably have no afferents below the tracheal anastomosis, have reported tightness after inhaling methacholine (Banner et al., 1988). The magnitude of sensation evoked by experimentally induced bronchoconstriction is greater than that evoked by a similar increase in external resistance in the same subjects (Schwartzstein et al., 1991; Taguchi et al., 1991). In one of these studies, normally asymptomatic asthmatic subjects also reported that the quality of the sensation differed between the two interventions: bronchoconstriction produced a predominant sensation of tightness, whereas external loading produced a sense of "effort or work" (Schwartzstein et al., 1991). These experiments strongly suggest that the breathlessness of asthma is not merely a result of the increased work of breathing, but this area clearly requires more definitive experiments.

IV. The Sense of Air Hunger: Chemoreceptors

Disturbances in arterial blood gases form one of the most powerful stimuli to breathe. It has long been known that sufficiently high chemical stimulus to breathe also elicits an uncomfortable sensation (Hill and Flack, 1908). The nature of this sensation and the afferent pathways by which it reaches the forebrain have not been well agreed, however. Various descriptors that may apply are listed in Table 1 (please note that "dyspnea" is not among them, because it is never volunteered by subjects having no clinical or respiratory training). The variety of descriptors probably reflects differences in the use of language as well as different shades of sensory quality evoked by the many experimental (and experiential) conditions. Further discussion of the language problem is found in Chap. 5. We have chosen to use the term "air hunger" (Wright and Branscomb, 1954) to describe the sensation of urge to breathe that is evoked by chemical stimuli because it does not carry unwanted connotations and because it seems specific to the situation in suggesting

Table 1 Language Used by Subjects in Connection with Chemoreceptor Stimulation[a]

Air hunger	Short of breath
Urge to breathe	Winded
Out of breath	Puffed (British usage)
Can't catch breath	Starved for air
Can't get breath	Suffocating
Breathless (British usage)	

[a]Note that these terms are probably not exactly synonymous.

a drive to action comparable to thirst and hunger (as discussed later). Although few authors have used the term "air hunger," we sometimes use it in discussing their findings when it appears to us that the experimental intervention used is likely to have evoked this same sensation. The sense of air hunger may be modified by other factors. Some aspects of the experience that may affect the quality and intensity of the evoked sensation apart from the intensity of stimulus are the nature of stimulus (e.g., hypercapnia, hypoxia, and exercise), other accompanying stimuli (e.g., increases or decreases in ventilation, temperature and humidity of inhaled gas, physical work, and added resistance), and affective conditions (e.g., the degree of control the subject has and the subject's expectations).

A. Afferent Pathways

Referring again to Fig. 1, four possible pathways exist by which air hunger may reach consciousness: (1) direct sensory pathways from the chemoreceptors to the forebrain (Kukorelli et al., 1969), (2) blood gas-sensitive neurons in the midbrain or forebrain, such as those described in the reticular formation (Dell, 1958), (3) projection of medullary respiratory center motor activity (corollary discharge) to the forebrain (Chen et al., 1992), and (4) projection of respiratory mechanoreceptors to the forebrain; these receptors would then indirectly give information on respiratory center activity (Campbell et al., 1967).

Hypothesis 4 received strong support from a set of experiments published in the late 1960s in which respiratory muscle contraction was completely abolished by curarization in two normal subjects (Campbell et al., 1967). These subjects reported that the "distressing sensation which limits breath hold" was absent during paralysis; they consequently allowed the anesthetist to stop ventilation for a period four times as long as their maximum breath hold under control conditions. Owing to criticism that the breath holds were not unusually long considering the blood gas levels encountered (the anesthetist had hyperventilated the subjects with a high-oxygen mix), the experiment was repeated on one of the subjects (the principal author) during hypercapnia, with similar results (Campbell et al., 1969). The authors concluded that the activity of respiratory muscles was essential to evoke air hunger. Evidence contradicting hypothesis 4 existed, although it was largely circumstantial or anecdotal. Two other subjects totally paralyzed with neuromuscular block commented in passing that they experienced respiratory discomfort when ventilation was reduced (Smith et al., 1947; Stevens et al., 1976). Patients paralyzed by poliomyelitis reported shortness of breath when end-tidal carbon dioxide partial pressure ($P_{ET_{CO_2}}$) was raised (Patterson et al., 1962; Opie et al., 1959). Several studies showed that the sense of discomfort associated with breath hold or hypercapnia was reduced by breathing; to us, this seemed incompatible with the idea that increased respiratory muscle contraction *causes* air hunger (Hill and Flack, 1908; Fowler, 1954; Remmers et al., 1968). More recent studies showed that voluntary hyperventilation did not cause breathlessness unless it was accompanied by hypercapnia (Adams et al., 1985; Freedman et al., 1987; Lane et al., 1987; Schwartzstein et al., 1987). However the direct evidence of Campbell et al. (1967, 1969) was difficult to controvert; the central role of respiratory muscle afferents in the origin of dyspnea was widely accepted (e.g., Burki, 1987; Whitelaw et al., 1987; Killian and Jones, 1988; Altose, 1991; Homma et al., 1991).

A test of this hypothesis required a situation in which blood gases could be altered without concomitant change in afferent traffic from the respiratory muscles. Again, ventilator-dependent C1–2 quadriplegics provided an ideal opportunity for study (Banzett et al., 1989). Ventilation could be maintained absolutely constant while arterial P_{CO_2} was varied by altering inspired CO_2 concentration. The subject could then be blinded to the experimental maneuver. Because we were not sure what quality of sensation hypercapnia would evoke under these circumstances, we first allowed the subjects to provide their own descriptions. When $P_{ET_{CO_2}}$ was raised in these subjects, they reported sensing an "urge to breathe," "shortness of breath," or "starved for air." Forced-choice procedures revealed that they could reliably detect changes of 7 mm Hg in $P_{ET_{CO_2}}$, although this should not be taken as an absolute limit. All subjects agreed that the feeling was much like the sensation at the end of a long breath hold, but most said it was somewhat different from the out-of-breath sensation of heavy exercise. They all thought that air hunger was a good descriptor, although none had volunteered it. Subsequent studies have borne out this initial set of descriptors (Simon et al., 1989; Banzett et al., 1990; Manning et al., 1992). The sensation was often quite unpleasant and in some subjects intolerable. It thus appeared that respiratory muscle activity is not necessary to evoke the sense of respiratory discomfort that accompanies hypercapnia.

Further study was needed, because the clinical cases of quadriplegia studied might have had undetected activity in some respiratory muscles, potentially invoking mechanoreceptors (mechanism 4). We therefore studied subjects similar to those in the study of Campbell et al., respiratory physiologists completely paralyzed by a neuromuscular blocking agent. The study design differed so that we might completely blind the subject to manipulation of the independent variable and we might achieve conditions closer to steady state. Constant positive-pressure mechanical ventilation was maintained while inspired CO_2 concentration was raised and lowered in random order, each level being held for about 4 minutes. At 40 s intervals subjects rated air hunger (a term on which all agreed following preliminary experiments without paralysis). In all subjects air hunger was positively correlated with $P_{ET_{CO_2}}$, and in three of four the correlation was highly significant (see Fig. 2). Subjects again likened the sensation to that of breath hold and again found it to be quite unpleasant at times: "like you're going to die because you're not getting enough air," in the words of one subject. The intensity of sensation at a given $P_{ET_{CO_2}}$ was not measurably affected by paralysis. Hypothesis 4 was therefore more strongly rejected: respiratory muscle activity is not

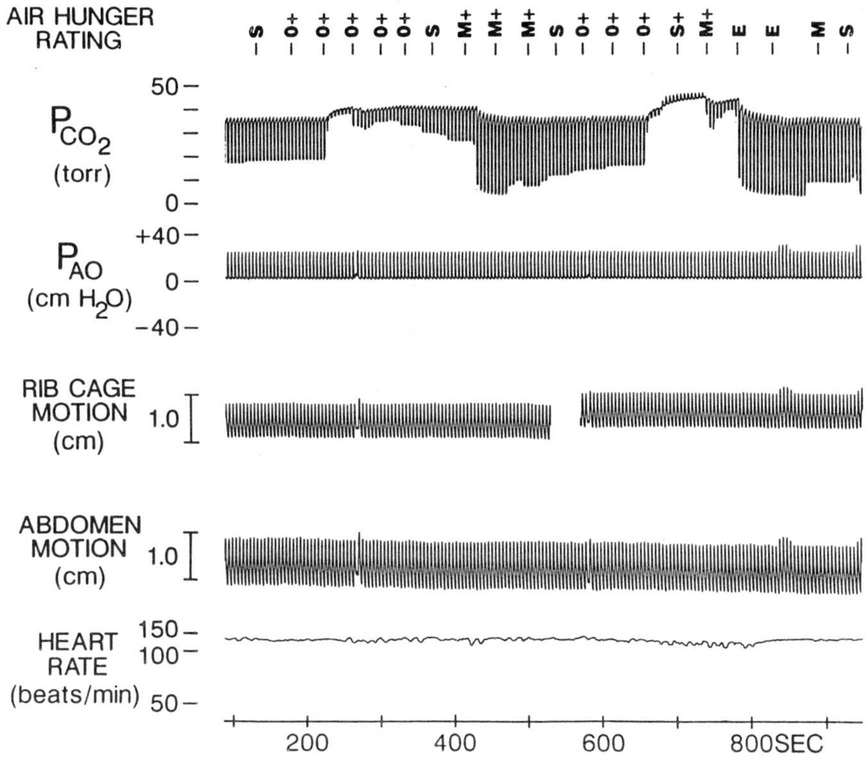

Figure 2 Time course of physiologic variables in the paralysis experiment (Banzett et al, 1990, subject RB). During this time, the subject was completely paralyzed with the curare analog Vecuronium, with the exception of one arm whose circulation was occluded with a tourniquet to allow signaling of sensation. Constant mechanical ventilation, $P_{ET_{CO2}}$ altered by changing inspirated P_{CO2}. Ratings defined as 0 = no air hunger, S = clearly perceptible air hunger causing only minor discomfort, M = air hunger bearable for about 4–5 min., E = intolerable air hunger, requiring immediate change in $F_{I_{CO2}}$. '+' indicates intermediate levels. Note the following features: (1) Steady pressure and magnetometer traces, compared to fig. 2, suggest complete muscular relaxation throughout. (The gap and subsequent upward shift in rib cage motion at 530–570 sec represent accidental change in instrument zero position; the transient increase in pressure and motions at 840–850 sec resulted from a brief increase in ventilator tidal volume.) (2) Attempted inspiratory pressure maneuvers at 260 and 580 sec show no sign of muscle contraction. (4) Inspired P_{CO2} exceeds $P_{ET_{CO2}}$ from 680 to 740 sec.

essential to generate the sense of air hunger. Surprisingly, we found that relatively modest elevations in PET_{CO_2} (about 5 mm Hg) produced intolerable discomfort during fixed ventilation, both before and after paralysis. Because these experiments overturned a long-held notion of the origin of breathlessness, they were viewed with skepticism by many. One objection raised was that the chest wall motion produced by mechanical ventilation might somehow permit perception of air hunger during paralysis, making the breath-hold experiment fundamentally different. Another group of workers performed essentially similar experiments to ours, as well as retesting the breath-hold studies of Campbell et al. (Gandevia et al., 1993). The results of the inspired CO_2 experiments were very similar to ours: subjects reported "severe discomfort associated with breathing," with a modest rise in PET_{CO_2} (to about 45 mm Hg). They also reported similar sensations during maximal breath hold, was of a similar duration to that seen in the unparalyzed state. The quality of the sensation and the PET_{CO_2} that evoked "severe" ratings were unchanged by total paralysis with atracurium, results directly contrary to the findings of Campbell et al. These authors, too, concluded that respiratory muscles are not needed for the normal sensations of breathlessness.

There remain, therefore, three candidate neural pathways for air hunger: (1) direct projection to the forebrain from the accepted respiratory chemoreceptors, (2) CO_2-sensitive neurons in the forebrain or midbrain, and (3) corollary discharge from brain stem respiratory centers. Electrophysiological evidence from animal studies suggests that all pathways exist (Dell, 1958; Kukorelli et al., 1969; Chen et al., 1991, 1992), but such studies cannot tell us which of these are actually used in perception. The relevant animal neurophysiological studies are discussed in Chap. 2. What can we deduce about these three neural pathways from studies in humans?

As mentioned, it is postulated that corollary discharge informs the sensory cortex of the intensity of motor commands. A sense of effort is said to result from corollary discharge accompanying limb muscle activation (McCloskey, 1983). Wright and Branscombe (1954) proposed that motor activity of the respiratory centers gives rise to air hunger (implicitly by projection of corollary discharge to the forebrain). This theory is attractive because it provides convenient integration of the many afferent inputs that influence sensation. Almost all existing experimental evidence is consistent with this theory, but a number of important points have not been explored. Does a copy of automatic respiratory center motor command project to perceptual areas of the forebrain? If so, what quality of sensation does it evoke?

The notion that corollary discharge arising from voluntary limb activation gives rise to a sense of effort is fairly well accepted, but the conclusion is far from certain even in this well-studied system (McCloskey, 1983; Lansing and Banzett, 1993). Less is known about sense of effort in the respiratory system. When subjects whose respiratory muscles are weakened by fatigue, partial paralysis, or complete paralysis were asked to produce inspiratory pressures against an occluded airway, they overestimated the magnitude of pressure produced, suggesting that the increased central command necessary to voluntarily produce a given muscle force is factored into their judgment of pressure production (Campbell et al., 1980; Killian et al., 1984; Gandevia et al., 1993). The authors deduced that a respiratory sense of effort was present and that it was the same as the sense of breathlessness; they did not, however, address the origin of the command. When completely paralyzed subjects in a different experiment were asked to produce maximal inspiratory pressures, however, they reported experiencing no sense of effort localized to respiratory structures (Lansing and Banzett, 1993). More research is needed to resolve these discrepancies. In any case, these experiments address only the sensation of effort that may arise from voluntary, cortically originated respiratory efforts; they do not speak to the problem of corollary discharge that arises in the medulla. When increased ventilation is produced voluntarily subjects are likely to report effort, but similar levels of ventilation driven by hypercapnia are more likely to be reported as an "unpleasant urge to breathe" but with *less* perceived effort (Demediuk et al., 1992).

It is not easy to construct experiments in the human to determine the role of corollary discharge arising from the automatic respiratory centers. One approach is to examine sensation in subjects who lack automatic breathing. Congenital central hypoventilation syndrome is a rare condition characterized by failure to breathe while asleep and absence of ventilatory response to changes in blood gases. The exact nature of the lesion is unknown, but there are two likely hypotheses: that the medullary respiratory centers are nonfunctional, or that the common final path of chemoreceptor input to the centers is interrupted, such that the centers are not sufficiently facilitated to carry on during sleep. Subjects having this condition did not report feeling air hunger during hypercapnia, which does not stimulate their breathing (Shea et al., 1993b). Their maximal breath-hold times were well beyond normal limits, requiring the experimenter to stop breath holds for safety. These patients seem to have a relatively normal ventilatory response to exercise (Paton et al., 1993; Shea et al., 1993a), and there was some suggestion that they experienced shortness of breath when breathing hard during heavy exercise (Shea et al., 1993b). These data suggest that respiratory center outflow is necessary to evoke air hunger, but an alternative explanation is that the chemoreceptor pathway to the cortex has been interrupted together with those to the medulla. In any case, these results contradict the idea that air hunger arises from higher brain neurons sensitive to CO_2 (hypothesis 2), thereby narrowing the likely pathways to those mentioned in hypotheses 1 and 3.

B. Adequate Stimuli and Relationship to Intensity of Sensation

The most common laboratory stimuli used to evoke the sensation of air hunger have been hypercapnia and breath holding (combined hypoxia and hypercapnia).

Experiments with eucapnic hypoxia suggest that it produces similar sensations (Adams et al., 1985). Exercise produces a slightly different quality of sensation, usually described as short of breath or out of breath (Simon et al., 1989), which probably comprises air hunger modified by the accompaniment of heavy breathing and muscular work. (Because this sensation is an entirely expected event during exercise, many healthy subjects fail to report it unless specifically asked.) To a useful first approximation, the intensity of this uncomfortable urge to breathe is related to the level of *involuntary* ventilatory drive, regardless of the particular stimulus (Lane et al., 1987, 1990), although some stimuli, such as hypoxia, may have a sensory effect slightly larger or smaller than their effect on ventilation would predict (Ward and Whipp, 1989; Lane et al., 1990).

Much work has been done on the sensory response to CO_2 because it is a safe and convenient stimulus. Less is known about the sensory responses to hypoxia or fixed acid. Breath-hold experiments have shown a synergistic effect between hypoxia and hypercapnia in terminating breath hold (reviewed by Mithoeffer, 1965). Although hypoxia alone causes an urge to breathe, little is known about the quality of sensation evoked. The sensory response to hypoxia is very dependent on the level explored: mild hypoxia is not a strong respiratory stimulus, but extreme hypoxia is likely to affect sensation by dulling mental processes. Indeed, sudden exposure to extremely low inspired oxygen pressure (Po_2) can cause loss of consciousness before respiratory symptoms give adequate warning. Even less is known about the sensory response to fixed acid. During anaerobic exercise, perception of breathlessness may correlate with the acute increase in lactic acidosis; however, direct tests of this proposal have not been made.

What is the quantitative relationship between the stimulus to breathe and air hunger? One problem is the variety of ways in which air hunger is assessed. On the one hand, there are behavioral measures, such as the breakpoint of a breath hold, whereas there are several forms of sensory scaling (see Chap. 3). In considering the relationship between air hunger and the stimulus to breathe, we examine experiments in which breathing is not allowed to change as chemical drive is altered; this encompasses three basic types of experiments: breath holding, voluntarily targeted ventilation, and fixed mechanical ventilation.

The breakpoint of breath holding indicates the tolerable limit of air hunger, and one may take the levels of blood gases at breakpoint as the chemical stimulus that causes this intolerable sensation (see examples in Table 2). When breakpoint is used to measure air hunger, only the upper limit of sensation is ascertained. Breath hold is far from a steady state: the Pco_2 at central chemoreceptors may not have time to reach equilibrium at breakpoint. The tolerable Pco_2 at breakpoint is strongly influenced by Po_2 principally through the action of the carotid bodies (Davidson et al., 1974). Another sort of breakpoint, limit of Pco_2 tolerated at fixed ventilation, has also been determined; these experiments allow more time for gas equilibrium, but breakpoint may be influenced by lung inflation (see later). This form of breakpoint has been determined during both active and passive ventila-

Table 2 Tolerable Limit of PA_{CO2}[a]

Tolerable PA_{CO_2}	PO_2	VL	$\dot{V}E$ (L/minute)	Condition	Subjects	Reference[b]
50	52	FRC	0	Breath hold	Normal	3
66	400+	FRC	0	Breath hold	Normal	3
47–57	58–79	TLC	0	Breath hold	Normal	2
53–63	300+	TLC	0	Breath hold	Normal	2
53	57	?	0	Breath hold	Normal	1
67	400+	?	0	Breath hold	Normal	1
48	60	FRC	0	Breath hold	Normal	4
66	360	FRC	0	Breath hold	Normal	4
48–57	400	TLC	0	Breath hold	Normal	6
40–45	50	TLC	0	Breath hold	Normal	6
56–63	400	TLC	0	Breath hold	CBX	6
50–54	35	TLC	0	Breath hold	CBX	6
48–51	400+		5	Voluntary targeted	Normal	5
51–60	400+		15	Voluntary targeted	Normal	5
41–46	400+		7–9	Passive ventilation	Normal	7
33–45[c]	400+		6–15	Passive ventilation	Quadriplegic	8
46–58	300+		9–12	Passive ventilation	Normal	10
47–52	60–70		9–12	Passive ventilation	Normal	10
46				Passive ventilation	Normal	9

[a]VL, lung volume; $\dot{V}E$, minute ventilation; TLC, total lung capacity; CBX, carotid bodies resected.
[b](1) Douglas and Haldane, 1909; (2) Ferris et al., 1946; (3) Otis et al., 1948; (4) Rahn et al., 1953; (5) Remmers et al., 1968; (6) Davidson et al., 1974; (7) Banzett, et al., 1990; (8) Manning et al., 1992; (9) Gandevia et al., 1993; (10) Banzett and Lansing, unpublished observations).
[c]These quadriplegic patients were chronically maintained at very low PET_{CO_2}, and thus the PCO_2 values represent increases of 13–29 mm Hg above "resting" levels.

tion. Table 2 lists blood or end-tidal PCO_2 values at breakpoint during breath hold and during fixed ventilation. The values for alveolar carbon dioxide pressure ($PACO_2$) at breakpoint in Table 2 vary from the low 40s to about 60. Some of this variation is probably a result of the failure of CO_2 to equilibrate in the region of the medullary chemoreceptors during relatively short maneuvers, such as breath hold. Some of the variability is caused by the effect of ventilation on the sensation of air hunger, as discussed later.

C. Dynamic Response of Air Hunger

How fast does air hunger change in response to a sudden change in stimulus? The answer to this question can reveal something about sensory processes and is necessary to assess experimental results. Adams et al. (1985) showed that rating of breathlessness in normal subjects can follow a sinusoidal change in PET_{CO_2} or

$P_{ET_{O_2}}$ at .05 cycles per minute but is unable to follow a 2 cycle per minute stimulus. In these experiments, breathing was allowed to increase in response to the stimulus, so that subjects could have received cues from their breathing motion, although they were told to disregard this sensation.

During fixed mechanical ventilation with hyperoxic gas mixtures, the time course of the response of air hunger ratings after a step change in $P_{ET_{CO_2}}$ appears to have about a 1 minute time constant (Banzett et al., 1990), consistent with the equilibration dynamics of the central chemoreceptors. These results are in accord with the cruder determinations of dynamic response that can be made using data from experiments on totally paralyzed subjects. When the $P_{ET_{CO_2}}$ changes are superimposed on slightly hypoxic mixtures, a faster response emerges (Banzett and Lansing, unpublished observations). The dynamic responses observed are consistent with the known dynamics of peripheral and central chemoreceptors, and there appears to be no significant central processing delay. Air hunger ratings respond very rapidly to changes in tidal volume, further evidence that central processing delays are insignificant (Manning et al., 1992; Flume et al., 1993).

D. Interaction of Ventilation with Air Hunger

Normally, an increase in breathing accompanies an increase in air hunger. What is the relationship between these events? We have already seen that the ventilatory increase does not cause air hunger. Does it augment or diminish air hunger? Does it change the quality of the sensation?

It has long been known that breathing instantly and dramatically reduces the air hunger felt at the end of a long breath hold, even if the inspired gas concentrations are such that no improvements in blood gases can result (Hill and Flack, 1908; Fowler, 1954). When subjects having held their breath to breakpoint are allowed to rebreathe from a bag containing low P_{O_2} and high P_{CO_2}, they feel immediate relief and are then able to resume breath holding for 10 s or so. Apparently there is no "memory" for this relieving effect, because isocapnic hyperventilation *before* breath hold does not extend breath-hold duration (Norfleet and Bradley, 1987). During targeted voluntary ventilation, the tolerable level of hypercapnia is lower if ventilation is voluntarily restrained to a target value below the ventilation subjects would normally achieve at that P_{CO_2} (Remmers et al., 1968; Chonan et al., 1987; Schwartzstein et al., 1989). Chonan et al. (1990) showed that voluntary decreases in breathing below the spontaneous level of $P_{ET_{CO_2}}$ 50 mm Hg sharply increased ratings of "difficulty in breathing" but that voluntary increases in breathing also caused a moderate increase in ratings. The latter finding appears to stand in contrast with the finding of Adams et al. (1985), who showed that voluntary increases in ventilation caused no increase in "breathlessness"; however, difficulty in breathing may have been interpreted by subjects to include both air hunger and effort, and thus the quality of sensation in the

Chonan experiment may have differed above and below the spontaneous ventilation, as noted by a few of their subjects. It thus appears that breathing diminishes air hunger, but what aspect of breathing is important? Lung inflation, chest wall motion, respiratory muscle contraction, the relief of willful effort needed to inhibit breathing, corollary discharge from respiratory centers, and the subject's sense of control are broad possibilities.

Opie et al. (1959) progressively raised $\text{P}_{\text{ET}_{CO_2}}$ in mechanically ventilated poliomyelitis patients and asked them to report how they felt. When ventilation was held at the subject's normal level and CO_2 was added to the inspired air, subjects volunteered comments (not reported verbatim) that the investigators interpreted as shortness of breath. On average, an 18 mm Hg rise in $\text{P}_{\text{ET}_{CO_2}}$ was required to elicit shortness of breath. In a second experiment ventilation was lowered and metabolic CO_2 was allowed to accumulate; in this circumstance subjects became short of breath after a much smaller (6 mm Hg) rise in $\text{P}_{\text{ET}_{CO_2}}$. This suggested that greater passive inflation of the lungs was effective in relieving air hunger. [Although the finding that local anesthetic block of the vagus prolonged breath hold seems to contradict this hypothesis, it must be remembered that the IX nerve, carrying chemoreceptor traffic, was also blocked in these experiments (Guz et al., 1966b).] Our laboratory examined this interaction of CO_2 and tidal volume in C1–2 ventilator-dependent quadriplegic subjects (Manning et al., 1992). The results were consistent with those reported by Opie et al.: when $\text{P}_{\text{ET}_{CO_2}}$ was held constant at a level evoking slight air hunger at the usual (large) ventilator tidal volume, subsequent reduction in the tidal volume by half evoked severe air hunger. This study, using a more sophisticated psychophysical design, not only confirmed earlier results but allowed us to identify pulmonary afferents as an important component of the response. In addition, the more detailed reports of subjective descriptions showed an interesting feature: the subjects did not distinguish between the quality of sensation evoked by elevated $\text{P}_{\text{ET}_{CO_2}}$ at constant tidal volume and that evoked by reduced tidal volume at constant $\text{P}_{\text{ET}_{CO_2}}$! Although, as expected, they reported accurately real reductions in tidal volume, they also perceived an illusive reduction in tidal volume when $\text{P}_{\text{ET}_{CO_2}}$ was raised at constant tidal volume.

Vibration of the rib cage can relieve air hunger (Manning et al., 1991), an effect the authors attributed to chest wall receptors, although the vibration may also have been transmitted to the lung. There is evidence that lung transplant recipients find less relief from the air hunger of breath hold when allowed to rebreathe alveolar gas (Flume et al., 1993) and that CO_2-induced breathlessness is increased by aerosol anesthesia of the lungs (Hamilton et al., 1987), although lung transplant patients did not report being more breathless during exercise (Kimoff et al., 1990). Most of these observations suggest that the sense of lung expansion is somehow mixed with the sense of increasing chemical drive before the signal reaches the level of consciousness. This phenomenon has a corollary in recent neurophysiological studies showing that ascending traffic from respiratory centers in the medulla is modified by vagal pulmonary afferents (Eldridge and Chen, 1992).

E. Respiratory Drive: Ventilation Appropriateness

The preceding observations suggest that if ventilation is low in relation to the drive to breathe, the sense of air hunger is intensified. The reader will notice some relation of this statement to the concept of length-tension inappropriateness proposed three decades ago by Campbell and coworkers. In its original form (Campbell et al., 1963), this concept proposed that breathlessness was caused by an imbalance between the drive to respiratory muscles and the resultant movement. The authors clearly stated that the site of integration was at the level of muscle mechanoreceptors and used the theory to explain virtually all forms of breathlessness. The term "length-tension inappropriateness" has been taken to have widely differing specific meanings since its first use, often quite different from its original meaning. Although the original statement comprised a testable hypothesis, subsequent usage of the term has often been so vague as not to be useful in designing experiments.

Our analysis of the existing data suggests a testable statement of the appropriateness concept that might better be termed ventilatory drive-ventilation appropriateness, namely, that if the level of breathing is inadequate for the level of drive, air hunger is greatly increased (as has been proposed by others). In particular, we propose that the perception of chemical drive, ascending via direct projections or via medullary activity (hypothesized mechanism 1 or 3), is modified by ascending sensations of ventilation from pulmonary afferents and perhaps from chest wall and upper airway afferents. This integration takes place at some level above the brain stem respiratory centers. This concept can be extended to encompass respiratory drive other than that originating in chemoreceptors, notably the ventilatory drive of exercise. This concept of ventilatory drive-ventilation appropriateness, however, is not intended to explain all forms of respiratory discomfort.

V. Conclusion

In the past few years we have moved away from the idea that respiratory muscle receptors provide essentially all respiratory sensation and have provided further evidence to heed the warning that any hypothesis purporting to explain all respiratory sensation should be viewed with suspicion. Respiratory sensations arising from the lungs and chemoreceptors may well provide useful information in healthy people (e.g., how deeply to inspire to sing that next phrase, when to come up from the bottom of the pool, or when to quit or moderate exercise), and are probably important in signaling cardiopulmonary disease (when to take a puff of bronchodilator or visit the doctor). Much remains to be learned.

References

Adams, L., Lane, R., Shea, S.A., Cockcroft, A., and Guz, A. (1985). Breathlessness during different forms of ventilatory stimulation: a study of mechanisms in normal subjects and respiratory patients. Clin. Sci. 69:663–672.

Adrian, E. (1933). Afferent impulses in the vagus and their effect on respiration. J. Physiol. (Lond.) 79:332–358.

Altose, M.D. (1991). Chest wall mechanisms in respiratory sensation. In Control of Breathing and Dyspnea. Edited by T. Takashima and N.S. Cherniack. Oxford, Pergamon Press, pp. 235–241.

Armstrong, D.J., and Luck, J.C. (1974). Accessibility of pulmonary stretch receptors from the pulmonary and bronchial circulations. J. Appl. Physiol. 36:706–710.

Bakers, J.H., and Tenney, S.M. (1970). The perception of some sensations associated with breathing. Respir. Physiol. 10:85–92.

Banner, N.R., Heaton, R., Hollingshead, L., Guz, A., and Yacoub, M.H. (1988). Bronchial reactivity to methacholine after combined heart-lung transplantation. Thorax 43: 955–959.

Banzett, R.B., Lansing, R.W., and Brown, R. (1987). High-level quadriplegics perceive lung volume change. J. Appl. Physiol. 62:567–573.

Banzett, R.B., Lansing, R.W., Reid, M.B., Adams, L., and Brown, R. (1989). "Air hunger" arising from increased P_{CO_2} in mechanically ventilated quadriplegics. Respir. Physiol. 76:53–67.

Banzett, R.B., Lansing, R.W., Brown, R., Topulos, G.P., Yager, D., Steele, S.M., Londoño, B., Loring, S.H., Reid, M.B., Adams, L., and Nations, C.S. (1990). "Air hunger" from increased P_{CO_2} persists after complete neuromuscular block in humans. Respir. Physiol. 81:1–17.

Bevan, J.A., and Murray, J.F. (1963). Evidence for a ventilation-modifying reflex from the pulmonary circulation in man. Proc. Soc. Exp. Biol. Med. 114:393–396.

Bitterman, H., Kerem, D.H., Shabati, Y., Gavriely, N., and Palti, Y. (1983). Respiration maintained by externally applied vibration and steady tracheal insufflation in the cat. Anesth. Analg. 62:33–38.

Breuer, J. and Hering, E. (1868). Self-steering of respiration through the Nervus Vagus. In Breathing: Hering-Breuer Centenary Symposium. Edited by R. Porter. Translated by Ullmann, E, London, J., and A. Churchill. pp. 365–394.

Burki, N.K. (1980). Dyspnea. Clin. Chest Med. 1:47–55.

Burki, N.K. (1987). Dyspnea. Lung 165:269–277.

Campbell, E.J., Freedman, S., Clark, T.J., Robson, J.G., and Norman, J. (1967). The effect of muscular paralysis induced by tubocurarine on the duration and sensation of breath-holding. Clin. Sci. 32:425–432.

Campbell, E.J., Godfrey, S., Clark, T.J., Freedman, S., and Norman, J. (1969). The effect of muscular paralysis induced by tubocurarine on the duration and sensation of breath-holding during hypercapnia. Clin. Sci. 36:323–328.

Campbell, E.J.M., and Howell, J.B.L. (1963). The sensation of breathlessness. Br. Med. Bull. 19:36–40.

Campbell, E.J.M., Gandevia, S.C., Killian, K.J., Mahutte, C.K., and Rigg, J.R.A. (1980). Changes in the perception of inspiratory resistive loads during partial curarization. J. Physiol. (Lond.) 309:93–100.

Chapman, K.R., and Rebuck, A.S. (1983). Inspiratory and expiratory resistive loading as a model of dyspnea in asthma. Respiration 44:425–432.

Chen, Z., Eldridge, F.L., and Wagner, P.G. (1991). Respiratory-associated rhythmic firing of midbrain neurones in cats: relation to level of respiratory drive. J. Physiol. 437:305–325.

Chen, Z., Eldridge, F.L., and Wagner, P.G. (1992). Respiratory-associated thalamic activity is related to level of respiratory drive. Respir. Physiol. 90:99–113.

Chonan, T., Mulholland, M.B., Cherniack, N.S., and Altose, M.D. (1987). Effects of voluntary constraining of thoracic displacement during hypercapnia. J. Appl. Physiol. 63:1822–1828.

Chonan, T., Mulholland, M.B., Altose, M.D., and Cherniack, N.S. (1990). Effects of changes in level and pattern of breathing on the sensation of dyspnea. J. Appl. Physiol. 69:1290–1295.

Coleridge, J.C.G., and Coleridge, H.M. (1984). Afferent vagal C fibre innervation of the lungs and airways and its functional significance. Rev. Physiol. Biochem. Pharmacol. 99:1–110.

Cross, B.A., Guz, A., Jain, S.K., Archer, S., Stevens, J., and Reynolds, F. (1976). The effect of anaesthesia of the airway in dog and man: a study of respiratory reflexes, sensations and lung mechanics. Clin. Sci. 50:439–454.

Davidson, J.T., Whipp, B.J., and Wasserman, K., Koyal, S.N., and Lugliani, R. (1974). Role of the carotid bodies in breath-holding. N. Engl. J. Med. 290:819–822.

Dell, P. (1958). Humoral effects on the brainstem reticular formations. In Reticular Formation of the Brain. Edited by H. Jasper, L. Proctor, R. Knighton, W. Noshay, and R. Costello. Boston, Little, Brown and Company. pp. 365–379.

Demediuk, B.H., Manning, H., Lilly, J., Fencl, V., Weinberger, S.E., Weiss, J.W., and Schwartzstein, R.M. (1992). Dissociation between dyspnea and respiratory effort. Am. Rev. Respir. Dis. 146:1222–1225.

DiMarco, A.F., Wolfson, D.A., Gottfried, S.B., and Altose, M.D. (1982). Sensation of inspired volume in normal subjects and quadriplegic patients. J. Appl. Physiol. 53:1481–1486.

Douglas, C.G., and Haldane, J.S. (1909). The regulation of normal breathing. J. Physiol. (Lond.) 38:420–440.

Easton, P.A., Jadue, C., Arnup, M.E., Meatherall, R.C., and Anthonisen, N.R. (1985). Effects of upper or lower airway anesthesia on hypercapnic ventilation in humans. J. Appl. Physiol. 59:1090–1097.

Eisele, J.H., and Jain, S.K., (1971). Circulatory and respiratory changes during unilateral and bilateral cranial nerve IX and X block in two asthmatics. Clin. Sci. 40:117–125.

Eldridge, F.L., and Chen, Z. (1992). Respiratory-associated rhythmic firing of midbrain neurons is modulated by vagal input. Respir. Physiol. 90:31–46.

Elliott, M.W., Adams, L., Cockcroft, A., MacRae, K.D., Murphy, K., and Guz, A. (1991). The language of breathlessness. Use of verbal descriptors by patients with cardiopulmonary disease. Am. Rev. Respir. Dis. 144:826–832.

Ferris, E.B., Engel G.L., Stevens, C.D., and Webb, J. (1946). Voluntary breathholding. III. The relation of the maximum time of breath-holding to the oxygen and carbon dioxide tensions of arterial blood, with a note on its clinical and physiological significance. J. Clin. Invest. 25:734–743.

Fillenz, M. and Widdicombe, J.G. (1972). Sensation mediated by respiratory receptors. In Handbook of Sensory Physiology. Edited by E. Heil. Berlin, Springer-Verlag. pp. 106–112.

Flume, P.A., Eldridge, F.L., and Edwards, L.J. (1993). Role of vagal input in the relief of the distress of breathholding: normals vs. pts. with double lung transplants. Am. Rev. Respir. Dis. 147:A550.

Folinsbee, L.J., Gliner, J.A., and Horvath, S.M. (1982). Perceptual cues used in reproduction of inspired volume. Perception Psychophysics 32:449–453.

Fowler, W.S. (1954). Breaking point of breath holding. J. Appl. Physiol. 6:539–545.

Fox, J., Kreisman, H., Colacone, A., and Wolkove, N. (1986). Respiratory volume perception through the nose and mouth determined noninvasively. J. Appl. Physiol. 61:436–439.

Freedman, S., Lane, R., and Guz, A. (1987). Breathlessness and respiratory mechanics during reflex or voluntary hyperventilation in patients with chronic airflow limitation. Clin. Sci. 73:311–318.

Fuller, R.W., Dixon, C.M.S., and Barnes, P.J. (1985). Bronchoconstrictor response to inhaled capsaicin in humans. J. Appl. Physiol. 58:1080–1084.

Gandevia, S.C., and Macefield, G. (1989) Projection of low-threshold afferents from human intercostal muscles to the cerebral cortex. Respir. Physiol. 77:203–214.

Gandevia, S.C., Killian, K.J., and Campbell, E.J. (1981). The effect of respiratory muscle fatigue on respiratory sensations. Clin. Sci. 60:463–466.

Gandevia, S.C., Killian, K., McKenzie, D.K., Crawford, M., Allen, G.M., Gorman, R.B., and Hales, J.P. (1993). Respiratory sensations, cardiovascular control, kinaesthesia and transcranial stimulation during paralysis in humans. J. Physiol. (Lond.) 470: 85–107.

Gliner, J.A., Folinsbee, L.J., and Horvath, S.M. (1981). Accuracy and precision of matching inspired lung volume. Perception Psychophysics 29:511–515.

Gottfried, S.B., Redline, S., and Altose, M.D. (1985). Respiratory sensation in chronic obstructive pulmonary disease. Am. Rev. Respir. Dis. 132:954–955.

Grippi, M.A., Pack, A.I., Davies, R.O., and Fishman, A.P. (1985). Adaptation to reflex effects of prolonged lung inflation. J. Appl. Physiol. 58:1360–1371.

Guz, A. (1970). Discussion. In Breathing: Hering-Breuer centenary symposium. Edited by R. Porter. London, Churchill. pp. 250.

Guz, A., and Trenchard, D.W. (1971). Pulmonary stretch receptor activity in man: a comparison with dog and cat. J. Physiol. (Lond.) 213:329–343.

Guz, A., Noble, M.I., Trenchard, D., Smith, A.J., and Makey, A.R. (1966a). The Hering-Breuer inflation reflex in man: studies of unilateral lung inflation and vagus nerve block. Respir. Physiol. 1:382–389.

Guz, A., Noble, M.I., Widdicombe, J.G., Trenchard, D., Mushin, W.W., and Makey, A.R. (1966b). The role of vagal and glossopharyngeal afferent nerves in respiratory sensation, control of breathing and arterial pressure regulation in conscious man. Clin. Sci. 30:161–170.

Hamilton, R.D., Winning, A.J., Perry, A., and Guz, A. (1987). Aerosol anesthesia increases hypercapnic ventilation and breathlessness in laryngectomized humans. J. Appl. Physiol. 63:2286–2292.

Head, H. (1889). On the regulation of respiration. J. Physiol. (Lond.) 10:1–70.

Hill, L., and Flack, F. (1908). The effect of excess of carbon dioxide and of want of oxygen upon the respiration and the circulation. J. Physiol. (Lond.) 37:77–111.

Homma, I., Kanamaru, A., and Sibuya, M. (1991). Mechanoreceptors and respiratory sensation. In Control of Breathing and Dyspnea. Edited by T. Takashima and N.S. Cherniack. Oxford, Pergamon Press. pp. 229–234.

Jain, S.K., Subramanian, S., Julka, D.B., and Guz, A. (1972). Search for evidence of lung chemoreflexes in man: study of respiratory and circulatory effects of phenyldiguanide and lobeline. Clin. Sci. 42:163–177.

Katz-Salamon, M. (1984). The ability of human subjects to detect small changes in breathing volume. Acta Physiol. Scand. 120:43–51.

Kazakov, U.N. (1966). Cortical projection of pulmonary receptors in the cat. Fiziol. Zh. SSSR 52:847–854.

Killian, K.J., and Jones, N.L. (1988). Respiratory muscles and dyspnea. Clin. Chest Med. 9:237–248.

Killian, K.J., Gandevia, S.C., Summers, E., and Campbell, E.J. (1984). Effect of increased lung volume on perception of breathlessness, effort, and tension. J. Appl. Physiol. 57:686–691.

Kimoff, R.J., Cheong, T.H., Cosio, M.G., Guerraty, A., and Levy, R.D. (1990). Pulmonary denervation in humans. Effects on dyspnea and ventilatory pattern during exercise. Am. Rev. Respir. Dis. 142:1034–1040.

Kostreva, D.R., Zuperku, E.J., Hess, G.L., Coon, R.L., and Kampine, J.P. (1975). Pulmonary afferent activity recorded from sympathetic nerves. J. Appl. Physiol. 39:37–40.

Kukorelli, T., Namenyi, J., and Adam, G. (1969). Visceral afferent projection areas in the cortex. II. Representation of the carotid sinus receptor area. Acta Physiol. Acad. Sci. Hung. 36:261–263.

Lane, R., Cockcroft, A., and Guz, A. (1987). Voluntary isocapnic hyperventilation and breathlessness during exercise in normal subjects. Clin. Sci. 73:519–523.

Lane, R., Adams, L., and Guz, A. (1990). The effects of hypoxia and hypercapnia on perceived breathlessness during exercise in humans. J. Physiol. (Lond.) 428:579–593.

Langrehr, D. (1964). Receptor-Afferenzen im Halsvagus des Menschen. Klin. Wochenschr. 42:239–244.

Lansing, R.W., and Banzett, R.B. (1993). What do paralyzed awake humans feel when they attempt to move? J. Motor Behav. 25:309–313.

Lansing, R.W., Banzett, R.B., Brown, R., and Reid, M. (1988). Airway anesthesia diminished tidal volume perception in a C1-C2 quadriplegic. FASEB J. 2:A1298.

Manning, H.L., Basner, R., Ringler, J., Rand, C., Fencl, V., Weinberger, S.E., Weiss, J.W., and Schwartzstein, R.M. (1991). Effect of chest wall vibration on breathlessness in normal subjects. J. Appl. Physiol. 71:175–181.

Manning, H.L., Shea, S.A., Schwartzstein, R.M., Lansing, R.W., Brown, R., and Banzett, R.B. (1992). Reduced tidal volume increases "air hunger" at fixed P_{CO_2} in ventilated quadriplegics. Respir. Physiol. 90:19–30.

Marshall, R., Stone, R., and Christie, R. (1954). The relationship of dyspnea to respiratory effort in normal subjects, mitral stenosis and emphysema. Clin. Sci. 13:625–631.

McCloskey, D. (1981). Corollary discharges: motor commands and perception. In Section 1: The nervous system. Edited by J. Brookhart, V. Mountcastle, and V. Brooks. Washington, D.C., American Physiological Society. pp. 1415–1447.

Mead, J., Smith, J.C., and Loring, S.H. (1985). Volume displacements of the chest wall and their mechanical significance. In The Thorax. Edited by C. Rousssos and P.T. Macklem. New York, Marcel Dekker. 1st ed. pp. 369–392.

Mithoefer, J.C. (1965). Breath holding. In Handbook of Physiology, Section 3: Respiration. Edited by W.O. Fenn and H. Rahn. Washington, D.C., American Physiological Society. pp. 1011–1025.

Morton, D.R., Klassen, K.P., and Curtis, G.M. (1950). The clinical physiology of the human bronchi. I. Pain of tracheobronchial origin. Surgery 28:699–704.

Newsom-Davis, J. (1979). Neural control of the diaphragm. B. Sensory aspects. High cervical cord transection (proceedings). Am. Rev. Respir. Dis. 119:69.

Norfleet, W.T., and Bradley, C.L. (1987). Can eucapnic hyperventilation prolong a subsequent breath-hold? Respir. Physiol. 70:369–376.

O'Brien, J.H., Pimpaneau, A., and Albe-Fessard, D. (1971). Evoked cortical responses to vagal, laryngeal and facial afferents in monkeys under chloralose anaesthesia. Electroenceph. Clin. Neurophysiol. 31:7–20.

Opie, L., Smith, A., and Spalding, J. (1959). Conscious appreciation of the effects produced by independent changes of ventilation volume and of end-tidal P_{CO_2} in paralysed patients. J. Physiol. (Lond.) 149:494–499.

Otis, A.B., Rahn, H., and Fenn, W.O. (1948). Alveolar gas changes during breath holding. Am. J. Physiol. 152:674–686.

Paton, J.Y., Swaminathan, S., Sargent, C.W., Hawksworth, A., and Keens, T.G. (1993). Ventilatory response to exercise in children with congenital central hypoventilation syndrome. Am. Rev. Respir. Dis. 147:1185–1191.

Patterson, J.L., Mullinax, P.F., Bain, T., Kreuger, J.J., and Richardson, D.W. (1962). Carbon dioxide-induced dyspnea in a patient with respiratory muscle paralysis. Am. J. Med. 32:811–816.

Petit, J.M., and Delhez, L. (1970). Some recent experimental data on the origin of dyspnea and ventilatory regulation in asthmatics (French). Acta Tuberc. Pneumol. Belg. 61:169–186.

Plassman, B.L., and Lansing, R.W. (1990). Perceptual cues used to reproduce an inspired lung volume. J. Appl. Physiol. 69:1123–1130.

Prys-Roberts, C. (1970). Discussion. In Breathing: Hering-Breuer centenary symposium. Edited by R. Porter. London, Churchill. pp. 249.

Rahn, H., Bahnson, H.T., Muxworthy, J.F., and Hagen, J.M. (1953). Adaptation to high altitude: changes in breath-holding time. J. Appl. Physiol. 6:154–157.

Redline, S., Gottfried, S.B., and Altose, M.D. (1991). Effects of changes in inspiratory muscle strength on the sensation of respiratory force. J. Appl. Physiol. 70:240–245.

Remmers, J.E., Brooks, J., and Tenney, S.M. (1968). Effect of controlled ventilation on the tolerable limit of hypercapnia. Respir. Physiol. 4:78–90.

Salamon, M., von Euler, C., and Franzen, O. (1976). Perception of mechanical factors in breathing. University of Uppsala Dept. of Psychology Report No. 189.

Sant'Ambrogio, F.B., and Sant'Ambrogio, G. (1982). Circulatory accessibility of nervous receptors localized in the tracheobronchial tree. Respir. Physiol. 49:49–73.

Sant'Ambrogio, G., Mathew, O.P., and Sant'Ambrogio, F.B. (1988). Characteristics of laryngeal cold receptors. Respir. Physiol. 71:287–297.

Schwartzstein, R.M., La Hive, K., Pope, A., Steinbrook, R.A., Leith, D.E., Weiss, J.W., Fencl, V., and Weinberger, S.E. (1987). Detection of hypercapnia by normal subjects. Clin. Sci. 73:333–335.

Schwartzstein, R.M., Simon, P.M., Weiss, J.W., Fencl, V., and Weinberger, S.E. (1989). Breathlessness induced by dissociation between ventilation and chemical drive. Am. Rev. Respir. Dis. 139:1231–1237.

Schwartzstein, R., Lilly, J., Israel, E., Basner, R., Sparrow, D., Weinberger, S., and Weiss, J.W. (1991). Breathlessness of asthma differs from that of external resistive loading. Am. Rev. Respir. Dis. 143:A596.

Shea, S.A., Andres, L.P., Shannon, D.C., and Banzett, R.B. (1993a). Ventilatory responses to exercise in humans lacking ventilatory chemosensitivity. J. Physiol. (Lond.). 468: 623–640.

Shea, S.A., Andres, L.P., Shannon, D.C., Guz, A., and Banzett, R.B. (1993b). Respiratory sensations in subjects who lack a ventilatory response to CO_2. Respir. Physiol. 93:203–219.
Simon, P.M., Schwartzstein, R.M., Weiss, J.W., Lahive, K., Fencl, V., Teghtsoonian, M., and Weinberger, S.E. (1989). Distinguishable sensations of breathlessness induced in normal volunteers. Am. Rev. Respir. Dis. 140:1021–1027.
Simon, P.M., Schwartzstein, R.M., Weiss, J.W., Fencl, V., Teghtsoonian, M., and Weinberger, S.E. (1990). Distinguishable types of dyspnea in patients with shortness of breath. Am. Rev. Respir. Dis. 142:1009–1014.
Smith, J., Kreisman, H., Colacone, A., Fox, J., and Wolkove, N. (1990). Sensation of inspired volumes and pressures in professional wind instrument players. J. Appl. Physiol. 68:2380–2383.
Smith, S.M., Brown, H.O., Toman, J.E.P., and Goodman, L.S. (1947). The lack of cerebral effects of *d*-tubocurarine. Anesthesiology 8:1–14.
Stanley, N.N., Altose, M.D., Cherniack, N.S., and Fishman, A.P. (1975). Changes in strength of lung inflation reflex during prolonged inflation. J. Appl. Physiol. 38:474–480.
Stevens, J.K., Emerson, R.C., Gerstein, G.L., Kallos, T., Neufeld, G.R., Nichols, C.W., and Rosenquist, A.C. (1976). Paralysis of the awake human: visual perceptions. Vision Res. 16:93–98.
Stubbing, D.G., Killian, K.J., and Campbell, E.J. (1981). The quantification of respiratory sensations by normal subjects. Respir. Physiol. 44:251–260.
Sullivan, T.Y., and Yu, P.L. (1983). Airway anesthesia effects on hypercapnic breathing pattern in humans. J. Appl. Physiol. 55:368–376.
Sullivan, T.Y., Muzzin, S., Hamilton, R.D., Adams, L., Shea, S.A., Horner, R.L., and Guz, A. (1991). Volume detection during voluntary and passive breathing. Respir. Physiol. 84:323–335.
Taguchi, O., Kikuchi, Y., Hida, W., Iwase, N., Satoh, M., Chonan, T., and Takishima, T. (1991). Effects of bronchoconstriction and external resistive loading on the sensation of dyspnea. J. Appl. Physiol. 71:2183–2190.
Ward, S.A., and Whipp, B.J. (1989). Effects of peripheral and central chemoreflex activation on the isopnoeic rating of breathing in exercising humans [published erratum in J. Physiol. (Lond.) 1990; 420:489]. J. Physiol. (Lond.) 411:27–43.
West, D.W., Ellis, C.G., and Campbell, E.J. (1975). Ability of man to detect increases in his breathing. J. Appl. Physiol. 39:372–376.
Whitelaw, W.A., McBride, B., and Ford, G.T. (1987). Effect of lung volume on breath holding. J. Appl. Physiol. 62:1962–1969.
Winning, A.J., Hamilton, R.D., Shea, S.A., Knott, C., and Guz, A. (1985). The effect of airway anaesthesia on the control of breathing and the sensation of breathlessness in man. Clin. Sci. 68:215–225.
Winning, A.J., Hamilton, R.D., Shea, S.A., and Guz, A. (1986). Respiratory and cardiovascular effects of central and peripheral intravenous injections of capsaicin in man: evidence for pulmonary chemosensitivity. Clin. Sci. 71:519–526.
Wolkove, N., Altose, M.D., Kelsen, S.G., Kondapalli, P.G., and Cherniack, N.S. (1981). Perception of changes in breathing in normal human subjects. J. Appl. Physiol. 50:78–83.
Wright, G.W., and Branscomb, B.V. (1954). The origin of the sensations of dyspnea? Trans. Am. Clin. Clin. Assoc. 66:116–125.
Zechman, F.W., Jr., and Wiley, R.L. (1986). Afferent inputs to breathing: respiratory sensation. In Section 3: The Respiratory System. Edited by N.S. Cherniack and J.G. Widdicombe. Bethesda, MD, American Physiological Society. pp. 449–474.

7

Sense of Effort and Dyspnea

KIERAN J. KILLIAN

McMaster University
Hamilton, Ontario, Canada

SIMON C. GANDEVIA

Prince of Wales Medical Research Institute
Randwick, Sydney, Australia

I. Introduction

For a number of years it has been our contention that effort intolerance and dyspnea are related and that the sense of effort is central to the mechanism of dyspnea (Gandevia et al., 1981; Killian and Campbell, 1983, 1985, 1991; Killian, 1992a, b). Effort is mechanistically credible and is consistent with a great deal of experimental and clinical data. Furthermore, it provides a useful way of looking at dyspnea with the power to explain and to predict the intensity of dyspnea in most clinical circumstances. Hence, our mandate is to address the sense of muscular effort and its relationship to dyspnea. To accomplish our objective we discuss (1) the history of muscular sensation; (2) muscle receptors; (3) the sensations associated with muscular activity and the relationship of the sense of effort to these sensations; (4) the meaning of the word dyspnea; and finally, (5) dyspnea as a quantitative entity and its relationship to the sense of effort.

II. Origin of the Muscle Senses

External bodies composed of the basic elements, fire, air, water, and earth emitted invisible emanations, gained access through special sense organs, and met with similar elements in the blood, thus giving rise to sensation. In this manner, the heart was thought to be the organ responsible for conscious sensation (Quin, 1992). The anatomical demonstration of nerves by Erasistratus and Herophilus (258 BCE), followed by the experimental demonstration of their function by Galen (130–200 CE), led to the idea that the brain was the origin of sensation. With a background of these competing mechanisms and the five basic senses proclaimed by Aristotle—vision, audition, taste, smell, and touch—the ability to sense muscular discomfort, force, and fatigue were explained within the confines of touch (Aristotle, 384–322 BCE). Descartes, Locke, Berkeley, Hume, Kant, Engel, Brown, Biran, Tiedemann, Gruithuisen, Mill, Spencer, and Bain questioned the adequacy of touch to explain these muscular sensations at a philosophical level. Their contribution to the muscle senses has been reviewed by Boring (1942) and more recently by Scheerer (1987).

The next major step in the evolution of the muscle senses came with the experimental demonstration of the separate neural pathways in the anterior (motor) and posterior (sensory) roots of the spinal cord by Magendie (1822) and Bell (1811–1823). Bell proclaimed "that neither bodies nor the images of bodies enter the brain" and suggested that the quality of the sensation was determined by the specificity of the nerve that is excited. He also argued that the efferent motor command to the muscle and the afferent activity arising in the muscle were essential to the muscle senses (Bell, 1833, 1869). Muller (1838) subsequently formalized sensory processes in a series of 10 laws. The most important were (1) the sensorium is directly aware of the sensory nerves; (2) sensory nerves are divided into five types corresponding to the special senses; (3) the same stimulus acting on different nerves gives rise to different qualities; different stimuli acting on the same nerve give rise to the same quality; (4) particular stimuli excite particular nerves (origin of the concept of adequate stimulus); and (5) the locus of specificity lies in the nerve or in its central termination in the brain. Muller, in specific reference to the muscle senses, directly acknowledged both afferent and efferent mechanisms: "The idea of weight and pressure in raising bodies or in resisting forces may in part arise from the consciousness of the amount of nervous energy transmitted from the brain rather than from a sensation in the muscles themselves." Thereafter, the muscle senses were accepted as the sixth sense and the sense of "innervation," and sensations arising in the muscles emerged as separate dimensions.

The measurement of sensation was initially considered impossible because of its introspective nature. Hence, the sense of innervation was largely a philosophical concept: consciousness is sensory, and one simply knows the intensity of the willed motor command when and by how much a particular muscle or group of muscles are activated. Arguments supporting the sense of innervation included the perceived heaviness of paretic limbs; the perceived movements of amputated limbs; and the perceived movement of anesthetic limbs. Vision played an important role in the evolution of the muscle senses. In the midnineteenth century, visual illusions were popular experimental models. The sense of innervation and afferent information arising in the ocular muscles were important to help explain the third dimension, or depth. Awareness of the motor command to the ocular muscles enabled the brain to know eye position, whereas feedback control was ill suited to stabilize the visual field in the presence of moving retinal images (Helmholtz, 1867). The sense of innervation was founded on this background and initially favored at a time when specific muscular receptors had not yet been characterized.

Experimental methods for the quantitative measurement of the relationship between physical stimuli and evoked sensation emerged. These studies required detection of "just noticeable" changes in stimulus magnitude. Weber applied the method to show that a lifted weight must increase by approximately 6% to achieve a just noticeable difference, whereas an increase of 33% is needed for a weight placed in a hand resting on a table to achieve a just noticeable difference (Weber, 1860). Psychophysical studies on weight discrimination proliferated, and it is not surprising that the sense of innervation continued to predominate.

Studies on weight discrimination were broadened to include the discrimination of joint movement with the pioneering studies of Goldscheider (1898). By 1880, the term "muscle senses" was replaced by the sense of movement (*kinesthesis*), as Bastian pointed out that the muscle senses were complex, involving sensations arising in muscles, tendons, joints, and skin (Bastian, 1880). After section of the posterior spinal roots in monkeys, Sherrington noted that the movement of the affected limb was severely impaired (Mott and Sherrington, 1895). The fine control of muscle movement was dependent on afferent activity arising in the recently demonstrated muscular receptors, Golgi tendon organs (named and found by Golgi), and muscle spindles (Sherrington, 1894). The concept of adequate and appropriate stimuli emerged (Sherrington, 1924a, b): "the main function of a receptor is therefore to lower the threshold excitability of the (reflex) arc for one kind of stimulus" (Sherrington, 1900). An inadequate or inappropriate stimulus would fail to elicit a reflex response or to generate a specific sensation.

The pioneering ablation studies of Flourens (1842) established the importance of the site of central termination of neural pathways and discrete localization was also demonstrated within the motor cortex by Leyton and Sherrington (1917). Using direct cortical stimulation in the human, Penfield and Boldrey (1937) constructed the cortical representations of the motor and sensory "homunculus." Hence, by the early part of this century muscular sensations depended on adequate and appropriate stimuli acting on muscular receptors resulting in afferent input terminating to specific sites in the brain.

Direct experimental studies on the neural aspects of sensory stimulation appeared with the availability of better amplifiers and the ability to record from single nerve fibers (Adrian, 1928). Because of the influence of Sherrington, the term "proprioception" replaced "kinesthesia." The neurophysiologists, braced by objective studies on peripheral receptors and the measurement of afferent neural activity, considered the sense of innervation speculative, unproven, and unnecessary and considered the arguments for its existence philosophical, psychological, and frankly inferior. The organization of the motor program was based on behavioral learning and memory, and the conscious surveillance of outgoing motor command was denied.

By the early part of the twentieth century, the sensory receptors stimulated by muscular contraction were known and the theory of the sense of innervation was receding. By having subjects match the magnitude of perceived muscular sensory stimuli using the paired upper limbs, McCloskey and his colleagues demonstrated that weight lifted by a nonfatigued arm was matched to a larger weight lifted by the fatigued arm (McCloskey et al., 1974; Gandevia and McCloskey, 1977a, 1978; Jones and Hunter, 1983). Reasoning that the descending motor commands would vary inversely with the size of the reflexly driven component of the contraction, they went on to demonstrate that the heaviness of a lifted weight decreased when tonic vibration reflexes were induced; vibration of the antagonist increased the perceived heaviness of weight (Gandevia and McCloskey, 1978; Jones and Hunter, 1983). Local curarization increased the perceived heaviness of lifted weights (Gandevia and McCloskey, 1977b; for review, see McCloskey, 1978, 1981; Gandevia, 1987; Cafarelli, 1988). The sense of innervation reemerged as the most plausible explanation for the sense of heaviness. Roland and Ladegaard-Pederson (Roland and Ladegaard-Pederson, 1977; Roland, 1978) extended these studies, showing that both effort and perceived tension can be discriminated separately during partial neuromuscular blockade. Perceived heaviness was plausibly analogous to effort and related to the sense of innervation; perceived tension was peripheral in origin and most likely related to tendon organ stimulation. The sense of effort, sense of tension, and sense of movement constitute discrete dimensions to the muscle senses. Although these could be separated, they were seldom explicitly acknowledged.

III. Proprioceptors and Their Cortical Projections

The primary muscular receptors (muscle spindle endings and Golgi tendon organs) and their central projections have provided a framework for the study of the muscle senses. In its simplest form, the sensory system consists of a physical stimulus acting on a sensory receptor (usually located peripherally). This translates the magnitude of the stimulus into a change in discharge frequency, which is then carried by nerve fibers to the central nervous system. At various levels within the central nervous system the input creates a central representation of the stimulus, which is then interpreted within the context of stimulation and in light of previous experience. Measurements can be applied to some of the individual processes using neurophysiological techniques, and psychophysical techniques can be applied to the final conscious sensory response and its relationship to the physical stimulus (Schmidt, 1981). Here, we briefly discuss muscular receptors.

A. Muscle Spindles

The muscle spindles were demonstrated in histological sections by Kolliker in 1862 and by Kuhne in 1863. In 1894, the spindle was recognized as a sensory organ by Sherrington, who provided a complete description of the spindle and its two afferent endings. Its separate and distinct motor supply was identified in 1927 (Boake, 1927; Hinsey, 1927; Hines and Towers, 1928). The function of the fusimotor system was dissected by Matthews and others, and in 1972 a comprehensive account of muscle spindles and their physiological properties was contained in a landmark publication, *Mammalian Muscle Receptors and Their Central Actions* (Matthews, 1972). Activation of spindle afferents by vibration was shown to yield an illusion of movement and a sense of displacement, finally establishing the role of the spindle in the sense of limb position and displacement (Goodwin et al., 1972). Projection of muscle spindle afferents to the sensorimotor cortex was shown in animal and human studies (Phillips et al., 1971; Gandevia and Burke, 1988). Many detailed reviews have subsequently appeared (Matthews, 1977, 1981a, b; Phillips and Porter, 1977).

B. Golgi Tendon Organs

Golgi tendon organs are thinly encapsulated bundles of small tendon fascicles demonstrated in histological sections at the junction of muscle and tendon by Golgi in 1880. Cattaneo showed that they were sensory end organs in 1888. Both findings were substantiated by Sherrington in 1894. Their structure was described in great detail by Huber and Dewitt in 1900. Initially they were thought to respond to high tension only and to be ill suited to the role of conscious perception of tension. However, Houk and Henneman (1967), stimulating single motor axons, showed that even single units were sufficient to stimulate tendon organs (for review see Jami, 1992). The projection of 1b afferents to the cortex, long suspected on the basis of nonselective nerve stimulation, was demonstrated formally by McIntyre et al. in 1984. Hence, all objections to the tendon organs as the source of the sense of muscle tension have been eliminated. In recent studies, greater emphasis has arisen of their capacity to follow dynamic changes in muscle force. The tendon organs were extensively reviewed by Jami in 1992.

C. Joint Receptors

Joint receptors, Ruffini type and paciniform type, were demonstrated by Rauber and Krause in 1874. No doubt has ever been expressed about their afferent nature. By the end of the nineteenth century, joint receptors were considered the source of the conscious appreciation of the position of the limbs in space (Goldscheider, 1898). Joint receptors tend to fire most at the extremes of joint movement and are not ideally suited to mediate movement over the normal operating range (Matthews, 1988). Extensive study of the senses of displacement and position have led to the idea that muscle spindles and joint and skin receptors can all provide information about joint position and movement (Goodwin et al., 1972; McCloskey, 1973; Cross and McCloskey, 1973; Gandevia and McCloskey, 1976; McCloskey, 1978; Ferrell et al., 1987; Ferrell and Smith, 1989; Gandevia et al., 1992).

D. Free Nerve Endings

Free nerve endings lying between muscle fibers are stimulated by osmolarity, potassium ions, adenosine, prostaglandins, lactate, and so on. They are considered important to the control of blood flow relative to the metabolic demands of muscle (Honig, 1979). Many free nerve endings are remote from vessels, and it is not hard to imagine that the role of these endings remains undefined; but chemical and mechanical stimulation may result in pain, especially that related to claudication and the discomfort associated with overuse. Afferent discharges from these receptors can reflexly affect the discharge of α motor neurons, influencing their responsiveness.

E. Nonmuscular Receptors

Receptors stimulated as a consequence of muscular activity also include skin receptors. The stimulation of these receptors is important in directing attention and providing a calibration for muscle afferent activity. A crude sense of position is probably also possible.

F. Central Mechanisms for Effort

The primary mechanism responsible for the sense of innervation is believed to involve a centrally generated signal related to the descending motor command (McCloskey, 1978, 1981; Woodcock et al., 1981). Indirect evidence suggests that such a mechanism involves the presence of signals arriving at or leaving the motor cortex (for review see Gandevia, 1982, 1987; Gandevia et al., 1992). The relevant command signal is generated "upstream" of the anterior horn cells in the spinal cord, but the mechanisms are complex and more than merely the global activation of cortical motoneurons. The exact mechanism through which motor programs are constructed and the sense of effort generated remain poorly understood.

IV. Dimensions of Muscular Sensation

Muscle contraction is initiated volitionally and through other means that can loosely be termed nonvolitional. Both require the generation of central motor programs and motor commands. Muscle contraction activates the muscle spindles (through lengthening and via the fusimotor system and joint receptors to provide a sense of displacement or movement) and stimulates tendon organs to yield a sense of tension. When muscles are fatigued, small-diameter muscle afferents (groups 3 and 4) are activated and may produce a sense of discomfort and/or pain. However, the sensations evoked by muscular contraction have many dimensions (effort, tension, movement, and pain), and these dimensions are not confined to the stimuli that activate the primary receptors. Some recognized sensations are based on the relationships between sensory "inputs." For example, resistance is dependent on the relationship between tension and the rate of displacement. Elastance is dependent on the relationship between tension and displacement (perception of the stiffness of springs). Weakness is dependent on the relationship between effort and tension for movement. The relationship between effort and displacement is an alternative. A sense of muscle "timing," together with derivatives of force and position, can also be sensed. Thus the sensation associated with everyday muscular activity can be dissected into many dimensions. Finally, there are the dimensions of appropriateness (effort is appropriate for activity, and tension is appropriate for movement). There is also a tolerance threshold for some of these sensory dimensions. This is likely to be based on sensory intensity and varies from subject to subject. Although we have been implicitly aware of these dimensions, their explicit demonstration in the act of breathing has come in a rather obscure fashion. Many sensory dimensions of breathing are unpleasant and are not explained by muscle senses, including pleuritic pain, tracheitis, and direct probing of the airways.

V. Respiratory Sensations

Normal breathing is generally insentient, and it is tempting to consider breathing sentient only in the presence of dyspnea or when attention has been directed to it. However, we have come to recognize that there are many dimensions of respiratory sensation. By simply directing attention to the act of breathing, we can sense, volume, pressure, load, effort, and a broad general appreciation of the appropriateness of the act of breathing (pressure versus volume as load; effort versus pressure as weakness; ventilation versus activity as appropriateness of breathing; and breathing need versus satiety).

Studies related to threshold detection of added elastic and resistive loads were central to the recognition of the existence of these various dimensions of respiratory sensation (Campbell et al., 1961; Bennett et al., 1962). Pressure changes alone, volume changes alone, and flow changes alone were mechanisms considered in the threshold detection of added loads. Changes in all these dimensions can be sensed but are not perceived as an added load. It was argued that the relationship between the primary muscular stimuli of tension (pressure) and displacement (volume/flow) leads to the sensation of resistive and elastic loads. That pressure (tension) and volume (displacement) were sentient was implicit but not explicitly stated in Campbell's original papers. Bakers and Tenney in 1970 demonstrated that pressure, volume, and ventilation can be discriminated and scaled.

Subjects asked to rate the magnitude of added "loads" actually rated the pressure, which is dependent on both the magnitude of the load and the magnitude of displacement (volume × elastance or flow × resistance) (Killian et al., 1980). It was subsequently demonstrated that subjects have the ability to scale the magnitude of respiratory muscle tension, the magnitude of effort, the magnitude of volume or ventilation, or the magnitude of the added load (Killian et al., 1980, 1984; Stubbing et al., 1981, 1983; Altose et al., 1985). Subjects can sense a number of dimensions related to the act of breathing. Parsimony dictates the likely receptors (tendon organs for pressure sensation; muscle spindles and joint receptors for ventilation), but the full neural mechanisms remain to be elucidated.

A. Terminology

Dyspnea and *breathlessness* have been used to describe discomfort associated with the act of breathing in any setting, even the discomfort associated with not breathing, that is, breath holding! There are reasons to consider dyspnea and breathlessness as separate sensations. *Apnea* was originally used to describe the cessation of breathing, and *dyspnea* was originally used to describe difficult or labored breathing. In the nineteenth century, "apnea" and "dyspnea" were widely used by respiratory physiologists to describe the extremes of respiratory muscle activity. The association of dyspnea with the perception of excessive respiratory muscle activity was automatically inferred. On the other hand, the association of apnea with breathlessness was not commonly inferred. Hence, its restricted usage to describe the perception of an increased urge or need to breathe (one would like to breathe more to achieve satiety) is a recent phenomenon. Such a feeling is common following short-term, very high intensity activity, such as stair climbing, is sometimes reported with acute airflow limitation or pulmonary edema, and is also experienced with breath holding. Breathlessness and this sense of need to breathe may be mediated by chemoreceptors or their central connections. Dyspnea and breathlessness share the quality of discomfort. Dyspnea appears to be mediated by the muscle senses (Gandevia et al., 1981; Killian and Campbell, 1983, 1985, 1991; Killian, 1992a, b; Gandevia and Burke, 1988). Breathlessness appears to be mediated by chemoreceptors or their central connections (Guz et al., 1981; Adams et al., 1985; Freedman et al., 1987; Lane et al., 1987a, b; Chonan et al., 1987, 1990; Schwartzstein et al., 1987, 1989; Cockroft et al., 1989). The separation of respiratory sensations in this way appears to have usefulness for clinical and physiological purposes and when considering neural mechanisms. They may also occur simultaneously, both contributing to discomfort in an additive to interactive manner. Hence, discomfort with breathing is one dimension of respiratory sensation in the same way that unpleasantness is one dimension of taste.

The ability to exercise to a normal exercise capacity without intolerable discomfort with breathing defines appropriateness, and the term "dyspnea" is clinically used only when dyspnea is experienced at a reduced exercise capacity. The same intensity of discomfort is experienced by normal subjects at maximal exercise, but the *dyspnea* is not usually used in this setting. Dyspnea has been quantified for many years by the exercise capacity attained within the limits imposed by the tolerance for discomfort associated with breathing; the Medical Research Council dyspnea scale is a formal example (1986). "Inappropriateness" used in this way antedated the general concept of inappropriateness propounded by Campbell and Howell (1963).

There is a class of sensations that includes the senses of hunger and thirst. For this class of sensations, alleviation of the problem relieves the discomfort. This class of sensations is ill defined and often confused by its somatic manifestations, such as the gastric contractions of hunger pain and the dry mouth of dehydration. A sense of need to breathe may be another member of this class of sensations and is easily exemplified by the experience of breath holding. Studies performed by Fowler (1954) on breath holding had a profound influence in this area. Subjects could prolong breath holding after breathing from a gas mixture that increased rather than decreased chemoreceptor activity. Thereafter, chemoreceptor activity was considered an unimportant component of dyspnea and became even more entrenched when Campbell in two separate studies reported prolongation of breath holding during total neuromuscular blockade, even suggesting that breath holding might be prolonged indefinitely following neuromuscular blockade (Campbell et al., 1967, 1969). Breath holding was considered limited by the tolerance of the individuals for the discomfort associated with the increasingly intense inspiratory muscle contractions.

The experimental induction of chemoreceptor stimulation with rebreathing results in hypercapnia and hypoxia and is accompanied by increased neuromuscular activity and perhaps an unsatiated need to breathe. How much of the discomfort experienced is a result of neuromuscular activity, how much is caused by a direct contribution of chemoreceptor activity, and how much is related to an unsatiated need to breathe have not been definitively answered. The intensity of discomfort experienced is excessive for the contractile activity of the respiratory muscles, and the excess discomfort has been attributed to chemoreceptor activity, perhaps accompanied by an insatiable need to breathe often referred to as breathlessness (Guz et al., 1981; Adams et al., 1985; Freedman et al., 1987; Lane et al., 1987a; Lane et al., 1987b; Chonan et al., 1987, 1990; Schwartzstein et al., 1987, 1989; Cockroft et al., 1989; Banzett et al., 1990; Gandevia et al., 1993).

B. Measurement of Dyspnea

During the performance of standardized progressive exercise protocols, subjects can rate the intensity of discomfort associated with breathing (Jones, 1988; Killian et al., 1992). Quantitative semantics using such terms as "slight," "moderate," and "severe" have commonly been used to measure sensations for the purposes of everyday communication (Borg, 1964; Borg and Hosman, 1970; Borg and Lindblad, 1976). This approach has been formalized in the Borg rating scale. The descriptive terms are tagged to numbers from 0 to 10 in a manner reflecting the absolute and relative magnitude of the terms as they are commonly used (Borg, 1972, 1985). The first Borg scale (6–20) was constructed for the measurement of perceived exertion such that perceived exertion increased linearly with heart rate (perceived exertion approximately equal to 10 times the heart rate). The original scale should not be confused with the current scale, which is a general scale that can be used for any sensation. Other scales are available and are discussed elsewhere in this book.

There are normal values for the rating of dyspnea during standardized progressive exercise. These are illustrated in Fig. 1 (Killian et al., 1992). To use these standards, the patient exercises on a bicycle ergometer with progressive increases in work rate of 100 kpm/minute every minute to maximal capacity. At each work rate the subject estimates the dyspnea by matching its perceptual magnitude to the semantic terms on the Borg scale. To compare magnitude across subjects, the actual work rate in kilopond-meter/minute is transformed and expressed as a percentage of the predicted maximal power output of the particular subject and the rating is then compared to that expected. Percentile responses are superimposed to indicate the variability in rating among normal subjects.

Diseases are often defined in structural terms, but their effects are expressed through impairment in physiological function. Dyspnea rated by patients with mild FEV_1 (forced expiratory volume in one second, 60–80% of predicted), moderate (FEV_1 40–60%), and severe ($FEV_1 < 40\%$) ventilatory impairment is shown in Fig. 2. The rating of discomfort is dependent on the contribution of

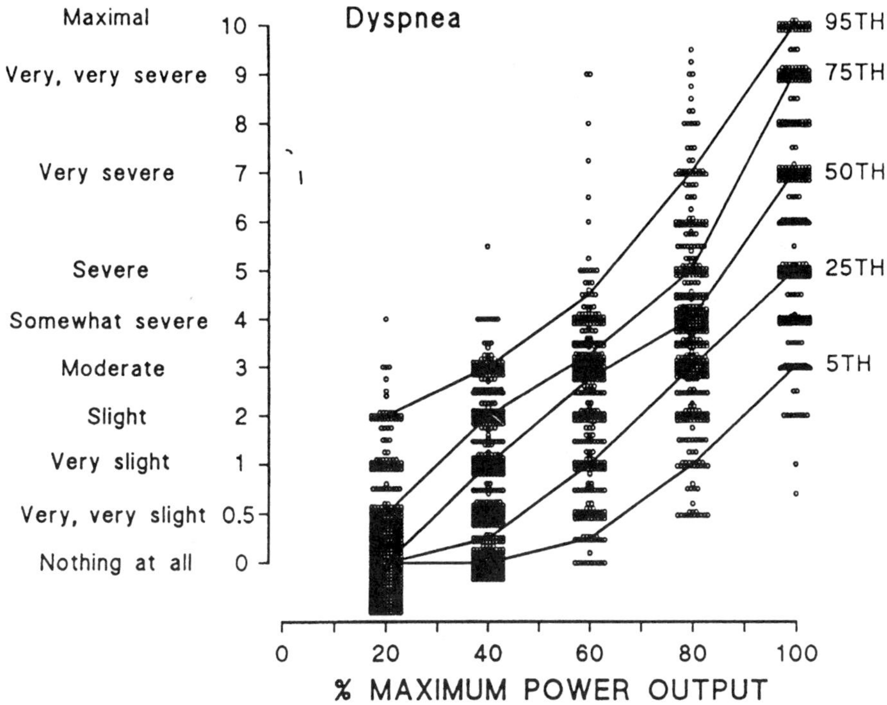

Figure 1 Individual ratings of perceived magnitude of dyspnea are plotted against power output, expressed as a percentage of maximal achieved. Percentile responses are superimposed to indicate the variability in rating in normal subjects.

independent factors, some of which can be quantified. An example is the following relationship.

$$\text{Dyspnea (Borg scale)} = 1.8 + 0.05 \times \text{power output (\% of predicted)} - 0.02\ \text{FEV}_1\ \text{(\% of predicted)} - 0.0005\ \text{MIP (\% of predicted)} = r = 0.70$$

where MIP is maximum inspiratory pressure. This approach can quantify the contribution of factors contributing to dyspnea as long as the numbers of subjects studied are large, the distribution of the factor wide, and the methods not subservient to the rating biases in individual subjects.

From a clinical perspective, dyspnea is often attributed to diseases of the heart, lungs, or neuromuscular systems, but these diseases express themselves by impairments in physiological function, which in turn express themselves in the generation of dyspnea. In disease, impairments of physiological function are often quantified indirectly. Isolation of the independent contributors to dyspnea must be

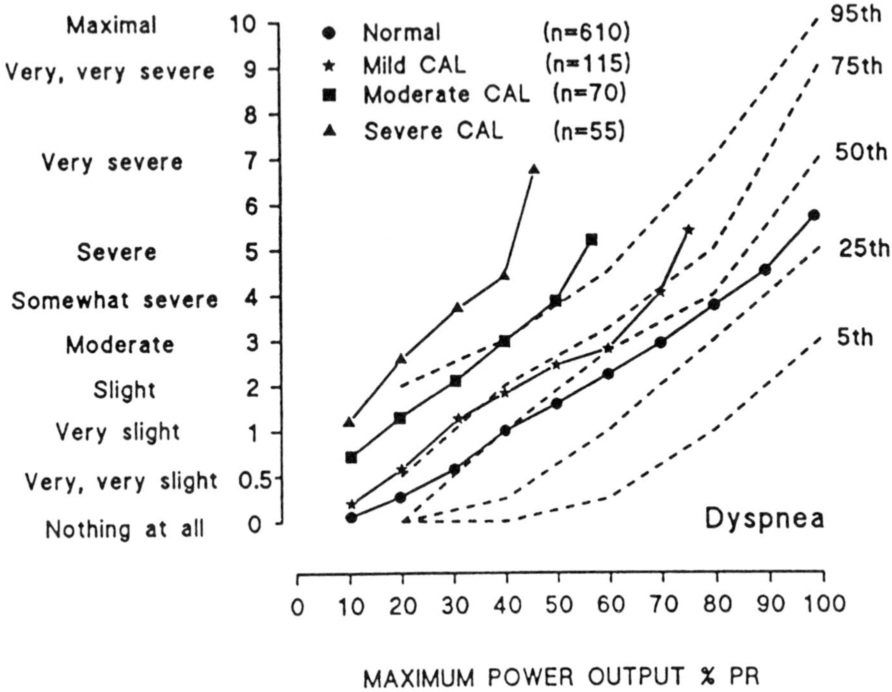

Figure 2 Dyspnea rated by normal subjects and patients with mild (FEV_1 60–80% of predicted), moderate (FEV_1 40–60% of predicted), and severe (FEV_1 < 40% of predicted) ventilatory impairment are shown superimposed on normal percentile responses; see Fig. 1.

analyzed in light of a sequence of unit processes involved in tissue respiration. The medullary respiratory centers coordinate the inputs from higher centers (behavioral factors operate in this way), chemoreceptors, chest wall, respiratory and other muscles, and the lungs. The final motor output activates respiratory muscles. Respiratory muscle activation is characterized by muscle shortening and the development of tension. Muscle shortening results in chest wall and lung expansion. Ventilation is proportional to inspiratory muscle shortening. Tension is dependent on the impedance (resistance, elastance, and inertance) of the ventilatory pump and ventilation. The ventilation required depends on metabolic demand and on the efficiency of gas exchange, and the net result is the achievement of gas exchange in proportion to metabolic demand with the maintenance of normoxemia and normocapnia. Figure 3 sequentially illustrates the interdependent physiological factors controlling ventilation. Illustrated on the left is an incomplete list of factors that modulate individual processes. The mass, strength, length, coor-

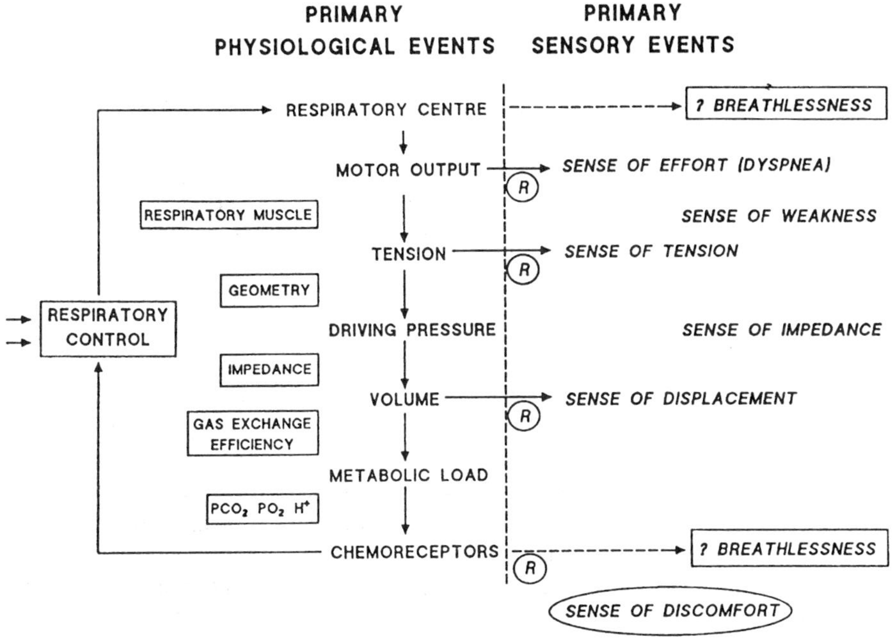

Figure 3 Interdependent interaction of physiological processes and the effects on sensory receptors (R).

dination, and endurance capacity of the respiratory muscles, the impedance of the ventilatory pump, and gas exchange efficiency are all variable across subjects in health and disease and ultimately contribute to sensation (see the right side of Fig. 3). These factors are interdependent, but they are also somewhat independent. Each is an independent contributor to sensory receptor stimulation and to the central motor output required to sustain the metabolic demands of the body, but a change in one is usually associated with changes in the others.

C. Is There a Central Unifying Factor to Dyspnea?

Clinically dyspnea is usually related to the presence and severity of diseases of the heart, lung, and neuromuscular systems. Concepts of respiratory, cardiac, and neuromuscular dyspnea have been useful, but the application of these principles to the problems encountered by the dyspneic patient has shortcomings. The introduction of sensory physiology to the problems encountered by the dyspneic patient provides a framework for the patient's management. It remains our contention that effort is of central importance, but the roles played by other sensory mechanisms are not dismissed.

The motor commands associated with the sense of effort cannot be measured in the same way that neural signals from human muscle afferents can be measured. Premovement potentials on the scalp overlying the motor cortex can be measured during voluntary breathing efforts but are absent during quiet breathing (Macefield and Gandevia, 1992). However, such an approach is unlikely to be very useful in the clinical setting to define the motor command associated with dyspnea. Crude assessments of motor command or effort are commonly derived from the relative level of motor activity. For example, electromyographic signals and levels of force or pressure can be expressed as a fraction of maximal voluntary levels of these parameters.

Physiologically, dyspnea and breathlessness are usually considered in relation to the hydrogen ion and gas status of the arterial blood and to the mechanics of breathing. However, the quality and quantity of the sensory information associated with dyspnea vary across subjects and disease states, as do the subjective and physiological responses. The sense of effort is common to almost all the clinical circumstances in which dyspnea occurs. Effort and dyspnea both increase as ventilation increases, as the load opposing the muscles increases, and as the respiratory muscles are weakened, whereas when ventilation or the load opposing the respiratory muscles is reduced or the respiratory muscles strengthened, dyspnea is relieved. Indeed, the persistence of dyspnea in a ventilated patient usually indicates a high intensity of respiratory muscle activity or inadequate ventilation. In reality, all the usual therapeutic measures to relieve dyspnea directly or indirectly reduce respiratory muscle effort. For example, bronchodilators reduce the dyspnea caused by acute bronchoconstriction in asthma. To conclude, dyspnea occurs frequently when respiratory motor commands are high, and thus inspiratory effort is likely to be an important determinant.

References

Adams, L., Lane, R., Shea, S.A., Cockcroft, A., and Guz, A. (1985). Breathlessness during different forms of ventilatory stimulation: a study of mechanisms in normal subjects and respiratory patients. Clin. Sci. 69:663–672.

Adrian, E.D. (1928). The Basis of Sensation. Christophers, London.

Altose, M.D., Leitner, J., and Cherniack, N.S. (1985). Effects of age and respiratory efforts on the perception of resistive ventilatory loads. J. Gerontol. 40:147–153.

Aristotle (1912). De partibus animalium. In: The Works of Aristotle, Vol. 5, Edited by J.A. Smith and W.D. Ross. Clarendon, Oxford.

Aristotle (1936). De anima (On the soul). In: Aristotle, Vol. 8/23, Loeb Classical Library. Heinemann, London.

Bakers, J.H.C.M., and Tenney, S.M. (1970). Perception of some sensations associated with breathing. Respir. Physiol. 10:85–92.

Banzett, R.B., Lansing, R.W., Brown, R., Topoulos, G.P., Yager, D., Steele, S.M., Londono, B., Loring, S.H., Reed, M.B., Adams, L., and Nations, C.S. (1990). "Air hunger" arising from increased P_{CO_2} persists after complete neuromuscular block in humans. Respir. Physiol. 81:1–18.

Bastian, C. (1880). The Brain as an Organ of the Mind, C. Keegan Paul & Co., London, pp. 540–544.

Bell, C. (1833). The hand: its mechanism and vital endowments as envincing design. Bridgewater Treatise on the Power, Wisdom and Goodness of God as Manifested in the Creation. In: Of the Muscular Sense. W. Pickering, London, pp. 191–207.

Bell, C. (1869). Idea of a new anatomy of the brain: submitted for the observations of his friends (1811). Reprinted in 1869, J. Anat. Physiol. 3:153–166.

Bennett, E.D., Jayson, M.I.V., Rubenstein, D., and Campbell, E.J.M. (1962). The ability of man to detect added non-elastic loads to breathing. Clin. Sci. 23:155–162.

Boeke, J. (1927). Die morphologische Grundlage der sympathischen Innervation der quergestreiften Muskelfasern. Z. Mikrosk. Anat. Forsch. 8:561–639.

Borg, G. (1964). On quantitative semantics in connection with psychophysics. Educational and Psychological Research Bulletin, University of Umea, 3.

Borg, G. (1972). A ratio scaling method for interindividual comparisons. Reports from the Institute of Applied Psychology, University of Stockholm, 27:1–12.

Borg, G. (1985). Psychophysical studies of effort and exertion: some historical, theoretical and empirical aspects. In: The Perception of Physical Exertion in Physical Work. Proceedings of an International Symposium Held at the Wenner-Gren Centre, Stockholm, Macmillan, London, pp. 3–12.

Borg, G., and Hosman, J. (1970). The metric properties of adverbs. Institute of Applied Psychology Report, University of Stockholm, 7.

Borg, G., and Lindblad, I. (1976). The determination of subjective intensities in verbal descriptions of symptoms. Institute of Applied Psychology Report, University of Stockholm, 75.

Boring, E.G. (1942). Sensation and Perception in the History of Experimental Psychology, Century Psychology Series. Appleton-Century-Crofts, New York.

Cafarelli, D. (1988). Force sensation in fresh and fatigued human skeletal muscle. Exerc. Sport Sci. Rev. 16:139–168.

Campbell, E.J.M., and Howell, J.B.L. (1963). The sensation of breathlessness. Br. Med. Bull. 19:36–40.

Campbell, E.J.M., Freedman, S., Smith, P.S., and Taylor, M.E. (1961). The ability of man to detect added elastic loads to breathing. Clin. Sci. 20:223–231.

Campbell, E.J.M., Freedman, S., Clark, T.J.H., Robson, J.G., and Jones, N.L. (1967). The effect of muscular paralysis induced by tubocurarine on the duration and sensation of breath-holding. Clin. Sci. 32:425–432.

Campbell, E.J.M., Godfrey, S., Clark, T.J.H., Freedman, S., and Jones, N.L. (1969). The effect of muscular paralysis induced by tubocurarine on the duration and sensation of breath-holding. Clin. Sci. 36:323–328.

Cattaneo, A. (1888). Organes Nerveux Terminaux Musculo-Tendineux Leurs Condition Normales et Leur Maniere de se Comporter Apres la Section des Racines Nerveuses et des Nerf Spinaux. Arch. Ital. Biol. 10:337–357.

Chonan, T., Mulholland, M.B., Cherniack, N.S., and Altose, M.D. (1987). Effects of

voluntary constraining of thoracic displacement during hypercapnia. J. Appl. Physiol. 63:1822–1828.
Chonan, T., Mulholland, M.B., Leitner, J., Altose, M.D., and Cherniack, N.S. (1990). Sensation of dyspnea during hypercapnia, exercise, and voluntary hyperventilation. J. Appl. Physiol. 68:2100–2106.
Cockroft, A., Adams, L., and Guz, A. (1989). Assessment of breathlessness. Q. J. Med. 72:669–676.
Cross, M.J., and McCloskey, D.I. (1973). Position sense following surgical removal of joints. Brain Res. 55:443–445.
Ferrell, W.R., and Smith, A. (1989). The effect of loading on position sense at the proximal interphalangeal joint of the human index finger. J. Physiol. (Lond.) 418:145–161.
Ferrell, W.R., Gandevia, S.C., and McCloskey, D.I. (1987). The role of joint receptors in human kinaesthesia when intramuscular receptors cannot contribute. J. Physiol. (Lond.) 386:63–71.
Flourens, M.J.P. (1842). Recherches experimentales sur les proprietes et les fonctions du systeme nerveux dans les animaux vertebres.
Fowler, W.S. (1954). Breaking point of breath-holding. J. Appl. Physiol. 6:539–545.
Freedman, S., Lane, R., and Guz, A. (1987). Breathlessness and respiratory mechanics during reflex or voluntary hyperventilation in patients with chronic airflow limitation. Clin. Sci. 73:311–318.
Gandevia, S.C. (1982). The perception of motor commands or effort during muscular paralysis. Brain 105:151–195.
Gandevia, S.C. (1987). Roles for perceived voluntary motor commands in motor controls. Trends Neurosci. 10:81–85.
Gandevia, S.C., and McCloskey, D.I. (1976). Joint sense, muscle sense, and their combination as position sense, measured at the distal interphalangeal joint of the middle finger. J. Appl. Physiol. 260:387–407.
Gandevia, S.C., and McCloskey, D.I. (1977a). Sensation of heaviness. Brain 100:345–354.
Gandevia, S.C., and McCloskey, D.I. (1977b). Changes in motor commands, as shown by changes in perceived heaviness, during partial curarization and peripheral muscle anaesthesia in man. J. Physiol. (Lond.) 272:673–689.
Gandevia, S.C., and McCloskey, D.I. (1978). Interpretation of perceived motor commands by reference to afferent signals. J. Physiol. (Lond.) 283:493–499.
Gandevia, S.C., Killian, K.J., and Campbell, E.J.M. (1981). The effect of respiratory muscle fatigue on respiratory sensations. Clin. Sci. 60:463–466.
Gandevia, S.C., and Burke, D. (1988). Projection to the cerebral cortex from proximal and distal muscles in the human upper limb. Brain 111:389–403.
Gandevia, S.C., McCloskey, D.I., and Burke, D. (1992). Kinaesthetic signals and muscle contraction. Trends Neurosci. 15:62–65.
Gandevia, S.C., Killian, K.J., McKenzie, D.K., Crawford, M., Allen, G.M., Gorman, R.B., Hales, J.P. (1993). Respiratory sensations, cardiovascular control, kinaesthesia and transcranial stimulation during paralysis in humans. J. Physiol. (Lond.) 470:85–107.
Goldscheider, A. (1898). 1. Uber den Muskelsinn und die Theorie der Ataxie. 2. Untersuchungen uber den Muskelsinn. In: Gesammelte Abhandlungen von A. Goldscheider, Vol. II. Barth, Leipzig, pp. 9–281.

Golgi, C. (1880). Sui Nervi dei Tendini dell'Uomo e di Altri Vertebrati e di un Nuovo Organo Nervoso Terminale Musculo-Tendineo, 1880. Reprinted in 1903, Vol. 1, Opera Omnia, Milan. In: Opera Omnia, Vol. 1. Ulrico Hoepli, Milan, pp. 171–198.
Goodwin, G.M., McCloskey, D.I., and Matthews, P.B.C. (1972). The contribution of muscle afferents to kinaesthesia shown by vibration induced illusions of movement and by the effects of paralysing joint afferents. Brain 95:705–748.
Guz, A., Adams, L., Minty, K., and Murphy, K. (1981). Breathlessness and ventilatory drives of exercise, hypercapnoea and hypoxia (abstract). Clin. Sci. 61:429–439.
Helmholtz, H. (1867). Handbuch der physiologischen optik. Voss, Leipzig.
Hines, M., and Tower, S.S. (1928). Studies on the innervation of skeletal muscles. II. Of muscle spindles in certain muscles of the kitten. Bull. Johns Hopkins Hosp. 42:264–307.
Hinsey, J.C. (1927). Some observations on the innervation of skeletal muscle of the cat. J. Comp. Neurol. 44:87–195.
Honig, C.R. (1979). Contributions of nerves and metabolites to exercise vasodilation: a unifying hypothesis. Am. J. Physiol. 236:H705–H719.
Houk, J., and Henneman, E. (1967). Responses of Golgi tendon organs to active contractions of the soleus muscle of the cat. J. Neurophysiol. 30:466–481.
Huber, G.C., and Dewitt, L.M.A. (1900). A contribution on the motor nerve-ending and on the nerve-endings in the muscle spindles. J. Comp. Neurol. 7:169–230.
Jami, L. (1992). Golgi tendon organs in mammalian skeletal muscle: functional properties and central actions. Physiol. Rev. 72:623–666.
Jones, L.A., and Hunter, I.W. (1983). Effect of fatigue on force sensation. Exp. Neurol. 81:640–650.
Jones, N.L. (1988). Clinical Exercise Testing. W.B. Saunders, Philadelphia.
Killian, K.J. (1992a). The nature of breathlessness and its measurement. In: Breathlessness 1991. Proceedings of the Campbell Symposium held in Hamilton, Ontario, May 1991. Edited by N.L. Jones and K.J. Killian. Decker Medical Publications, Hamilton, pp. 74–87.
Killian, K.J. (1992b). Symptoms Limiting Exercise. In: Breathlessness 1991. Proceedings of the Campbell Symposium held in Hamilton, Ontario, May 1991, Edited by N.L. Jones and K.J. Killian, Decker Medical Publications, Hamilton, pp. 132–142.
Killian, K.J., and Campbell, E.J.M. (1983). Dyspnea and exercise. Annu. Rev. Physiol., Vol. 45, 465–479.
Killian, K.J., and Campbell, E.J.M. (1985). Dyspnea. In: The Thorax, Part B. Edited by C. Roussos and P.T. Macklem. Marcel Dekker, New York, pp. 787–828.
Killian, K.J., and Campbell, E.J.M. (1991). Dyspnea. In: The Lung: Scientific Foundations, Edited by R.G. Crystal and J.B. West. Raven Press, New York, pp. 1433–1443.
Killian, K.J., Mahutte, C.K., Howell, J.B.L., and Campbell, E.J.M. (1980). Effect of timing, flow, lung volume and threshold pressures on resistive load detection. J. Appl. Physiol. 49:958–963.
Killian, K.J., Gandevia, S.C., Summers, E., and Campbell, E.J.M. (1984). Effect of increased lung volume on perception of breathlessness, effort, and tension. J. Appl. Physiol. 57:686–691.
Killian, K.J., Summers, E., Jones, N.L., and Campbell, E.J.M. (1992). Dyspnea and leg effort during incremental cycle ergometry. Am. Rev. Respir. Dis. 145:1339–1345.

Kolliker, G. (1862). Untersuchungen uber die letzten Endigungen der Nerven. Z. Wissensch. Zool. 12:149–164.

Krause, W. (1874). Histologische Notizen. Zentralbl. Med. Wissensch. 12:211–212.

Kuhne, W. (1863). Uber die Endigung der Nerven in the Muskeln. Virchows Arch. [A] 27:508–523.

Lane, R., Cockcroft, A., Adams, L., and Guz, A. (1987a). Arterial oxygen saturation and breathlessness in patients with chronic obstructive airways disease. Clin. Sci. 72:693–698.

Lane, R., Cockcroft, A., and Guz, A. (1987b). Voluntary isocapnic ventilation and breathlessness during exercise in normal subjects. Clin. Sci. 73:519–523.

Leyton, A.S.F., and Sherrington, C.S. (1917). Observations on the excitable cortex of the chimpanzee, oranj-utan and gorilla. Q. J. Exp. Physiol. 11:135–222.

Macefield, G., and Gandevia, S.C. (1992). Peripheral and central delays in the cortical projections from human truncal muscles. Brain 115:123–135.

Magendie, F. (1822). Experiences sur les fonctions des racines des nerfs rachidiens. J. Physiol. Exp. Pathol. 2:276–371.

Matthews, P.B.C. (1972). Mammalian Muscle Receptors and Their Central Actions. Edward Arnold, London.

Matthews, P.B.C. (1977). Muscle afferents and kinesthesia. Br. Med. Bull. 33:137–142.

Matthews, P.B.C. (1981a). Evolving views on the internal operation and functional role of the muscle spindle. J. Physiol. (Lond.) 320:1–30.

Matthews, P.B.C. (1981b). Muscle spindles: their messages and their fusimotor supply. In: Handbook of Physiology. The Nervous System, Vol. II. Motor Control. Edited by V.B. Brooks. American Physiological Society, Bethesda, MD. pp 189–228.

Matthews, P.B.C. (1988). Proprioceptors and their contribution to somatosensory mapping: complex messages require complex processing. Can. J. Physiol. Pharmacol. 66:430–438.

McCloskey, D.I. (1973). Differences between the senses of movement and position shown by the effects of loading and vibration of muscles in man. Brain Res. 61:119–131.

McCloskey, D.I. (1978). Kinesthetic sensibility. Physiol. Rev. 58:763–820.

McCloskey, D.I. (1981). Corollary discharges and motor commands. In: Handbook of Physiology. The Nervous System, Vol. II. Motor Control. Edited by V.B. Brooks. American Physiological Society, Bethesda, MD. pp 1415–1447.

McCloskey, D.I., Ebeling, P., and Goodwin, G.M. (1974). Estimation of weights and tensions and apparent involvement of a "sense of effort." Exp. Neurol. 42:220–232.

McIntyre, A.K., Proske, U., and Rawson, J.A. (1984). Cortical projection of afferent information from tendon organs in the cat. J. Physiol. (Lond.) 354:395–406.

Medical Research Council. (1986). MRC Respiratory Symptoms Questionnaire. London.

Mott, F.W., and Sherrington, C.S. (1895). Experiments upon the influence of sensory nerves upon movement and nutrition of the limbs. Proc. R. Soc. Lond. 57:481–488.

Muller, J. (1838). Zur vergleichenden Physiologie des Gesichtssinnes. In: Handbuch der Physiologie des Menschen II, Bk. 5, pp. 44–55.

Penfield, W.G., and Boldrey, E. (1937). Somatic motor and sensory representation in the cerebral cortex of man as studied by electrical stimulation. Brain 60:389.

Phillips, C.G., and Porter, R. (1977). Corticospinal Neurones. Their Role in Movement. Academic Press, London.

Phillips, C.G., Powell, T.P.S.W., and Wiesendanger, M. (1971). Projection from low threshold muscle afferents of hand and forearm to are 3a of baboon's cortex. J. Physiol. (Lond.) 271:419–446.

Quin, C.E. (1992). The centre thought to control sensory and motor activity in the early history of medicine. J. R. Soc. Med. 85:102–105.

Rauber, A. (1874). Uber die Vater'schen Korper der Gelenkakpsein. Zentralbl. Med. Wissensch. 12:305–306.

Roland, P.E. (1978). Sensory feedback to the cerebral cortex during voluntary movement in man. Behav. Brain Sci. 1:129–171.

Roland, P.E., and Ladegaard-Pederson, H. (1977). A quantitative analysis of sensation of tension and kinaesthesia in man. Evidence for peripherally originating muscular sense and for a sense of effort. Brain 100:671–692.

Scheerer, E. (1987). Muscle sense and innervation feelings: a chapter in the history of perception and action. In: Perspectives on Perception and Action. Edited by H. Heuer and A.F. Sanders. Lawrence Erlbaum Associates, Hillsdale, NJ, pp. 171–194.

Schmidt, R.F. (1981). Fundamentals of Sensory Physiology. Springer Verlag, New York.

Schwartzstein, R.M., LaHive, K., Pope A., Steinbrook, R.A., Leith, D.E., Weiss, J.W., Fencl, V., and Weinberger, S.E. (1987). Detection of hypercapnia by normal subjects. Clin. Sci. 73:333–335.

Schwartzstein, R.M., Simon, P.M., Weiss, J.W., Fencl, V., and Weinberger, S.E. (1989). Breathlessness induced by dissociation between ventilation and chemical drive. Am. Rev. Respir. Dis. 139:1231–1237.

Sherrington, C.S. (1894). On the anatomical constitution of nerves of skeletal muscle; with remarks on recurrent fibres in the ventral spinal nerve root. J. Physiol. (Lond.) 17: 211–258.

Sherrington, C.S. (1900). The muscular sense. In: Textbook of Physiology, Vol. 2. Edited by E.A. Shafer. T.J. Pentland, Edinburgh, pp. 1002–1025.

Sherrington, C.S. (1924a). Problems of muscular receptivity. Nature (Lond.) 113:892–894.

Sherrington, C.S. (1924b). Problems of muscular receptivity. Nature (Lond.) 113:929–932.

Stubbing, D.G., Killian, K.J., and Campbell, E.J.M. (1981). The quantification of respiratory sensations by normal subjects. Respir. Physiol. 44:251–260.

Stubbing, D.G., Ramsdale, E.H., Killian, K.J., and Campbell, E.J.M. (1983). Psychophysics of inspiratory muscle force. J. Appl. Physiol. 54:1216–1221.

Weber, E.H. (1860). Weber Fraction. De pulsu, resorptione, auditu et tactu. Annotationes anatomicae et physiologicae. Koehler, Leipzig.

Woodcock, A.A., Gross, E.R., Gelert, A., Shah, S., Johnson, M., and Geddes, D.M. (1981). Effects of dihydrocodeine, alcohol and caffeine on breathlessness and exercise tolerance in patients with chronic obstructive lung disease and normal blood gases. N. Engl. J. Med. 305:1611–1616.

8

Reflex Respiratory Stimulation and Respiratory Sensation

LEWIS ADAMS

Charing Cross and Westminster Medical School
University of London
London, England

I. Introduction

In considering the neurophysiological basis of respiratory sensations in conscious humans, a useful and conventional starting point is the respiratory control system itself. In the very simplest terms, neural networks within the brainstem generate an intrinsic respiratory rhythm with innervation of respiratory muscles via bulbospinal tracts. It is presumably these pathways that primarily subserve breathing during sleep and anesthesia. When conscious, it is generally assumed that the regular respiratory pattern that characterizes "unattended" breathing also has its basis in the automatic pathways, but that this activity can be modulated by activity from higher CNS structures. Such influences on breathing can range from subtle [e.g., opening the eyes causes modest increases in ventilation (Shea et al., 1987)] to profound (e.g., breath holding or maximum voluntary ventilation) and may be related to behavioral demands (e.g., defecation or speech), changes in emotional state (e.g., laughter or anxiety), or overt voluntary breathing acts. There are almost certainly corticospinal connections to respiratory muscles that are directly involved in volitional respiratory acts (Gandevia and Rothwell, 1987; Murphy et al., 1990), but the extent to which activation of such pathways influences respiratory-related neurons in the brainstem is unclear (Orem and Trotter, 1994). Moreover, the nature of the neurophysiological basis of changes in breathing associated with behavioral or emotional factors is not known.

Alongside the neural structures that give rise to efferent activity to respiratory muscles, there are receptors that provide afferent information with well-defined effects on the control of breathing. Peripheral and central chemoreceptors respond to perturbations in acid-base/blood gas status, pulmonary receptors provide feedback on mechanical and chemical changes within the airways and lung, and receptors within the respiratory muscles and rib cage monitor forces and displacements within the ventilatory "plant." In addition, there are other receptors in the upper airways, cardiovascular system, and musculoskeletal system that are likely to provide afferent input which can directly influence breathing.

In trying to elucidate the neural basis of respiratory sensations, it seems logical to take the view that they have their origin in structures within the respiratory apparatus (since that is where these sensations are felt). Thus, both chest wall and pulmonary receptors have been extensively studied with respect to their role in the genesis of respiratory sensations (for reviews, see Adams and Guz, 1991; Shea et al., 1994; Stulbarg and Adams, 1994; and Zechman and Wiley, 1986). There is good evidence that such receptors are important in the perception of lung volume, respiratory pressures and sensations of irritation or tightness in the airways and lungs (for a recent review, see Shea et al., 1994). These issues have been extensively dealt with in Chapters 4 and 6 of this volume. In addition, there is now sound experimental support for the view that the sensation of respiratory effort (associated with the perception of respiratory mechanical loads) derives primarily from the perception of the outgoing motor command to respiratory muscles (for reviews, see Gandevia, 1988; Adams and Guz, 1991; Shea et al., 1994). Based on the design of studies to test this hypothesis and by analogy with our understanding of perception of effort in other skeletal muscles, it seems likely that in this respect the efferent activity in question is that arising from motor cortical rather than brainstem structures, although this issue has not been directly addressed. This topic has been reviewed in Chapter 7.

Despite the obvious importance of lung/chest wall receptors in respiratory sensation, it has proved difficult to account for the important respiratory sensation of dyspnea (breathlessness) in terms of afferent activity from such receptors. Although a substantial amount of work has supported such a view, there is equally compelling evidence that their involvement in the genesis of dyspnea is dubious (for reviews, see Adams and Guz 1991; Shea et al., 1994). Much of this apparent conflict may be accounted for by differences in the way that various investigators have defined the term *dyspnea*. This matter is addressed comprehensively in Chapter 5.

In recent years, a view has arisen that the sensation of breathlessness may have its origin in respiratory-related neurons within the brainstem and that what is perceived by higher sensory areas as breathlessness depends on a corollary discharge of such neural activity (for review, see Adams and Guz, 1991). Moreover, there is accumulating evidence that rather than contributing to the breathless sensation, afferent information from respiratory mechanoreceptors may act to provide displacement-related relief of the sensation resulting from reflex activation of the brainstem respiratory areas (for review, see Shea et al., 1994). Recent studies in an animal model have provided intriguing neurophysiological evidence supporting such a view; this is reviewed in Chapter 2. A number of other chapters in this volume (notably Chapters 5, 6, 9, and 16) also address these issues with respect to experimental and clinical observations in human subjects. The main aim of the present chapter is to review in detail some of the evidence from studies in humans that reflex stimulation of breathing is associated with the genesis of the sensation of breathlessness. In reporting these studies, no distinction is made between the terms breathlessness and dyspnea; in addition, the sensation being investigated has generally been defined in terms of "an uncomfortable need to breathe," "an urge to breathe," or "air hunger." There is no assumption that the sensations assessed in these studies (often in healthy subjects undergoing reflex ventilatory stimulation) are analogous to those reported by patients who are breathless as a result of various pathophysiological states and in whom differences in psychological, emotional, and cognitive factors may result in very different perceptual experiences that are both unpleasant and characterized as breathlessness. These issues have been dealt with primarily in Chapters 3, 5, 6, 10, 11, 13, 15, and 16.

II. Ventilatory Stimulation, Ventilation, and Breathlessness

In spontaneously breathing healthy subjects, increases in ventilation resulting from increasingly more intense exercise, hypercapnia, or hypoxia are associated with a progressive rise in the intensity of the subjective sensation of breathlessness reported using a Visual Analogue Scale or Borg Scale (Adams et al., 1985a; Stark et al., 1981; Wilson and Jones, 1989). Similarly, if a hypercapnic or hypoxic stimulus is oscillated slowly (cycle time = 2 min), then breathlessness scores mirror the rises and falls in ventilation (Adams et al., 1985b). In addition, during steady-state exercise, both ventilation and breathlessness remain relatively constant, although there may be a small time-dependent increase in the latter (O'Neill et al., 1986). The recovery in breathlessness following exercise again matches that of ventilation (Stark et al., 1981). Patients with respiratory disease show qualitatively similar patterns of increase in breathlessness during ventilatory stimulation with exercise and hypercapnia although, not surprisingly, much greater levels of breathlessness are reported at much lower levels of ventilation compared with healthy subjects (Stark et al., 1982; Winning et al., 1988).

The studies just outlined do not allow us to know to what extent the perception of breathlessness depends upon the degree of reflex ventilatory stimulation or the accompanying mechanical ventilatory response, since these factors are highly correlated. On the other hand, common experience tells us that volitionally induced increases in ventilation at rest are not accompanied by the same sensations of breathlessness that are experienced during exercise, hypercapnia, or hypoxia. This has been demonstrated in normal subjects under experimental conditions. Thus, hypercapnic ventilatory stimulation induced a substantial increase in breathlessness, whereas the same level of ventilation produced voluntarily by the same subjects (with end-tidal P_{CO_2} held at a normocapnic level) was associated with minimal breathlessness (Adams et al., 1985b). In this study, the potential confounding effect on breathlessness of attention to a motor task was controlled for by having subjects undertake a manual tracking task during hypercapnia; the reported levels of breathlessness were the same whether or not subjects were distracted by needing to attend to a motor act. However, this observation has not been confirmed by another group who reported equivalent increases in breathlessness for the same levels of ventilation resulting from either exercise or voluntary hyperventilation (Chonan et al., 1990). Differences in the definition of breathlessness in these two studies may account for the different findings. Support for the idea that breathlessness in normal subjects is crucially dependent on automatic rather voluntary ventilatory stimulation comes from an elegant study by Lane et al. (1987b). These authors induced breathlessness with exercise and then, in two separate tests, asked subjects to target their breathing to a higher level. In the first condition, normocapnia was maintained by increasing inspired CO_2 concentration, and in the second condition, exercise workload was increased to a level that was metabolically appropriate for the higher ventilation. Subjects consistently reported less breathlessness for the same level of ventilation when a portion of the ventilation was produced voluntarily.

A study in patients with respiratory disease (mean FEV_1 = 35% predicted) gave results similar to those reported by Lane et al. (1987b) for healthy subjects. Mean levels of breathlessness of 52% (on a visual analogue scale) during hypercapnia fell to 5% when the same level of ventilation was achieved voluntarily. In this study, levels of breathlessness increased markedly when hypercapnia was surreptitiously induced while patients were performing a volitional breathing task in the absence of any differences in ventilation (Adams et al., 1985b). The question of whether differences in reported breathlessness between reflexly stimulated and voluntary breathing could be explained in terms of mechanical factors was addressed by Freedman et al. (1987) in chronic obstructive pulmonary disease (COPD) patients; no important differences in respiratory mechanics could be demonstrated between the two forms of ventilatory stimulation, although the marked differences in reported breathlessness were confirmed.

Direct evidence in humans supporting the thesis that the sensation of breathlessness derives primarily from reflex respiratory stimulation comes from recent experiments in conscious normal humans undergoing complete neuromuscular blockade. During fixed mechanical ventilation, small amounts of CO_2 added to the ventilator induced an urge to breathe in the presumed presence of increased activation of respiratory-related neurons in the brainstem but without any change in proprioceptive feedback from the lungs, respiratory muscle, or rib cage receptors (Banzett et al., 1990; Gandevia et al., 1993). These finding are consistent with those made in patients with C1–C3 spinal cord lesions (Banzett et al., 1989) and respiratory muscle paralysis (Opie et al., 1959), in whom hypercapnia induces sensations of breathlessness in the absence of any ventilatory response.

III. Reflex Ventilatory Stimuli and Breathlessness

A. Exercise

In most people (whether healthy or not), the sensation of breathlessness is an experience that is most commonly associated with exercise. In itself this is interesting because if this sensation does depend on activation of respiratory-related areas in the brainstem (see previous discussion), then this indicates that such areas are involved in control of breathing during exercise. In view of our continuing uncertainty about the mechanisms of respiratory control during exercise, it seems worthwhile to make this observation as it suggests that the neural basis of isocapnic exercise hyperpnea is at least different from that for isocapnic voluntary hyperventilation, although in both cases (unless exercise is severe) acid-base/blood gas status remains essentially unchanged. It is possible that both ventilatory and breathlessness responses to exercise occur secondarily to activation of locomotor areas in the brain (Eldridge and Waldrop, 1991), although the temporary persistence of both hyperpnea and breathlessness following the cessation of exercise (Stark et al., 1981) (proportional to the off-transient gas exchange dynamics) does not intuitively support this view. With respect to this question, it is of interest to examine the ventilatory and sensory responses to exercise in individuals who have abnormalities in automatic respiratory control as assessed by failure to maintain breathing during sleep and by reduced or absent ventilatory chemosensitivity. Recent studies in a group of young people with congenital chronic hypoventilation syndrome (Ondine's curse) have identified both ventilatory (Paton et al., 1993; Shea et al., 1993a) and breathlessness (Shea et al. 1993b) responses to exercise even though these individuals were able to hold their breath for extended periods without experiencing any respiratory discomfort. On the other hand, an earlier study in such children reported marked hypoventilation during exercise in the absence of any appreciable respiratory discomfort (Hyland et al., 1978). More studies are needed in individuals with dysfunction of automatic respiratory control mechanisms to provide further insight into their role in the genesis of breathlessness.

B. Hypercapnia

When normal subjects are exposed to a hypercapnic ventilatory stimulus at rest, they report greater intensities of breathlessness for a given degree of ventilatory stimulation compared with exercise (Stark et al., 1981; Adams et al., 1985a). One obvious explanation for this observation would be that stimulation of CO_2 chemoreceptors per se is perceived as breathlessness over and above that associated with the degree of ventilatory stimulation. However, another possibility is that the higher ratings during hypercapnia could be a reflection of the fewer sensory distractions and greater unfamiliarity associated with this type of ventilatory stimulation. In an attempt to address this question, Ward and Whipp (1989) and Lane et al. (1990) performed studies in which similar levels of steady-state ventilation were achieved either with exercise alone or with a lower level of exercise combined with hypercapnia. Both studies found that there was no difference in the perceived intensity of breathlessness in the two experimental conditions. These observations do not support a role for hypercapnia per se in the genesis of the breathless sensation and again are consistent with the idea that the degree of reflex activation of ventilation, whether by exercise or CO_2, is important in determining the intensity of breathlessness.

Using another approach to assess whether peripheral CO_2 chemoreceptor activity per se might give rise to the perception of breathlessness, Adams et al. (1985b) induced oscillating hypercapnic ventilatory stimulation in normal subjects at constant amplitude but at two different frequencies. For equivalent increases in end-tidal P_{CO_2}, less breathlessness was reported when the peripheral stimulus was oscillated more quickly. Under these experimental conditions, the intensity of breathlessness was found to correlate with the prevailing level of ventilation. While these results do not indicate that afferent activity resulting from peripheral chemoreception of CO_2 is directly perceived as a sensation of breathlessness, they do not allow any discrimination between central chemoreceptor excitation and the resultant increased activity of the respiratory complex as possible sources of neural information that can give rise to the sensation of breathlessness.

C. Hypoxia

As with hypercapnia, progressive hypoxia in normal subjects is associated with a greater degree of breathlessness than exercise at equivalent levels of ventilation

(Adams et al., 1985b). As in the case of hypercapnia, Lane et al. (1990) demonstrated that when ventilation was stimulated to a steady state with a combination of exercise and hypoxia (with normocapnia maintained), the level of breathlessness induced was the same as that reported at the same ventilation resulting from exercise alone. Again this finding is consistent with the view that hypoxia does not have a specific role in the genesis of breathlessness. However, in contrast to those findings, Ward and Whipp (1989) clearly demonstrated that unlike hypercapnia, hypoxia during exercise did produce higher ratings of breathlessness than exercise alone for the same amount of ventilatory stimulation, suggesting that hypoxia may have a "dyspnogenic" effect over and above its reflex stimulation of ventilation.

Studies in the non–steady state have also shown that during heavy exercise at constant workload, "step" increases and decreases in hypoxia result in abrupt increases and decreases in breathlessness well before the full ventilatory response to a change in arterial oxygen saturation has time to develop (Chronos et al., 1988), supporting a role for hypoxic chemostimulation per se in the genesis of breathlessness. On the other hand, at rest, rapid oscillation of a hypoxic stimulus induced a lower level of ventilation and less breathlessness than when similar amplitude fluctuations in arterial oxygen saturation were induced more slowly (Adams et al., 1985b); this observation argues against a direct influence of peripheral hypoxic chemostimulation on the perception of the breathless sensation.

It is difficult to reconcile some of the apparently conflicting findings relating to the question of whether hypoxia gives rise to the sensation of breathlessness "in excess" of its role as a ventilatory stimulus. Observations made during oxygen administration in hypoxic patients fail to clarify the issue. In patients with obstructive respiratory disease, Swinburn et al. (1984) prevented the usual fall in arterial oxygen saturation by administration of oxygen during exercise and found that the improvement in breathlessness at any workload could be accounted for in terms of oxygen-induced fall in ventilation. On the other hand, Lane et al. (1987a), in a similar group of patients, identified a component of the improvement in breathlessness with oxygen that could not be explained by the lower ventilation; a similar finding has been made in patients with restrictive lung disease (Swinburn et al., 1989).

D. Acidosis

In assessing the onset of breathlessness during progressive exercise in normal subjects, Chronos et al. (1988) noted an apparent association between this and the onset of lactic acidosis. Moreover, for a given degree of exercise-induced ventilation, the intensity of respiratory discomfort seems to be inversely correlated with physical fitness (Adams et al., 1986), which may reflect individual differences in the level of exercise at which anaerobiosis becomes established. On the other hand, clinical experience suggests that acidosis associated with clinical states (e.g., diabetic ketoacidosis) can induce marked ventilatory stimulation in the absence of associated sensations of breathlessness. The fact that this condition is typically associated with both hypocapnia (resulting in the diminution of another important ventilatory drive) and drowsiness may help to explain the apparent absence of the anticipated sensation of breathlessness. Lane and Adams (1993) have examined the role of acidosis in the genesis of breathlessness in normal subjects. These authors failed to show any difference in breathlessness during exercise in the presence of experimentally induced normocapnic metabolic acidosis compared with ordinary higher intensity exercise inducing the same level of ventilation.

IV. Conclusions

Taken together, the research discussed in this chapter is consistent with the view that breathlessness is a sensory experience related to the degree of activation of structures in the central nervous system (probably the brainstem) which are concerned with the automatic or reflex control of breathing. In this respect, the neurophysiological basis of this sensation may, in general terms, be analogous to that for other visceral sensations, such as hunger, thirst, and nausea. So far, research in this area suggests that, at least in healthy subjects, the conventional ventilatory stimuli of hypercapnia, hypoxia, acidosis, and exercise induce an intensity of breathlessness that depends more on the level of ventilation achieved than the exact nature of the ventilatory stimulus; the notable exception is voluntarily controlled ventilatory stimulation. On this point, Table 1 summarizes the results from a series of studies by our group in which the effect of a second ventilatory stimulus during exercise on intensity of the sensation of an urge to breathe was assessed.

In comparing these data on the intensity of breathlessness, it is not assumed that the exact quality of the reported sensation is identical with different ventilatory stimuli, although our own experience is that hypercapnia- and hypoxia-induced breathlessness is similar in quality to that associated with exercise if there is an unconstrained ventilatory response (Adams et al., 1985a). Moreover, it is not clear to what extent these studies in normal subjects are relevant with respect to the far wider perspective of breathlessness as a clinical symptom. Patients with respiratory disease can present with severe breathlessness with minimal disturbances in acid-base/blood gas status. Moreover, breathlessness is a common feature of clinical states as varied as heart disease, anemia, and anxiety, in which respiratory function is likely to be near normal. Clearly, the sensation of breathlessness is a complex sensory phenomenon depending on the central processing of

Table 1 Average Results from Three Studies in Normal Subjects in Which Exercise Was Paired with a Second Ventilatory Stimulus to Achieve the Same Levels of Ventilation as with Exercise Alone

Experimental condition	Number of subjects	Workload (watts)	$P_{ET}CO_2$ (mmHg)	SaO_2 (%)	Breathlessness at 50 L/min (%VAS)
Exercise alone[1]	18	150	44	96	38
Exercise + hypercapnia[1]	18	110	54	96	37
Exercise + hypoxia[1]	18	105	45	89	36
Exercise alone[2]	6	110	40	96	31
Exercise + acidosis[2]	6	85	41	96	29
Exercise alone[3]	9	130	39	96	29
Exercise + volition[3]	9	85	38	96	9

The mean intensity of the sensation of breathlessness at a mean ventilation of 50 L/min was assessed using a Visual Analogue Scale (VAS). Mean levels of workload, end-tidal P_{CO_2} ($P_{ET}CO_2$), and ear oximetry estimates of arterial oxygen saturation (SaO_2) at which measurements were made are shown. Results are taken from [1]Lane et al., 1990; [2]Lane and Adams, 1993; [3]Lane et al., 1987b.

both respiratory-related (arising from both within and outside the CNS) and nonrespiratory neural activity arising from other CNS structures.

References

1. Adams, L., and Guz, A. (1991). Dyspnea on exertion. In: Exercise: Pulmonary Physiology and Pathophysiology. Edited by B.J. Whipp and K. Wasserman. Marcel Dekker, New York, pp. 449–494.
2. Adams, L., Chronos, N., Lane, R., and Guz, A. (1985a). The measurement of breathlessness induced in normal subjects: validity of two scaling techniques. Clin. Sci. 69:7–16.
3. Adams, L., Lane, R., Shea, S.A., Cockcroft, A., and Guz, A. (1985b). Breathlessness during different forms of ventilatory stimulation: a study of mechanisms in normal subjects and respiratory patients. Clin. Sci. 69:663–672.
4. Adams, L., Chronos, N., Lane, R., and Guz, A. (1986). The measurement of breathlessness induced in normal subjects: individual differences. Clin. Sci. 70:131–140.
5. Banzett, R.B., Lansing, R.W., Reid, M.G., Adams, L., and Brown, R. (1989). 'Air hunger' arising from increased PCO_2 in mechanically ventilated quadriplegics. Respir. Physiol. 76:53–68.
6. Banzett, R.B., Lansing, R.W., Brown, R., Topulos, G.P., Yager, D., Steele, S.M., Londono, B., Loring, S.H., Reid, M.B., Adams, L., and Nations, C.S. (1990). 'Air hunger' from increased PCO_2 persists after complete neuromuscular block in humans. Respir. Physiol. 81:1–17.

7. Chonan, T., Mulholland, M.B., Leitner, J., Altose, M.D., and Cherniack, N.S. (1990). Sensation of dyspnea during hypercapnia, exercise, and voluntary hyperventilation. J. Appl. Physiol. 68:2100–2106.
8. Chronos, N., Adams, L., and Guz, A. (1988). Effect of hyperoxia and hypoxia on exercise-induced breathlessness in normal subjects. Clin. Sci. 74:531–537.
9. Eldridge, F.L. and Waldrop, T.G. (1991). Neural control of breathing during exercise. In: Exercise: Pulmonary Physiology and Pathophysiology. Edited by B.J. Whipp and K. Wasserman. Marcel Dekker, New York, 309–370.
10. Freedman, S., Lane, R., and Guz, A. (1987). Breathlessness and respiratory mechanics during reflex or voluntary hyperventilation in patients with chronic airflow limitation. Clin. Sci. 73:311–318.
11. Gandevia, S.C. (1988). Neural mechanisms underlying the sensation of breathlessness: kinesthetic parallels between respiratory and limb muscles. Aust. N. Z. J. Med. 18:83–91.
12. Gandevia, S.C., and Rothwell, J. (1987). Activation of the human diaphragm from the motor cortex. J. Physiol. 384:109–118.
13. Gandevia, S.C., Killian, K., McKenzie, D.K., Crawford, M., Allen, G.M., Gorman, R.B., and Hales, J.P. (1993). Respiratory sensation, cardiovascular control and kinaesthesia during complete paralysis in normal subjects. J. Physiol. 470:85–108.
14. Hyland, R.H., Jones, N.L., Powles, A.C.P., Lenkie, S.C.M., Vanderlinden, R.G., and Epstein, S.W. (1978). Primary alveolar hypoventilation treated with nocturnal electrophrenic respiration. Am. Rev. Respir. Dis. 117:165–172.
15. Lane, R., and Adams, L. (1993). The effects of metabolic acidosis on perceived breathlessness during exercise in humans. J. Physiol. 461:47–61.
16. Lane, R., Cockcroft, A., Adams, L., and Guz, A. (1987a). Arterial oxygen saturation and breathlessness in patients with chronic obstructive airways disease. Clin. Sci. 72:693–698.
17. Lane, R., Cockcroft, A., and Guz, A. (1987b). Voluntary isocapnic hyperventilation and breathlessness during exercise in normal subjects. Clin. Sci. 73:519–523.
18. Lane, R., Adams, L., and Guz, A. (1990). The effects of hypoxia and hypercapnia on perceived breathlessness during exercise in humans. J. Physiol. 428:579–593.
19. Murphy, K., Mier, A., Adams, L., and Guz, A. (1990). Putative cerebral cortical involvement in the ventilatory response to inhaled CO_2 in conscious man. J. Physiol. 420:1–18.
20. O'Neill, P.A., Stark, R.D., Allen, S., and Stretton, T.B. (1986). The relationship between breathlessness and ventilation during steady state exercise. Clin. Respir. Physiol. 22:247–250.
21. Opie, L.H., Smith, A.C., and Spalding, J.M.K. (1959). Conscious appreciation of the effects produced by independent changes of ventilation volume and end-tidal PCO_2 in paralysed patients. J. Physiol. 149:494–499.
22. Orem, J., and Trotter, R. (1994). Behavioral control of breathing. NIPS 9:228–232.
23. Paton, J.Y., Swaminathan, S., Sargent, C.W., Hawksworth, A., and Keens, T.G. (1993). Ventilatory response to exercise in children with congenital central hypoventilation syndrome. Am. Rev. Respir. Dis. 147:1185–1191.

24. Shea, S.A., Walter, J., Pelley, C., Murphy, K., and Guz, A. (1987). The effect of visual and auditory stimuli upon resting ventilation in man. Respir. Physiol. 68:345–357.
25. Shea, S.A., Andres, L.P., Shannon, D.C., and Banzett, R.B. (1993). Ventilatory response to exercise in humans lacking ventilatory chemosensitivity. J. Physiol. 468:623–640.
26. Shea, S.A., Andres, L.P., Shannon, D., Guz, A., and Banzett, R.B. (1993b). Respiratory sensations in subjects who lack a ventilatory response to CO_2. Respir. Physiol. 93:203–219.
27. Shea, S.A., Banzett, R.B., and Lansing, R.W. (1994). Respiratory sensations and their role in the control of breathing. In: Regulation of Breathing, Edited by J.A. Dempsey and A.I. Pack. Marcel Dekker, New York, 923–957.
28. Stark, R.D., Gambles, S.A., and Lewis, J.A. (1981). Methods to assess breathlessness in healthy subjects: a critical evaluation and application to analyse the acute effects of diazepam and promethazine on breathlessness induced by exercise or by exposure to raised levels of carbon dioxide. Clin. Sci. 61:429–439.
29. Stark, R.D., Gambles, S.A., and Chatterjee, S.S. (1982). An exercise test to assess clinical dyspnoea: estimation of reproducibilty and sensitivity. Br. J. Dis. Chest 76:269–278.
30. Stulbarg, M.S., and Adams, L. (1994). Manifestations of respiratory disease: Dyspnea. In: Textbook of Respiratory Medicine (Vol. 1). Edited by J.F. Murray and J.A. Nadel. Saunders, Philadelphia, 511–528.
31. Swinburn, C.R., Wakefield, J.M., and Jones, P.W. (1984). Relationship between ventilation and breathlessness during exercise in chronic obstructive airways disease is not altered by prevention of hypoxemia. Clin. Sci. 67:515–519.
32. Swinburn, C., Mould, H., Stone, T., Corris, P., and Gibson, G. (1989). The effect of supplemental oxygen on breathlessness and ventilation in hypoxaemic patients with interstitial lung disease. Thorax 44:861P.
33. Ward, S.A., and Whipp, B.J. (1989). Effects of peripheral and central chemoreceptor activation on the isopneic rating of breathing in exercise in humans. J. Physiol. 411:27–43.
34. Wilson, R.C., and Jones, P.W. (1989). A comparison of the visual analogue scale and modified Borg scale for the measurement of dyspnoea during exercise. Clin. Sci. 76:277–282.
35. Winning, A.J., Hamilton, R.D., and Guz, A. (1988). Ventilation and breathlessness on maximal exercise in patients with interstitial lung disease after local anaesthetic aerosol inhalation. Clin. Sci. 74:275–281.
36. Zechman, F.W., and Wiley, L. (1986). Afferent inputs to breathing: In Handbook of Physiology. The Respiratory System: Volume 2, Part 2. Edited by N.S. Cherniack and J.G. Widdicombe. American Physiological Society, Bethesda, MD, 449–474.

9

Respiratory Sensation as a Respiratory Controller

NEIL S. CHERNIACK

School of Medicine
Case Western Reserve University
Cleveland, Ohio

I. Introduction

Breathing is an involuntary act that employs nervous pathways to drive a thoracoabdominal pump, thereby ventilating the lungs, drawing O_2 into the body and expelling CO_2. Ventilation rates vary among individuals and even in the same person depending on a multiplicity of chemical, mechanical, and thermal factors. The thoracoabdominal pump is itself complicated, and a given ventilation rate can be achieved by different mixes of stroke volume (tidal volume) and breathing frequency and by the use of different muscles, particularly the diaphragm, the intercostals, and the abdominals. Given the multiplicity of inputs and the rich possibilities for attaining a specific ventilation, how does the body decide how to breathe? One possibility is that ventilation arises from the summing of the action of different reflex pathways. Another notion is that ventilation is determined in a more sophisticated manner that involves higher brain centers as well as reflexes and optimizes in some way the operation of the thoracoabdominal pump (Longobardo et al., 1980; Mead, 1960; Otis, 1958; Poon, 1987; Yamashiro et al., 1975; Yamashiro and Grodins, 1971, 1973).

Because breathing uses energy that under stressful circumstances and certainly in the presence of lung disease can be quite substantial (Poon, 1987), a common idea is that ventilation patterns and perhaps even the level of breathing are set to satisfy the conflicting needs to preserve arterial pressure of carbon dioxide (P_{CO_2}) and oxygen (P_{O_2}) near desired levels and to minimize energy expenditure over time (i.e., in a steady state). Besides steady-stage gas exchange and energy usage, ventilation could be optimized with respect to other factors that impact on bodily functions; these include optimization of the dynamic properties of respiratory function (by minimizing fluctuations in gas tensions and the time required to return gas tensions to usual levels after a disturbance (Longobardo et al., 1980), or perhaps even more simply, the respiratory controller acts to minimize the sensations, particularly any discomfort, associated with breathing (Cherniack, 1986).

It is clear that the involuntary act of breathing can be modified substantially by willful actions. A common example of these are the profound effects on breathing produced by speaking or singing. The anatomical pathways that allow this voluntary control to be exerted are being identified, although very little is known concerning the neurophysiological mechanisms involved (Davenport et al., 1985, 1986; Orem and Netick, 1986). Physiological studies indicate that conscious individuals can estimate with fair accuracy the position, tension, and force exerted by their respiratory muscle, their degree of movement, their level of ventilation, the mechanical forces impeding airflow into and out of the lungs, and, directly, the effort involved in breathing (Altose, 1985). In addition, conscious individuals can perceive changes in the demand for ventilation and perhaps may even be able to identify the sources responsible for the increase in demand (Chonan et al., 1990b; Gottfried et al., 1981; Killian et al., 1981, 1982; Wolkove et al., 1981). It is possible that by using this information conscious individuals can modify the actions of the respiratory controller and readjust reflect actions on breathing.

That breathing usually occurs without awareness seems desirable because it allows attention to be directed to more complex interactions with the environment. Under some circumstances, when breathing is stimulated or the thoracoabdominal pump is stressed, breathing commands attention and is accompanied by feelings of distress or dyspnea. In these circumstances conscious control of breathing may intervene to alter either ventilation levels or patterns to reduce the awareness and/or discomfort caused by breathing; in this way, respiratory sensations may be used to optimize the performance of the respiratory system (Cherniack, 1986; Cherniack and Altose, 1987).

This chapter reviews ideas of respiratory optimization and examines the hypothesis that respiratory sensations can modify breathing, perhaps to minimize discomfort or even to reinforce other goals of the respiratory system, such as reduction in energy expenditure and maintenance of adequate gas exchange.

II. Types of Breathing and Their Interrelationships

It is useful at this point to distinguish involuntary (reflex) regulation from voluntary (cortically controlled) and from automatically driven breathing. Breathing in humans in non–rapid eye movement (non-REM) sleep occurs as the result of the activity of a central pattern generator consisting normally of a network of respiratory neurons. It is clear from studies in animals that the generation of the respiratory rhythm can occur without input from peripheral receptors. In non-REM sleep this intrinsic pattern proceeds nearly regularly with only minor interruptions, responding predictably to chemical and mechanical stimuli as well as to changes in metabolic rate and temperature (Phillipson and Bowes, 1986; Strohl et al., 1986).

Breathing is more flexible in wakefulness. Conscious humans can modify their breathing to allow communication and can learn to adjust breathing during work to perform tasks with less waste of energy. During much of our waking hours, intrinsically set and reflexly modified breathing is constantly interrupted by voluntary acts, and relatively little time is actually spent when breathing is exclusively under involuntary control.

Despite these voluntary interventions in breathing, we usually remain unaware of our breathing while we are awake. We have learned over time to adjust automatically (albeit voluntarily) our breathing during speech, for example, so breathing occurs without conscious appreciation. Sears (1971) proposed that even voluntary (cortically controlled) breathing can become automatic and that voluntary changes in breathing can like other willful acts (even those as complex as driving a car or playing a piano) become automatic, that is, habitual, and requiring little or no attention. Similar responses occur in other motor acts when parts of the body are hurt. A sprained ankle, for example, produces a transient limp to reduce pain during walking, but when chronic arthritis affects the hip, initially deliberate attempts to alter the gait to relieve discomfort can lead to modification of the usual walking rhythm so that discomfort is automatically reduced. The gait change, initially deliberate, now occurs habitually without conscious awareness.

Dyspnea (shortness of breath) can lead to immediate responses to improve breathing. These can be as gross as aborting an experiment in which one is forced to breathe through an obstruction or escaping from a space contaminated by CO_2. Adjustments could conceivably be more subtle, however, producing long-lasting modifications in breathing that could ultimately lead to prolonged hyperventilation or even to a decrease in breathing efforts to reduce discomfort when the cause of the dyspnea cannot be easily eliminated (as when there is chronic stable respiratory disease).

These examples also suggest that there are two phases in the voluntary reaction to dyspnea, an initial phase in which the strategy is to overcome a new respiratory problem by breathing harder, and a later phase, if dyspnea persists, to adopt breathing patterns that reduce breathing efforts.

III. Optimization in Respiratory Control

Many investigators have suggested that the respiratory controller has other priorities besides maintenance of normal levels of blood gas tensions and that the actual behavior of the system represents a compromise determined to optimize certain key features of breathing.

For example, Widdicombe and Nadel (1963) pointed out that although an increase in airway caliber and hence a decrease in airway resistance would enhance the ability of the controller to ventilate the lungs using less energy, greater caliber enlarges airway volume and brings about an undesirable increase in dead space with a reduction in alveolar ventilation. They suggested that the actual control of respiratory resistance represents some compromise between these two desirable objectives, minimal airway resistance and minimal dead space.

Similarly, at a given frequency of stimulation, there is an optimal length at which the diaphragm produces maximum force (Bradley et al., 1986; Breslin et al., 1990; Cherniack, 1959; Field et al., 1982). It has been suggested that accessory respiratory muscles are brought into play to maintain diaphragm length and force of contraction at nearly maximal levels. It is of interest that recent studies indicate that dyspnea seems to develop as accessory muscle usage increases (Bradley et al., 1986).

Longobardo et al. (1980) suggested that the respiratory system controller is set at a level of sensitivity that reconciles conflicting needs to maintain arterial blood gases tightly, which is facilitated by high controller gains, and a need to prevent wide swings in arterial tensions, which can result from too great a controller sensitivity.

A major impetus for the development of theories of optimization has been the well-known observation that hypercapnia develops in chronic obstructive pulmonary disease (COPD) considerably before the maximum ventilation capacity is reached (Lane and Howell, 1970). In concordance with experiments that showed that the O_2 cost of breathing was greatly increased in COPD (Cherniack, 1959), it was proposed that at some stage of deteriorating pulmonary function the O_2 cost of ventilating the lungs may exceed the additional improvement in oxygenation that could result from the ventilation increase (Rebuck and Slutsky, 1986). At that point ventilation increases are checked, allowing arterial P_{CO_2} to rise and arterial P_{O_2} to fall. In severe disturbances of lung function, elevated levels of P_{CO_2} could in fact have a beneficial effect (Longobardo et al., 1980), because with hypercapnia P_{CO_2} could be maintained stable by relatively small adjustment in ventilation requiring less O_2 expenditure. Adverse effects on pH would be reduced by bicarbonate retention by the kidney, and changes in cardiac output and redistributions of blood flow and enhanced erythropoesis might restore O_2 delivery to vital tissues.

Further support for respiratory work as an optimizing factor arose from the experiments of Milic-Emili and Tyler (1963). They studied normal subjects made to inhale CO_2 through different grades of resistance. They found that as the severity of the resistance became greater, the ventilatory response to CO_2 diminished but the inspiratory work of breathing remained fixed. This suggested that a fixed amount of inspiratory work was associated with each level of P_{CO_2}. However, later experiments indicated that even with substantial increases in external airway resistance, ventilatory responses to CO_2 could be maintained in conscious humans, indicating that the work of breathing may not be an overriding factor in setting ventilation levels (Altose et al., 1977; Sorli et al., 1978).

More recently, Poon proposed that ventilation is regulated to minimize some sum of both the deviation of P_{CO_2} from desirable levels and the work of breathing, and he developed equations describing the principles that might guide such a system (Poon, 1982). His own experiments seem to support the correctness of this supposition (Poon, 1982; Poon and Greene, 1985).

Longobardo et al. (1980) suggests that another priority of the respiratory system is to restore normal blood gas levels rapidly in acute situations. It has been proposed for a long time that the respiratory system acts as a first-line, rapidly responding system to preserve acid-base homeostasis. In a theoretical study, they suggested that minimizing the energy cost of expelling a given amount of CO_2 from the body in a given time (which they called figure of merit) is a priority of the respiratory system. Their study indicated that although speed of restoration was improved by increasing the ventilatory response to CO_2 (controller gain), the energy usage of the respiratory muscles to achieve rapid response increased, albeit gradually in normal subjects. The figure of merit was maximal at a controller gain of about 2–3 (the value observed in most normal individuals) and decreased at both higher and lower gains. Moreover, when the energy consumed in breathing increased, as in lung disease, the figure of merit reached a maximum value at lower levels of ventilatory response to CO_2. With higher respiratory energy cost, the point of maximal figure of merit was more obvious, and changes in its value occurred more sharply above and below the peak. They also pointed out that their figure of merit depended not only on the respiratory system but on the response of the circulatory system as well, which limited the delivery of CO_2 to the lungs. As cardiac output increased, the figure of merit was greater at higher levels of controller gain. Giordano et al. showed in experiments in animals that the expulsion of CO_2 could be altered by shifts in controller gain and was greater when the resting CO_2 was higher (Giordano et al., 1979).

Otis (1958) showed that at any given level of ventilation the work of breathing decreases as tidal volume is reduced and respiratory frequency increased. If account is taken of dead space effects, however, this decrease in work is offset by increasing dead space ventilation. Less alveolar ventilation occurs as breathing becomes more rapid and shallow. Otis could show then that to maintain a given level of alveolar P_{CO_2} there is an optimum frequency and tidal volume that minimize the work of breathing. Moreover, he predicted that as airway resistance increased, work could be lessened by increasing tidal volume and by reducing the breathing frequency. On the other hand, minimum work principles dictated a shallower tidal volume than normal and a more rapid breathing rate when the elastic forces opposing ventilation became greater.

Yamashiro demonstrated that if changes in functional residual capacity are considered in the calculation of respiratory work, the principle of work minimization can account for the changes in breathing frequency, inspiratory and expiratory time, and airflow trajectory as ventilation rises in normal subjects from rest to exercise (Yamashiro et al., 1975; Yamashiro and Grodins, 1971, 1973).

Contrary to the work hypothesis, however, Mead (1960) observed that in conscious guinea pigs breathing patterns seem to be adopted that minimize the integral of inspiratory force development over time rather than work; Milic-Emili believed both work and the pressure integral may be used as optimizing criteria in setting respiratory patterns (Bates and Milic-Emili, 1980). Moreover, Sorli et al. (1978) reported that patients with chronic obstructive lung disease who develop hypercapnia when in respiratory failure breathe with a smaller tidal volume and shorter inspiratory time than normals and that inspiratory time lengthens and tidal volumes grow greater as the obstruction is relieved and respiratory failure disappears. Although this observation seems contrary to the predictions that breathing should be deeper and slower with greater airway resistance, it is possible that chronic obstructive lung disease can heighten both the elastic and resistive forces opposing breathing, and the relative balance of these forces were unclear in the patients studied. It is of interest that respiratory sensations intensify with the effort used for each breath and with time (Killian et al., 1982). Thus it is possible that the hypercapnia observed in respiratory failure is caused by a controller strategy to reduce respiratory sensations.

Other important arguments against an optimizing work principle that acts generally are measurements in healthy persons showing that the work of breathing is exceedingly small and even large changes in pattern of ventilation entail little increase in energy costs (Yamashiro et al., 1975); nonetheless, energy costs can become very high in disease (Cherniack, 1959). Moreover, clinical observations indicate that many patients with lung disease seem to preserve normal arterial blood gases by considerably increasing their work of breathing (Sorli et al., 1978).

An additional difficulty with the work theory of optimization is that no mechanism has been identified that would allow the respiratory system to be aware of the energy cost of its muscles. Because of the many different muscles involved in breathing, the biological mechanism that would allow such a calculation to be made seems extraordinarily complex and difficult.

At the present time, although it is recognized that the work or energy cost of breathing can affect ventilatory responses, it is not clear that it plays a significant role in optimizing ventilation levels, controller gain, or breathing patterns either in normal subjects or in patients with lung disease.

Observations suggesting that force minimization is an important optimizing principle are of considerable interest because the pattern of breathing that minimizes force is not greatly different from that which minimizes work (Mead, 1960). Force of contraction can be quantified by conscious individuals, as can the effort required to drive the muscles of breathing (Killian et al., 1982), and could in part depend on signals to the brain from tendon organs in muscles, but the mechanism that allows the integration of signals from different muscles remains a problem.

The idea that muscle fatigue limits ventilatory responses, which has emerged in several studies, suggests another link to respiratory sensations (Kongragonta et al., 1988; Macklem and Roussos, 1977; Roussos and Macklem, 1977). Peripheral fatigue (fatigue at level of the muscles themselves or at the myoneural junction) could clearly interfere with the effectiveness of respiratory efforts, but it is not obvious that it occurs in humans except under extreme circumstances. Some investigators have observed "central fatigue," that is, a reduction in the activity of nerves supplying respiratory muscles as the respiratory load is made more severe or with time as a very great load is maintained (Bellemare and Bigland-Ritchie, 1987). This central response to loads could be considered restricted by the controller to prevent damage to the respiratory muscles. It is known that with muscle fatigue the sense of effort increases (Gandevia et al., 1981). Hence, respiratory sensations could play a significant role in initiating central fatigue. Central fatigue may have as its biological basis increased endorphin formation, which occurs during breathing on severe loads, which in turn reduces respiratory responses. Scardella and coworkers (1986) have shown that hypercapnia eventually occurs in conscious goats required to breathe through massive restrictive loads for long periods of time but that hypercapnia can be delayed or reversed by the administration of naloxone, an endorphin antagonist.

IV. Effect of Respiratory Sensation on Breathing

It is not difficult to demonstrate that higher brain centers can modify breathing in normal humans (Fink, 1961; Fink et al., 1963). Sleep, for example, changes the distribution of nervous output to the respiratory muscles and tends to decrease overall ventilation levels (Strohl et al., 1986). These effects are believed to be a sleep modification of higher brain center operation, not a direct effect on the respiratory sensory receptors themselves. A number of environmental effects alter respiration even in the waking state, presumably by acting on the cortex. Light has a stimulating effect on breathing; sounds, both musical and noise, alter respiratory patterns and can affect ventilatory levels (Shea et al., 1987). Even the performance of mental arithmetic influences breathing (Rigg et al., 1977).

It is also clear that respiratory diseases can induce voluntary changes in breathing. In chronic obstructive pulmonary disease, for example, pursed-lips breathing and certain characteristic changes in posture that are adopted by patients (even breathing quietly) seem to be behavioral adjustments that facilitate gas exchange or improve respiratory muscle function (Barach, 1974; Gandevia and Macefield, 1989; Mueller et al., 1970; Sharp et al., 1980). Initially these strategies are probably learned by trial and error, but with time they occur habitually.

Stimulation of respiratory muscle proprioceptors is known to produce cortical effects, and pathways have been identified that allow the cortex to superimpose its commands on the reflex activity of the respiratory muscles (Davenport et al., 1985, 1986; Lipski et al., 1986; Orem and Netick, 1986). Respiratory effort can be perceived even in the presence of little or no input from peripheral receptors, however (McCloskey, 1978; McCloskey et al., 1974), and can be quantified (Altose et al., 1985). The midbrain or hypothalamus may be structures involved in transmitting this sense of effort to the cortex (Chen et al., 1991). Moreover, it has been proposed that dyspnea occurs when effort becomes sufficiently intense (Altose, 1985; Cherniack and Altose, 1987).

The intriguing question is whether respiratory sensations can affect the motor traffic to the respiratory muscles. A number of studies bear on this question. It has been shown that a normal conscious human can appreciate changes in the resistance to airflow caused by external devices (Chonan et al., 1990a; Gottfried et al., 1981; Wolkove et al., 1981). In addition, humans are able to detect changes in either resistive or elastic loads and to distinguish between them (Chonan et al., 1990; Gottfried et al., 1981; Wolkove et al., 1981). This ability appears to require the capability to recognize separately volume and flow signals and to relate them to respiratory force produced or effort exerted. Respiratory loads can also be graded according to their severity (Altose, 1985; Killian et al., 1981). Killian has suggested that the ability to grade loads involves a summation of inputs that signal changes in respiratory force and its duration, with force predominating (Killian et al., 1981). The process may be even more complex: Altose et al. (1985) showed that resistance could be graded by normal subjects even when the force exerted by the respiratory muscles was kept constant and sensory intensity corrected for force duration. Recently it was demonstrated that conscious animals can also detect resistance changes (Davenport et al., 1991). This is a particularly important observation because it opens the possibility of examining the anatomical and neurophysiological basis of resistive sensations in more detail than has been possible with human experimentation alone. Orem's work in conscious cats has also demonstrated the usefulness of animal models in determining the anatomical pathways relating the reflex to the voluntary control of breathing (Orem and Netick, 1986).

Tack et al. (1981, 1982, 1983) found that the perceived intensity of respiratory movements varies with age and seems to involve complex integration of flow, volume, and force signals. They demonstrated in conscious humans asked to duplicate tidal volumes on resistive and elastic loads of different severity that sensation was related to the product of both force and volume signals, each raised to a different power. In both elderly and young subjects the force signal seemed to contribute more to the sensory intensity than the volume signal, but force was even more dominant in the older than in the younger subjects. It is of interest that sensory intensity was related to a work signal because both are determined by multiplication of pressure and volume signals. However, the Tack study clearly showed that the relationship between sensory intensity and work was indirect.

Altose et al. (1977) showed that hypercapnic patients with obstructive lung disease had poor immediate responses to loads as measured by the occlusion pressure technique, and Gottfried et al. found that patients with COPD seemed to be less aware of changes in the relative size of resistive loads than healthy subjects. Gottfried et al. also demonstrated that there was a good relationship between the exponent of magnitude estimation for resistive loads and the slope of the ventilatory response to CO_2 while on the load (Gottfried et al., 1978, 1981). This suggested that the greater intensity of the sensation produced by loads, the greater is the respiratory response.

Santiago and coworkers (1981), like Altose, found that many patients with COPD (unlike normal subjects) failed to demonstrate an increased occlusion pressure response during CO_2 rebreathing while on loads. They also found that these depressed responses could be reversed and made more normal by the administration of naloxone, but others have not found this (Simon et al., 1989a). In addition to possible differences in endorphin production and release, the older age of COPD patients may contribute to depressed responses on loads because age has been reported to diminish load perception (Tack et al., 1981, 1982, 1983).

It may be important that the studies by the Altose, Gottfried, and Edelman groups were done under constrained and rather artificial circumstances that limited the ability of the subjects to use different strategies. The motor response to load was measured during hypercapnic rebreathing, so that the rate of rise in CO_2 was independent of the ventilation rate and the exposure to the load was brief. Moreover, the behavior adapted under these circumstances depends on both the effect of the load itself and the response to CO_2, which does not depend on the sensitivity of chemoreceptors alone. Personality clearly affects the response to CO_2, as do many other internal and environmental signals (Aitken, 1962; Dudley and Pitts-Poarch, 1980; Saunders et al., 1972). The predominance of evidence indicates that conscious individuals temporarily increase respiratory force when exposed to loads (resistive or elastic), but not much is known about responses when exposure to loads is more prolonged.

Oliven et al. (1983) attempted to address the relationship between respiratory sensations and motor output in a somewhat different way. Because the sensory intensity of a load depends in large part on the effort required to ventilate the lungs, they measured the ability of subjects to grade changes in force production during isometric contractions of the respiratory muscles using the technique of magnitude production. Like others, they found that the exponent for magnitude production of force differed among the subjects studied. They then placed the subjects, normal subjects and patients with COPD, on a resistive load for 10 minutes or for as long as the subjects could tolerate loaded breathing. They found that many of the subjects during this time period allowed P_{CO_2} to rise, but by varying amounts. The rise in P_{CO_2} was related inversely to the changes in tidal volume adopted during resistive load breathing. Although some subjects reduced their tidal volume but others increased it, the rise in P_{CO_2} was significantly related to the change in tidal volume. Subjects who increased their tidal volume had smaller or no elevations in P_{CO_2}, but subjects who decreased tidal volume raised their P_{CO_2} more. More importantly, there was a statistically significant direct relationship between the observed exponent in the magnitude production of force study and the increase in P_{CO_2} and a significant inverse relationship to the decrease in tidal volume. Oliven and coworkers (1987) reasoned that a smaller tidal volume requires less respiratory muscle force than larger tidal volumes. The subjects who were most acutely aware of force changes (whom they believed were those subjects with the largest exponents for magnitude production) reduced their tidal volume the most, allowing them to use less force. They therefore believed that in this less constrained study of respiratory responses, subjects chose to minimize the effects of respiratory sensations by reducing tidal volume even at the price of raising arterial P_{CO_2}. The differences in the response to the loads could not be explained by differences in the subjects' ventilatory responses to CO_2. They observed in another study a similar relationship between increases in P_{CO_2} caused by inhalation of a bronchoconstrictor and the exponent for sensory intensity of force.

Like the experiments described earlier, the interpretation of the results of the study by Oliven et al. is complicated. Even though variations in pulmonary performance as measured by routine pulmonary function testing also failed to explain the variations in response, potential differences in the use of respiratory muscles during loaded breathing were not measured.

More recent studies of respiratory sensation have used the Borg scale or the visual analog scale to evaluate sensory phenomenon among individuals rather than magnitude estimation or production techniques. Chonan et al. (1990a) used a visual analog scale to study the changes in breathing effort when healthy humans either increased or decreased ventilation from normal levels. The CO_2 content of the inspired air was adjusted so that P_{CO_2} levels remained constant despite the variations in ventilation required by the experiment. They observed that the perceived effort in breathing increased both when ventilation rose and when it declined from spontaneously adopted values, although the rate at which the sensation of effort increased was greater when ventilation fell than when ventilation rose. They believed that these results supported the ideas that a sense of comfort might reinforce physiological mechanisms that normally set the level of quiet breathing. The increase in effort experienced when the subjects decreased their breathing was believed to be attributable to signals arising from muscle spindles. Schwartzenstein et al. (1989), who performed similar experiments, largely confirmed the Chonan group's results but found an appreciable number of subjects who reported no change in the sense of effort when asked to increase their breathing voluntarily. Adams et al. (1985) found no change in dyspnea (which was defined as an unpleasant sensation) when breathing was voluntarily increased, although dyspnea was heightened when ventilation was stimulated either by exercise or by CO_2 inhalation.

Chonan et al. (1990b) also provided suggestive data that the usually adopted pattern of breathing is also the pattern that minimizes awareness of breathing. Keeping minute ventilation constant, subjects who either increased or decreased tidal volume complained of greater respiratory effort. Chonan et al. believe that signals from muscle spindles may account for the discomfort experienced with a reduction in tidal volume and changes in tendon organ signals when tidal volume was increased.

Although these experiments lend support to the idea that resting breathing occurs at levels of ventilation and breathing patterns that conform to those that produce the least discomfort, they do not prove a causal relationship.

The contribution of signals from chemoreceptors to respiratory sensations remains unclear. Banzett et al. seem to have demonstrated that changes in CO_2 can be sensed even in the absence of muscle movement, contrary to earlier experiments (Banzett et al., 1989, 1990; Campbell et al., 1967; Castele et al., 1985; Patterson et al., 1962; Schwartzstein et al., 1987). A number of studies by other investigators likewise show that CO_2 increases can be dyspnogenic even if greater respiratory muscle activity is prevented. Chonan et al. (1987) and Remmers et al. (1968) both showed that the increase in sensory intensity caused by rebreathing CO_2 is greater when ventilation is voluntarily restrained. What is not clear is whether a collateral sense of motor outflow to the muscles is responsible for CO_2 sensing, that is, whether increased neural traffic to the respiratory muscles can be detected regardless of its origin or whether the detection of CO_2 changes depends specifically on a greater sensory input from chemoreceptors.

Chonan et al. (1990) also examined the relative effects of different respiratory stimuli, namely voluntary hyperventilation, exercise, and hypercapnia. They found that the change in sensory intensity relative to ventilation changes was greater with CO_2 than with either exercise or voluntary hyperventilation. Chonan et al. concluded that CO_2 was a separate stimulus that increased respiratory effort independently of proprioceptive input. Adams et al. (1985) and Ward and Whipp (1989), however, found no difference in the degree of dyspnea produced by a given ventilation level whether it was produced by exercise or by hypercapnia or by a combination of the two. Ward and Whipp, however, thought that hypoxia may have an independent dyspnogenic effect.

Because changes in CO_2 and/or O_2 may affect the brain formation of neuropeptides that influence sensation, it is not unreasonable to believe that CO_2 and perhaps hypoxia specifically affects sensation, but a conclusive test of this possibility remains elusive (Neubauer et al., 1990).

V. Respiratory Sensation as an Optimizer of the Respiratory Controller

There is accumulating, but not yet overwhelming, evidence that respiratory sensations alter respiratory output significantly even over long periods of time.

The potential effects of respiratory sensations appear complicated. Respiratory sensations may act in quite opposite directions on respiratory activity. Intense respiratory sensations may initially intensify respiratory efforts (Gottfried et al., 1981). This seems to be an important factor in the acute response of many individuals to impaired pulmonary performances and, in some individuals, may be a long-lasting strategy. In other individuals it seems likely that, at least over the long term, respiratory sensations act to adjust the controller to minimize sensory effects (Oliven et al., 1987). The sorting out of these possibilities requires more standard methods of defining and scaling respiratory sensations. For example, there are unclear relationships among measurement of sensory intensity derived from magnitude estimation and production studies, visual analog and Borg scales, and the level of dyspnea reported on scales that are more clearly related to daily activities (Mahler et al., 1984, 1989; Muza et al., 1990; Stevens, 1957; Stubbing et al., 1981).

At this point it seems unlikely that in normal individuals a priority to reduce respiratory sensory input plays more than a supporting role to physiological reflexes, but its importance as a control system priority in patients with disease could be far greater.

Could sensations be particularly important when the need for energy conservation is great? Is it possible that respiratory sensations and the need to minimize them contribute to reducing energy expenditure? The data are fragmentary and are thus far inconclusive. Poon has suggested that respiration is regulated under all circumstances to keep the sum of the deviation in CO_2 from normal and ventilation itself at some minimum value (Poon, 1982; Poon and Greene, 1985). This concept is novel and ambitious because it attempts to develop some quantitative balance between the need to maintain adequate gas exchange and the need to reduce the effort required to achieve homeostasis (Oku et al., 1991). Previous theories have been based on the idea of hierarchy of control, either work or gas exchange being dominant.

Respiratory sensations could provide the biological basis for the Poon hypothesis. It is clear that ventilation change can be sensed and graded, even though whether they are always dyspnogenic regardless of how they are produced remains unsettled. However, whether CO_2 changes can be independently sensed is still controversial (Adams et al., 1985; Ward and Whipp, 1989). If it can be shown that minimization of sensation is an optimizing principle, then this same principle could also roughly at least optimize work and gas exchange in the way Poon hypothesizes.

More definitive investigations require a better description of sensation with regard to both intensity and quality. Progress in identifying different qualities of respiratory sensation is being made (Simon et al., 1989b). More information about the types of respiratory sensations certainly would help us, whether it is only the intensity of sensation that potentially affects breathing or whether the quality of the sensation has a separate effect.

References

Adams, L., Lane, R., Shea, S.A., Cockcroft, A., and Guz, A. (1985). Breathlessness during different forms of ventilatory stimulation: a study of mechanisms in normal subjects and respiratory patients. Clin. Sci. 69:663–672.

Aitken, R.C.B. (1962). Measurement of feelings using visual analogue scales. Proc. R. Soc. Med. 62:989–993.

Altose, M.D. (1985). Assessment and management of breathlessness. Chest 88:S77–S83.

Altose, M.D., McCauley, W.C., Kelsen, S.G., and Cherniack, N.S. (1977). Effects of hypercapnia and inspiratory flow-resistive loading on respiratory activity in chronic airways obstruction. J. Clin. Invest. 59:500–507.

Altose, M.D., Leitner, J., and Cherniack, N.S. (1985). Effects of age and respiratory effort on perception of resistive ventilatory loads. J. Gerontol. 40:147–153.

Banzett, R.B., Lansing, R.W., Reid, M.B., Adams, L., and Brown, R. (1989). "Air hunger" arising from increased P_{CO_2} in mechanically ventilated quadriplegics. Respir. Physiol. 76:53–68.

Banzett, R.B., Lansing, R.W., Brown, R., Topulos, G.P., Yager, D., Steele, S.M., Londono, B., Loring, S.H., Reid, M.B., Adams, L., and Nations, C.S. (1990). "Air hunger" from increased P_{CO_2} persists after complete neuromuscular blockade in humans. Respir. Physiol. 81:1–18.

Barach, A.L. (1974). Chronic obstructive lung disease. Postural relief of dyspnea. Arch. Physical Med. Rehab. 55:494–504.

Bates, J.H.T., and Milic-Emili, J. (1980). Breathing patterns and concepts of minimum respiratory work and minimum effort. In: Neurobiology of the Control of Breathing. Edited by C. von Euler and H. Lagercrantz. Raven Press, New York, pp. 243–249.

Bellemare, F., and Bigland-Ritchie, B. (1987). Central components of diaphragmatic fatigue assessed by phrenic nerve stimulation. J. Appl. Physiol. 62:1307–1316.

Bradley, T.D., Chartrand, D.A., Fitting, J.W., Killian, K.J., and Grassino, A. (1986). The relation of inspiratory effort sensation to fatiguing patterns of the diaphragm. Am. Rev. Respir. Dis. 134:119–124.

Breslin, E.H., Garoutte, B.C., Kohlman-Carrieri, V., and Celli, B.R. (1990). Correlations between dyspnea, diaphragm and sternomastoid recruitment during inspiratory resistive breathing in normal subjects. Chest 98:298–302.

Campbell, E.J.M., Godfrey, S., Clark, T.J.H., Freedman, S., and Norman, J. (1967). The effect of muscular paralysis induced by tubocurarine on the duration and sensation of breath-holding during hypercapnia. Clin. Sci. 36:323–328.

Castele, R.G., Connors, A.F., and Altose, M.D. (1985). Effects of changes in CO_2 partial pressure on the sensation of respiratory drive. J. Appl. Physiol. 59:1747–1751.

Chen, Z., Eldridge, F., and Wagner, P.G. (1991). Respiratory-associated rhythmic firing of midbrain neurones in cats: relation to level of respiratory drive. J. Physiol. (Lond.) 437:305–325.

Cherniack, N.S. (1986). Potential role of optimization in alveolar hypoventilation and respiratory instability. In: Neurobiology of the Control of Breathing. Edited by C. von Euler and H. Lagercrantz. Raven Press, New York, pp. 45–50.

Cherniack, N.S., and Altose, M.D. (1987). Mechanisms of dyspnea. Clin. Chest Med. 8:207–219.

Cherniack, R.M. (1959). The oxygen consumption and efficiency of the respiratory muscles in health and emphysema. J. Clin. Invest. 38:494–499.

Chonan, T., Mulholland, M.B., Cherniack, N.S., and Altose, M.D. (1987). Effects of voluntary constraining of thoracic displacement during hypercapnia. J. Appl. Physiol. 63:1822–1828.

Chonan, T., Mulholland, M.B., Altose, M.D., and Cherniack, N.S. (1990a). Effect of changes in level and pattern of breathing on the sensation of dyspnea. J. Appl. Physiol. 69:1290–1295.

Chonan, T., Mulholland, M.B., Leitner, J., Altose, M.D., and Cherniack, N.S. (1990b). Sensation of dyspnea during hypercapnia, exercise and voluntary hyperventilation. J. Appl. Physiol. 68:2100–2106.

Davenport, P.W., Thompson, F.J., Reep, R.L., and Freed, A.N. (1985). Projection of phrenic nerve afferents to the cat sensorimotor cortex. Brain Res. 328:150–153.

Davenport, P.W., Friedman, W.A., Thompson, F.J., and Franzen, O. (1986). Respiratory related cortical potentials evoked by inspiratory occlusion in humans. J. Appl. Physiol. 60:1843–1848.

Davenport, P.W., Dalziel, D.J., Webb, B., Bellah, J.R., and Vierck, C.J. Jr. (1991). Inspiratory resistive load detection in conscious dogs. J. Appl. Physiol. 70:1284–1289.

Dudley, D.L., and Pitts-Poarch, A.P. (1980). Psychophysiologic aspects of respiratory control. Clin. Chest Med. 1:131–143.

Field, S., Kelley, S.M., and Macklem, P.T. (1982). The oxygen cost of breathing in patients with cardiorespiratory disease. Am. Rev. Respir. Dis. 126:9–13.

Fink, B.R. (1961). Influence of cerebral activity in wakefulness on regulation of breathing. J. Appl. Physiol. 16:15–20.

Fink, B.R., Hanks, E.C., Ngai, S.H., and Papper, E.M. (1963). Central regulation of respiration during anesthesia and wakefulness. Ann. N.Y. Acad. Sci. 109:892–900.

Gandevia, S.C., and Macefield, G. (1989). Projection of low-threshold afferents from human intercostal muscles in the cerebral cortex. Respir. Physiol. 77:203–214.

Gandevia, S.C., Killian, K.J., and Campbell, E.J.M. (1981). The effect of respiratory muscle fatigue on respiratory sensation. Clin. Sci. 60:463–466.

Giordano, A., Longobardo, G.S., and Cherniack, N.S. (1979). Transient CO_2 elimination and storage as a function of the ventilatory response to CO_2. Respir. Physiol. 37: 219–237.

Gottfried, S.B., Altose, M.D., Kelsen, S.G., Fogarty, C.M., and Cherniack, N.S. (1978). The perception of changes in airflow resistance in normal subjects and patients with chronic airways obstruction. Chest 73:286–288.

Gottfried, S.B., Altose, M.D., Kelsen, S.G., and Cherniack, N.S. (1981). Perception of changes in airflow resistance in obstructive pulmonary disorders. Am. Rev. Respir. Dis. 124:566–570.

Killian, K.J., Mahotte, C.K., and Campbell, E.J.M. (1981). Magnitude scaling of externally added loads in breathing. Am. Rev. Respir. Dis. 123:12–15.

Killian, K.J., Bucens, D.D., and Campbell, E.J.M. (1982). Effect of breathing patterns on the perceived magnitude of added loads to breathing. J. Appl. Physiol. 52:578–584.

Kongragonta, V.R., Druz, W.S., and Sharp, J. (1988). Dyspnea and diaphragmatic fatigue in patients with chronic obstructive pulmonary disease. Am. Rev. Respir. Dis. 137: 662–667.

Lane, D.J., and Howell, J.B.L. (1970). Relationship between sensitivity to carbon dioxide and clinical features in patients with chronic airways obstruction. Thorax 25:150–159.

Lipski, J., Bektas, A., and Porter, R. (1986). Short latency inputs to phrenic motoneurons from the sensorimotor cortex in the cat. Exp. Brain Res. 61:280–289.

Longobardo, G.S., Cherniack, N.S., and Damokosh-Giordano, A. (1980). Possible optimization of respiratory controller sensitivity. Ann. Biomed. Eng. 8:143–158.

Macklem, P.T., and Roussos, C.S. (1977). Respiratory muscle fatigue; a cause of respiratory failure. Clin. Sci. Mol. Med. 53:419–422.

Mahler, D.A., Weinberg, D.H., Well, C.K., and Feinstein, A.R. (1984). The measurement of dyspnea: contents, interobserver agreement, and physiologic correlates of two new clinical indexes. Chest 85:751–758.

Mahler, D.A., Harver, A., Rosiello, R.A., and Daubenspeck, J.A. (1989). Measurement of respiratory sensation in interstitial lung disease: evaluation of clinical dyspnea ratings and magnitude scaling. Chest 96:767–771.

McCloskey, D.I. (1978). Kinesthetic sensibility. Physiol. Rev. 58:763–820.

McCloskey, D.I., Ebeling, P., and Goodwin, G.M. (1974). Estimation of weights and tension and apparent involvement of a "sense of effort." Exp. Neurol. 42:220–232.

Mead, J. (1960). Control of respiratory frequency. J. Appl. Physiol. 15:325–336.

Milic-Emili, J., and Tyler, J.M. (1963). Relation between work output of respiratory muscles and end-tidal CO_2 tension. J. Appl. Physiol. 18:497–504.

Mueller, R., Petty, T., and Filley, G. (1970). Ventilation and arterial blood gas changes induced by pursed lip breathing. J. Appl. Physiol. 28:784–789.

Muza, R.M., Silverman, M.T., Grover, G.C., Hellerstein, H.K., and Kelsen, S.G. (1990). Comparison of scales used to quantitate the sense of effort in patients with chronic obstructive pulmonary disease. Am. Rev. Respir. Dis. 141:909–913.

Neubauer, J.A., Melton, J.E., and Edelman, N.H. (1990). Modulation of respiration during brain hypoxia. J. Appl. Physiol. 68:441–451.

Oku, Y., Saidel, G.M., Chonan, T., Altose, M.D., and Cherniack, N.S. (1991). Sensation and control of breathing: a dynamic model. Ann. Biomed. Eng. 19:251–272.

Oliven, A., Kelsen, S.G., Deal, E.C., and Cherniack, N.S. (1983). Mechanisms underlying CO_2 retention during flow resistive loading in patients with chronic obstructive pulmonary disease. J. Clin. Invest. 7:1442–1449.

Oliven, A., Cherniack, N.S., Deal, E.C., and Kelsen, S.G. (1987). The effect of acute bronchoconstriction on respiratory activity in patients with chronic obstructive pulmonary disease. Am. Rev. Respir. Dis. 131:236–241.

Orem, J., and Netick, A. (1986). Behavioral control of breathing in the cat. Brain Res. 366:238–253.

Otis, A.B. (1958). The work of breathing. Physiol. Rev. 34:449–458.

Patterson, J.L., Mullinax, P.F., Bain, T., Kreager, J.J., and Richardson, D.W. (1962). Carbon dioxide-induced dyspnea in a patient with respiratory muscle paralysis. Am. J. Med. 32:811–816.

Phillipson, E.A., and Bowes, G. (1986). Control of breathing during sleep. In: Handbook of Physiology: The Respiratory System. Edited by N.S. Cherniack and J.G. Widdicombe. American Physiological Society, Bethesda, MD, pp. 649–689.

Poon, C.S. (1982). Optimal control of ventilation in hypoxia, hypercapnia and exercise. In : Modelling and Control of Breathing. Edited by B.J. Whipp and D.M. Wiberg. Elsevier, New York, pp. 189–196.

Poon, C.S. (1987). Ventilatory control in hypercapnia and exercise: optimization hypothesis. J. Appl. Physiol. 62:2447–2459.

Poon, C.S., and Greene, J.G. (1985). Control of exercise hyperpnea during hypercapnia in humans. J. Appl. Physiol. 59:792–797.

Rebuck, A.S., and Slutsky, A.S. (1986). Control of breathing in diseases of the respiratory tract and lungs. In: Handbook of Physiology: Control of Breathing. Edited by N.S. Cherniack and J.G. Widdicombe. American Physiological Society, Bethesda, MD, pp. 771–792.

Remmers, J.E., Brook, J.G., III,and Tenney, S.M. (1968). Effect of controlled ventilation on the tolerable limit of hypercapnia. Respir. Physiol. 4:78–90.

Rigg, J.R.A., Inman, E.M., Saunders, N.A., Leeder, S.R., and Jones, N.L. (1977). Interaction of mental factors with hypercapnic ventilatory drive in man. Clin. Sci. Mol. Med. 52:269–275.

Roussos, C., and Macklem, P.T. (1977). Diaphragmatic fatigue in man. J. Appl. Physiol. 43:187–197.

Santiago, T.V., Remolina, C., Scoles, V., III, and Edelman, N.H. (1981). Endorphins and the control of breathing. N. Engl. J. Med. 304:1190–1195.
Saunders, N.A., Heilpern, S., and Rebuck, A.S. (1972). Relation between personality and ventilatory response to carbon dioxide in normal subjects: a role in asthma. Br. Med. J. 1:719–721.
Scardella, A.T., Parisi, R.A., Phair, D.K., Santiago, T.V., and Edelman, N.H. (1986). The role of endogenous opioids in the ventilatory response to acute flow-resistive loads. Am. Rev. Respir. Dis. 133:26–31.
Schwartzstein, R.M.,Lahive, K., Pope, A., Steinbrook, R.A., Leith, D.E., Weiss, J.W., Fencl, V., and Weinberger, S.E. (1987). Detection of hypercapnia by normal subjects. Clin. Sci. 73:333–335.
Schwartzstein, R.M., Simon, P.M., Weiss, J.W., Fencl, V., and Weinberger, S.E. (1989). Breathlessness induced by dissociation between ventilation and chemical drive. Am. Rev. Respir. Dis. 139:1231–1237.
Sears, T.A. (1971) Breathing: a sensori-motor act. Sci. Basis Med. Annu. Rev. 129–147.
Sharp, J.T., Druz, W.S., Moisan, T., Foster, J., and Machnach, W.C. (1980). Postural relief of dyspnea in severe chronic obstructive pulmonary disease. Am. Rev. Respir. Dis. 122:201–211.
Shea, S.A., Walter, J., Pelley, C., Murphy, K., and Guz, A. (1987). The effect of visual and auditory stimuli upon resting ventilation in man. Respir. Physiol. 68:345–357.
Simon, P.M., Pope, A., Lahive, K., Steinbrook, R.A., Schwartzstein, R.M., Weiss, S.W., Fencl, V., and Weinberger, S.E. (1989a). Naloxone does not alter response to hypercapnia or resistive loading in chronic obstructive pulmonary disease. Am. Rev. Respir. Dis. 139:134–138.
Simon, P.M., Schwartzstein, R.M., Weiss, J.W., Lahive, K., Fencl, V., Teghtsoonian, M., and Weinberger, S.E. (1989b). Distinguishable sensations of breathlessness induced in normal volunteers. Am. Rev. Respir. Dis. 140:1021–1027.
Sorli, J., Grassino, A., Lorange, G., and Milic-Emili, J. (1978). Control of breathing. In: Breathing: Hering-Breuer Centenary Symposium. Edited by R. Porter. Churchill, London, pp. 159–175.
Stevens, S.S. (1957). On the psychophysical law. Psychol. Rev. 64:153–181.
Strohl, K.P., Cherniack, N.S., and Gothe, B. (1986). Physiological basis of therapy for sleep apnea. Am. Rev. Respir. Dis. 134:791–802.
Stubbing, D.G., Killian, K.J., and Campbell, E.J.M. (1981). The quantification of respiratory sensations by normal subjects. Respir. Physiol. 44:251–260.
Tack, M., Altose, M.D., and Cherniack, N.S. (1981). Effect of aging on respiratory sensations produced by elastic loads. J. Appl. Physiol. 50:844–850.
Tack, M., Altose, M.D., and Cherniack, N.S. (1982). Effect of aging on the perception of resistive ventilatory loads. Am. Rev. Respir. Dis. 126:463–467.
Tack, M., Altose, M.D., and Cherniack, N.S. (1983). Effects of aging on sensation of respiratory force and displacement. J. Appl. Physiol. 55:1433–1440.
Ward, S.A., and Whipp, B.J. (1989). Effects of peripheral and central chemoreflex activation of the isopnoeic rating of breathing in exercising human. J. Physiol. (Lond.) 411:27–43.

Widdicombe, J.C., and Nadel, J.A. (1963). Airway volume, airway resistance, and the work force of breathing. J. Appl. Physiol. 18:863–868.
Wolkove, N., Altose, M.D., Kelsen, S.G., Kondapalli, P.G., and Cherniack, N.S. (1981). Perception of changes in breathing in normal human subjects. J. Appl. Physiol. 50: 78–83.
Yamashiro, S.M., and Grodins, F.S. (1971). Optimal regulation of respiratory overflow. J. Appl. Physiol. 30:597–602.
Yamashiro, S.M., and Grodins, F.S. (1973). Respiratory cycle optimization in exercise. J. Appl. Physiol. 35:522–525.
Yamashiro, S.M., Daubenspeck, J.A., Lauritsen, T.N., and Grodins, F.S. (1975). Total work rate of breathing optimization in CO_2 inhalation and exercise. J. Appl. Physiol. 38:702–709.

10

Breathlessness in Chronic Obstructive Pulmonary Disease

DONALD A. MAHLER

Dartmouth Medical School
Lebanon, New Hampshire

I. Introduction

The major complaint of patients with chronic obstructive pulmonary disease (COPD) is dyspnea on exertion. This symptom usually worsens slowly over time (months to years) because of disease progression and/or the decline in lung function with aging. In many cases the patient ignores or denies any impact of dyspnea on performance of daily activities. Rather, he or she attributes difficulty in breathing to "getting old" and/or "being out of shape." However, breathlessness almost always represents cardiorespiratory dysfunction or deconditioning and is not simply a consequence of aging (Manning et al., 1992).

Patients usually have great difficulty describing the experience of dyspnea. Recent studies by Simon and colleagues (1989, 1990) and Elliott et al. (1991) indicate that breathlessness can encompass multiple sensations. Simon et al. (1990) reported that patients with COPD (mean ± standard deviation, SD, age, 65 ± 10 years) selected the descriptors "work" and "hunger" to characterize their shortness of breath (Table 1). In addition, some patients with COPD report that breathing difficulty is appreciated more during inspiration than expiration (Suero and Woolf, 1970; O'Connell and Campbell, 1976). This observation may relate to the pathophysiological consequences of hyperinflation associated with severe

Table 1 Descriptors of Breathlessness Reported by 16 Patients with COPD

Work	Hunger
My breathing requires effort.	I feel a hunger for more air.
My breathing requires more work.	I cannot get enough air.

Source: From Simon et al., 1990.

airflow obstruction. Hyperinflation leads to increased elastic recoil, increased intrinsic—or auto—positive end-expiratory pressure, and shortening of the vertical muscle fibers of the diaphragm. To inspire an adequate tidal volume, the patient with severe COPD must generate sufficient negative pleural pressure to overcome the added elastic load using predominantly the diaphragm muscle, which is operating at a mechanical disadvantage.

Rochester et al. (1991) suggested that chronic airflow obstruction exerts a dual effect on respiratory muscle function. Initially, added resistive and/or elastic loads may lead to musculature hypertrophy and augmented strength. Similowski et al. (1991) showed that patients with severe COPD may have normal strength of the diaphragm. With progression of disease, atrophy and decreased respiratory muscle strength may develop.

Alterations in the pattern of ventilatory muscle recruitment may occur in response to respiratory muscle dysfunction. For example, Martinez et al. (1990) reported that with increasing airflow obstruction there is a change from pleural pressure (Ppl) being generated by the diaphragm to a situation in which most of the Ppl is developed by the rib cage inspiratory muscles along with a substantial contribution by the muscles of expiration. The authors speculate that dyspnea relates to the shift in the pattern of ventilatory muscle recruitment from the diaphragm to the rib cage inspiratory muscles.

Furthermore, it is commonly reported that patients with COPD experience dyspnea while performing relatively simple tasks involving the upper extremities (Celli et al., 1986). Upper torso muscles have both rib cage and humeral-shoulder girdle attachments that provide combined respiratory and postural actions depending on the fixation point for motion. When a patient with severe COPD performs unsupported arm activities, such as washing, lifting, and combing hair, the contribution of the upper chest musculature to ventilation may be reduced. Even trivial tasks may require increased work or effort of the diaphragm and other respiratory muscles and thereby lead to dyspnea.

Patients with severe COPD develop two major breathing strategies during exertion in an effort to compensate for impaired ventilatory mechanics: dynamic hyperinflation and prolongation of expiration. Dynamic hyperinflation is manifest as an increase in end-expiratory lung volume; this creates an inspiratory threshold load and a mechanical disadvantage for the diaphragm (O'Donnell and Webb, 1993). Prolongation of expiration requires an increase in mean inspiratory flow to sustain a greater minute ventilation during exercise. These alterations in the mechanics of breathing create added demands on the respiratory muscles, particularly the diaphragm, and contribute to perceived intensity of breathlessness (O'Donnell and Webb, 1993).

This brief description focuses on the role of the respiratory muscles as a major factor contributing to breathlessness in COPD. Certainly, chemoreceptors, mechanoreceptors, and processing and integration of neural impulses within the central nervous system can also modulate the sensation of breathlessness in chronic airflow obstruction. These and other potential mechanisms contributing to respiratory sensation are reviewed extensively in previous chapters of this volume. However, it is plausible that abnormalities in the mechanics of breathing associated with severe COPD adversely affect the properties and function of the diaphragm and other respiratory muscles and thereby contribute to a sense or feeling of increased work and air hunger during breathing.

II. Clinical Assessment

A. History

The patient should be questioned about specific qualities of the breathlessness experience. Although many patients have difficulty describing what it feels like to be breathless, it is possible to provide a list of descriptor phrases from which the patient selects the appropriate characteristics (see Chap. 6) (Simon et al., 1990; Elliott et al., 1991). With a selection process it may then be possible to establish more closely a clinical diagnosis for the cause of breathlessness.

Physical activity has an important impact on the severity of dyspnea. Pertinent questions include the following. What impact does breathlessness have on your ability to work, participate in recreation, and perform activities of daily living? What activities or tasks have you stopped because of breathlessness? Although some patients may report being less breathless over a time period, one possible explanation is that the individual has reduced his or her daily activities. Furthermore, any change in functional status caused by the severity of breathlessness may be difficult for the symptomatic patient to recognize but may be obvious to family members and friends. Therefore, it is helpful to question the spouse or significant other to gain additional insight and/or confirm the patient's observations.

Body position can also influence breathlessness (Mahler, 1990a). For example, many patients with advanced COPD describe orthopnea, that is, dyspnea in the recumbent position. This symptom arises from alterations in gravitational forces in the recumbent position. There is elevation of the diaphragm and reduction in functional residual capacity (FRC) in the supine position. Although this leads to an increase in the length of the costal fibers of the diaphragm, an increase in Ppl is required to overcome the hydrostatic pressure of the abdomen. Abdominal "loading" may ensue in the supine position and contribute to breathing difficult. In addition, patients with COPD may have coronary artery disease caused by cigarette smoking as at least one risk factor. Left ventricular failure should also be considered as a cause for orthopnea in patients with COPD.

A small number of patients with severe COPD report some relief of dyspnea upon lying supine (Sharp et al., 1980). Postural improvement in breathlessness was related to enhanced diaphragmatic function; that is, the increased length of the vertical muscle fibers of the diaphragm was more beneficial than any increase in abdominal hydrostatic pressure (Sharp et al., 1980). Some patients with COPD may occasionally describe dyspnea in one lateral position but not in the contralateral position (trepopnea). The probable mechanism for trepopnea is regional ventilation-perfusion mismatching, which can then lead to positional hypoxemia and breathlessness.

Many patients with COPD report that breathing is the "worst" in the morning upon awakening from sleep (5–7 a.m.). Although marked diurnal fluctuation in lung function has been reported in patients with asthma, there is little information on diurnal changes in respiratory function in the COPD population. Morrison et al. (1992) found "no appreciable diurnal rhythm" (>20 L/minute) in peak expiratory flow rate in 20 selected patients with severe COPD over a 3 week period. Nocturnal hypoxemia, accumulation of secretions, and nadir levels of bronchodilator medications are probably the major factors contributing to breathlessness in the early morning. In fact, patients often complain that it takes several hours "to get going" in the morning because of being limited by dyspnea.

Pratter and colleagues (1989) examined the utility of a structured history and physical examination (using a 125-item questionnaire) to diagnose the causes of chronic dyspnea in a pulmonary subspeciality clinic. They found that a previous history of COPD was unreliable! The positive predictive value was only 45% (Pratter et al., 1989). This observation emphasizes the need for physiological testing to establish a specific diagnosis of COPD or an alternative cause of chronic dyspnea.

B. Physical Examination

Physical findings of the chest are usually normal in patients with COPD unless the forced expiratory volume in one second (FEV_1) is less than 50% of the predicted value (Stubbing et al., 1982). Physical signs of advanced COPD are listed in Table 2. The use of pursed-lips breathing is highly specific for obstructive airway disease. Many patients with severe airflow obstruction prefer the leaning forward

Table 2 Physical Abnormalities in Advanced Chronic Obstructive Pulmonary Disease

1. Tachypnea
2. Difficulty in completing sentences
3. Pursed-lips breathing
4. Use of accessory muscles of respiration (e.g., inspiratory contractions of the sternocleidomastoid muscles)
5. Leaning forward position with forearms resting on distal thighs
6. An increase in anterior-posterior chest diameter
7. Downward displacement of the diaphragm
8. Tracheal descent with inspiration
9. Recession of supraclavicular fossae during inspiration
10. Abnormal cardiac position (point of maximal impulse located in subxiphoid area)
11. Jugular venous distension
12. Diminished intensity of breath sounds
13. Wheezing during quiet breathing
14. Early-inspiratory crackles at lung bases
15. Prolonged expiratory time (>6 s during forced vital capacity maneuver)
16. Right ventricular heave; an increase in the pulmonic component of the second heart sound, right ventricular S3 gallop, and a murmur of tricuspid insufficiency indicate pulmonary hypertension

Source: From Mahler, 1992.

position with forearms resting on the thighs to provide some relief of breathlessness and to optimize diaphragmatic function (Sharp et al., 1980).

Auscultation of the chest is the most important part of the physical examination for evaluating COPD. Diminished intensity of breath sounds is probably the most reliable physical sign, especially in emphysema (Schneider and Anderson, 1965; Bohadana et al., 1978). Early inspiratory crackles at the posterior lung bases may be heard in some patients with COPD. The timing of crackles early in inspiration strongly suggests COPD, whereas middle to late inspiratory crackles are most common in interstitial lung disease and congestive heart failure (Nath and Capel, 1974). Forced expiratory time can be measured by placing the stethoscope over the trachea and listening to audible airflow while timing the duration; this is a simple technique to detect airflow obstruction (>6 s). Wheezing during tidal breathing is a frequent sign of airway obstruction, although obstruction can be present without wheezing.

The neck veins should be inspected to estimate right ventricular pressure. If the patient is positioned with his or her upper body elevated to an angle of 45°, the height of the jugular venous pulse at end expiration above the sternal notch can be used to quantify right ventricular filling pressure. A level greater than 4.5 cm indicates elevated right ventricular pressure (Hill, 1987). The heart sounds may be faint, especially in patients with severe hyperinflation. A right ventricular heave, an increase in the pulmonic component of the second heart sound, a right ventricular S3 gallop, and a murmur of tricuspid regurgitation reflect pulmonary hypertension and/or cor pulmonale.

C. Laboratory Testing

Pulmonary function testing is indicated to diagnose obstructive airway disease. A decreased FEV_1 and FEV_1/forced vital capacity (FVC) ratio, together with a consistent history (especially cigarette smoking), physical examination, and possibly other confirmatory laboratory data, is required to diagnose COPD (Medical Section of the American Lung Association, 1991).

Although additional testing is *not* necessary for the diagnosis of COPD, certain physiological tests may be useful to understand further the severity of breathlessness. For example, severe COPD is generally associated with an increase in FRC, which influences the relative position of the diaphragm. Both bronchoconstriction and physical exertion cause dynamic hyperinflation, which places the diaphragm at a mechanical (length-tension) disadvantage. Consequent altered mechanics of breathing may directly or indirectly contribute to increased dyspnea. Accordingly, it may be helpful to measure lung volumes, including FRC and total lung capacity (TLC), to determine the severity of hyperinflation.

Respiratory muscle function influences the severity of breathlessness at rest as well as during exercise (O'Connell and Campbell, 1976; LeBlanc et al., 1986; Mahler and Wells, 1988; Rochester, 1991). Measurement of both inspiratory ($P_{I_{max}}$) and expiratory ($P_{E_{max}}$) mouth pressures provides a noninvasive estimate of respiratory muscle strength. In severe COPD, $P_{I_{max}}$ may be reduced as a result of hyperinflation, whereas $P_{E_{max}}$ should remain normal (Rochester, 1991). Diminished values for both $P_{I_{max}}$ and $P_{E_{max}}$ suggest either inadequate effort or global respiratory muscle weakness. Generalized muscular weakness and malnourishment may develop with advancing age and progressive COPD; these conditions may then contribute to respiratory muscle weakness.

Oxygen saturation (SaO_2 should be measured by oximetry in all patients with moderate to severe COPD to estimate adequacy of oxygenation. As previously described (Chap. 10), hypoxemia stimulates ventilation and increases the intensity of breathlessness (Lane et al., 1987). Measurement of arterial blood gas tensions may also be appropriate to examine the partial pressure of carbon dioxide (Pa_{CO_2}) and to determine acid-base status.

Cardiopulmonary exercise testing (CPEX) attempts to simulate or reproduce daily activities that provoke breathlessness and other symptoms and can provide valuable clinical information about the specific cause of the patient's functional limitation. Although patients with COPD had reduced work capacity compared with age-matched normal subjects, the median intensity was 6 (severe to very severe) for dyspnea and 7 (very severe) for leg effort at peak exercise in both groups (Killian et al., 1992). In general, patients with mild to moderate COPD report higher values for leg discomfort or effort than dyspnea (Mahler and Harver, 1988; Killian et al., 1992), whereas dyspnea was the most frequent limiting symptom in patients with severe COPD (Killian et al., 1992). These findings emphasize the contributing role of deconditioning as a factor complicating exercise intolerance in patients with COPD.

The results of CPEX can be used (1) to determine exercise capacity and corresponding level of dyspnea; (2) to evaluate for oxygen desaturation; (3) to look for cardiac arrhythmia or ischemia; and (4) to prescribe exercise at a specific intensity (percentage) of exercise capacity and/or a specific rating of dyspnea.

D. Measurement of Dyspnea

The severity of dyspnea is not, unfortunately, routinely measured in medical practice. Nevertheless, I believe that it is important to quantify the intensity of breathing difficulty for three reasons: (1) dyspnea is the patient's major complaint, and clinical ratings represent a distinct dimension not provided by pulmonary function tests (Mahler and Harver, 1992) or magnitude estimation of respiratory loads (Mahler et al., 1987); (2) clinical dyspnea ratings influence and predict general health status to a greater extent than do physiological measurements (Mahler et al, 1992); and (3) a baseline value is necessary to measure response to specific therapy.

Several clinical instruments are available and have been shown to meet the criteria of validity, reliability and responsiveness (Mahler and Harver, 1990). Either the visual analog scale (VAS) (Aitken, 1969) or the 0–10 category ratio (CR-10) scale (Borg, 1982) is an appropriate tool to assess the acute, or short-term, efficacy of a particular medication or intervention (Fig. 1). The patient usually selects a rating on the VAS or CR-10 scale based on a specific task, such as walking, or over a specific time period, for example, the past 24 h.

Multidimensional instruments are preferred for a more comprehensive evaluation of dyspnea over a longer period of time. The baseline and transition dyspnea indexes (Mahler et al., 1984) and the dyspnea component of the chronic respiratory questionnaire (CRQ) (Guyatt et al., 1987) are established tools that can demonstrate clinically important changes in dyspnea as a result of therapy (Table 3). These instruments are relatively brief to complete and involve minimal expense.

An alternative approach is to measure breathlessness during steady-state or incremental CPEX to obtain more direct estimates of the stimulus-response (dyspnea) relationship (Killian et al., 1992; Mahler, 1992). Studies in normal subjects and patients with COPD have used the VAS and/or the CR-10 scale to rate dyspnea during exercise tests (Adams et al., 1985; Muza et al., 1990; Mador and

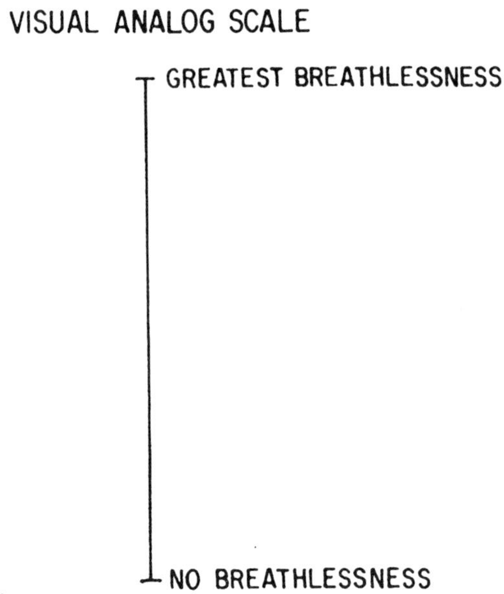

(A)

CATEGORY RATIO SCALE

0	Nothing at all
0.5	Very, very slight (just noticeable)
1	Very slight
2	Slight (light)
3	Moderate
4	Somewhat severe
5	Severe (heavy)
6	
7	Very severe
8	
9	
10	Very, very severe (almost max)
•	Maximal

(B)

Kufel, 1992; Mahler et al, 1991; Wilson and Jones, 1989). Wilson and Jones (1991) reported that normal subjects can differentiate between the intensity and distress of breathlessness during CPEX. It is important to provide clear and concise instructions to subjects and patients to obtain appropriate ratings. The slope and intercept of the $\dot{V}_E$ (minute ventilation)-dyspnea or work-dyspnea relationship obtained from an incremental CPEX can be calculated to summarize the data.

III. Treatment of Breathlessness

What are the major goals of therapy for patients with COPD? The traditional focus has been on improvement in lung function, particularly FVC and FEV_1 (Burrows and Earle, 1969). However, the dyspneic patient usually seeks medical care for symptom relief and for improvement in daily activities. Therefore, the health care provider should measure both physiological and symptom outcomes when prescribing treatment and again for evaluating the responses.

The goals of therapy for patients with COPD are to decrease the frequency, intensity, and distress of dyspnea and to improve functional status. However, standard treatments for patients with COPD have not always considered dyspnea as an outcome (Medical Section of the American Lung Association, 1991). For example, smoking cessation is essential to alter the deteriorating course of COPD. It is reasonable to assume (although unproven) that dyspnea will not be as severe in a patient if the individual stops smoking cigarettes. Another consideration is corticosteroid therapy. Most recommendations have emphasized the importance of demonstrating physiological improvement with a 2–4 week trial of prednisone because of the risk of various side effects with prolonged treatment (Mendella et al., 1982). However, should the health care provider stop oral corticosteroid therapy after a short-term trial if a patient reports less breathlessness and experiences enhanced performance of daily activities but there is no change in lung function? Finally, diuretic therapy is often effective in reducing the sense of dyspnea in patients with COPD who have right heart failure. These observations indicate that further studies are needed to evaluate the efficacy of various "standard" therapies on the relief of dyspnea.

A. Breathing Strategies

Pursed-Lips Breathing

Many patients with COPD spontaneously adopt pursed-lips breathing (PLB) to reduce dyspnea. With PLB there is an increase in tidal volume and a decrease in respiratory rate (Mueller et al., 1970), which results in an improvement in oxygen

---

Figure 1 (A) The visual analog scale (VAS) and (B) the 0–10 category ratio scale are instruments used to measure the severity of breathlessness.

Table 3 Multidimensional Clinical Instruments for Measuring Dyspnea[a]

Components and scores for the baseline and transition dyspnea indexes (from Mahler et al., 1984)	
Baseline dyspnea index	
Functional impairment	0–4
Magnitude of task	0–4
Magnitude of effort	*0–4*
Baseline focal score	0–12
Transition dyspnea index	
Change in functional impairment	−3 to 3
Change in magnitude of task	−3 to 3
Change in magnitude of effort	*−3 to 3*
Transition focal score	−9 to 9
Dyspnea component of chronic respiratory questionnaire (from Guyatt et al., 1987): activity (individual specific)	
A	1–7
B	1–7
C	1–7
D	1–7
E	*1–7*
CRQ dyspnea score	5–35

[a]For the baseline dyspnea index (BDI), specific criteria are listed for each of the five different grades for the three components. For the transition dyspnea index (TDI), specific criteria are listed for each of the seven different grades (changes) for the three components. An interviewer selects the grade for the BDI and TDI based on the responses of the patient to routine questions as part of a standard history. For the dyspnea component of the chronic respiratory questionnaire, the patient determines the five most important activities (A–E) that cause dyspnea and affect daily life by self-selection and by using a list of 26 activities. The patient indicates the severity based on a 1 (extremely short of breath) to 7 (not at all short of breath) scale.

saturation (Tiep et al., 1986). Breslin (1992) reported a change in the pattern of chest wall muscle recruitment (an increase in rib cage and accessory muscle recruitment during inspiration and expiration, an increase in abdominal muscle recruitment during expiration, and a decrease in inspiratory time/total respiratory time), along with improve ventilation, with PLB. Enhanced efficiency in respiratory muscle force generation and/or improved ventilation may contribute to less dyspnea in patients who use PLB. An alterative explanation is that PLB modulates receptors in the upper airway, for example, the oral mucosa, independently of changes in ventilation and pattern of breathing to reduce the severity of dyspnea (Simon et al., 1991). Finally, the greater sense of control, that is, less anxiety and panic, over breathing distress reported by patients using PLB could also relieve breathlessness.

All patients with COPD who experience dyspnea should be instructed in PLB. Standard instructions are available (Table 4). Tiep et al. (1986) has recommended that oximetry be used as an adjunct to PLB technique for temporarily improving oxygenation and lending physiological support for its clinical application.

Posture

Certain body positions may relieve dyspnea in patients with severe COPD. The leaning forward position with support of the upper extremities placed on the thighs or on a table appears to improve the length-tension relationship of the diaphragm and thereby reduce breathing difficulty (Sharp et al., 1980). Also, stabilization of the upper extremities allows specific humeral-shoulder girdle muscles to contribute to respiration rather than postural function. Occasionally, some patients with COPD may experience a reduction in dyspnea when lying supine.

Relaxation

Progressive muscle relaxation (PMR) is a technique that can be used to decrease the anxiety associated with breathlessness and to help the patient gain control during periods of breathing distress. Components of relaxation techniques include a quiet environment, a comfortable position, a passive attitude, a word or imagery repeated or thought of in a systematic manner, paced, slow breathing through pursed lips, and systematic tensing and relaxing of parts of the body (Bernstein and Borkovec, 1973). Refroe (1988) observed that PMR was more effective than no therapy in reducing dyspnea and anxiety for patients with COPD at each of four sessions. It is reasonable to encourage the symptomatic patient to practice relaxation every day to prepare for episodes of breathing difficulty. Other psychophysiological techniques that can be used to relieve dyspnea are visual imagery, biofeedback, and meditation (Sexton, 1987).

B. Chest Physiotherapy

Chest percussion, forced coughing, and incentive spirometry are components of chest physiotherapy used to promote expectoration of lower respiratory tract

Table 4 Patient Instructions for Pursed-Lips Breathing

1.	Breathe in through your nose slowly and deeply.
2.	Purse your lips as if to whistle.
3.	Breathe out slowly through pursed lips, taking twice as long to exhale as to inhale.

secretions and to prevent atelectasis. The modalities are more commonly prescribed for patients with predominantly chronic bronchitis. Although many patients report improvement in breathing after expectoration of sputum, the efficacy of chest physiotherapy on relieving dyspnea has not been formally evaluated.

C. Coping and Self-Care

Various coping and self-care strategies are helpful to control and, it is hoped, to lessen the impact of dyspnea on daily activities (Table 5) (Kohlman-Carrieri and Janson-Bjerklie, 1990). *Coping* refers to the patient's response to a new or different situation that requires modification of old strategies or development of new strategies. *Self-care* concerns repetitive use of strategies or efforts that have been effective in the past. Successful coping with breathlessness requires an individualized approach specific to life situations.

D. Environmental Control

Extreme ambient air conditions frequently contribute to complaints of dyspnea in patients with COPD. Hot, humid weather presumably causes breathlessness because airborne irritants and pollutants become more concentrated in the ambient air. Cold and dry weather may trigger bronchoconstriction. Many patients attempt to avoid these conditions by modifying their activities and by staying indoors, where it is possible to control the indoor environment.

In addition, patients with severe COPD frequently describe "breathing easier" when there is air movement. These individuals may sit by an open window to experience a breeze of air or have a fan blow air toward the face. Schwartzstein

Table 5 Coping and Self-care Strategies for Reducing Dyspnea

1.	Desensitization
2.	Relaxation and psychophysical techniques
3.	Activity modification and energy conservation
4.	Eating and meal preparation
5.	Social support
6.	Increased knowledge and education
7.	Symptom monitoring
8.	Contracting for goals
9.	Attitudes and life change
10.	Self-management of medications

Source: Adapted from Kohlman-Carrieri and Janson-Bjerklie, 1990.

et al. (1987) found that healthy individuals reported less dyspnea breathing hypercapnic air through an inspiratory resistance when cold air was directed against the cheek. Furthermore, Spence et al. (1993) reported that breathing cold air reduced the severity of breathlessness in patients with stable but severe COPD. Based on these findings, it is possible that receptors on the face or in the oral mucosa are involved in the perception of dyspnea.

E. Bronchodilators

Dull and Alexander (1984) previously suggested that the acute response to an inhaled bronchodilator can be used to predict the efficacy of chronic administration of a bronchodilator. However, there are at least two major arguments against this recommendation. First, reproducibility of bronchodilator response is poor (Guyatt et al., 1988). Second, acute response to an inhaled β-agonist does not identify patients with COPD who achieve a physiological and/or symptomatic benefit with bronchodilator therapy (Guyatt et al., 1988; Berger and Smith, 1988; Morrison et al., 1992). The concept of "fixed" or "nonreversible" airflow obstruction is a misnomer (Drazen and Gerard, 1989), and therapeutic decisions should not be made on the basis of acute bronchodilator responsiveness (Anthonisen et al., 1986). Accordingly, bronchodilator medication(s) should be prescribed for all symptomatic patients with COPD with the goals of relieving dyspnea and enhancing functional status (Pratter and Irwin, 1988; Mahler, 1990b).

β-2-Adrenergic Agonist

Many patients with COPD report subjective relief of breathlessness after use of an inhaled β-2-adrenergic medication. Dullinger and colleagues (1986) observed a significant improvement in dyspnea on the VAS after 1 week of inhaled metaproterenol given every 3 h while awake compared with an inhaled placebo. Similarly, Guyatt et al. (1987b) found less breathlessness on a VAS at completion of a 6 minute walking test with 2 puffs of albuterol four times a day for 2 weeks. In each study significant bronchodilation was observed with inhaled β_2-adrenergic therapy in the patients with COPD.

Anticholinergic Therapy

Hay and colleagues (1992) evaluated the acute effects of a single administration of 2 puffs of inhaled oxitropium compared with placebo in a double-blind, crossover trial in 32 patients with severe COPD. Ratings of dyspnea during cycle ergometry were reduced with anticholinergic medication along with a corresponding small increase in FEV_1 (0.16 ± 0.70 L). Certainly, additional studies are necessary to evaluate the long-term benefits of anticholinergic therapy on the severity of breathlessness in patients with COPD.

Theophylline

A total of six randomized, placebo-controlled, crossover studies have investigated the effects of sustained-release theophylline for 1–8 weeks on ratings of dyspnea using a standard instrument for measuring dyspnea in patients with COPD. All these clinical trials included patient populations with "nonreversible" airway obstruction based on either $\leqslant 15\%$ (Mahler et al., 1985; Chrystyn et al., 1988; Murciano et al., 1989) or $\leqslant 25\%$ (Eaton et al., 1982; Dullinger et al., 1986; Guyatt et al., 1987b) improvement in FEV_1 after an inhaled β_2-adrenergic agonist.

A significant improvement in dyspnea ratings (four studies) or a positive trend (two studies) was observed with theophylline therapy using either the VAS or the baseline and transition dyspnea indexes to quantify the severity of the symptom (Mahler, 1990b). Theophylline contributed to modest bronchodilation, with an increase in FEV_1 ranging between 10 and 15% (Mahler, 1990b). In addition, Chrystyn et al. (1988) reported that both trapped gas volume (the difference between TLC measured by body plethysmography and that measured by helium dilution) and FRC showed a progressive linear decrease with increasing serum theophylline concentrations. These investigators proposed that declines in trapped gas volume and FRC would improve the mechanical advantage of the diaphragm and chest wall muscles without necessarily affecting muscular contractility or fatiguability. Murciano and colleagues (1989) examined the effect of theophylline on respiratory muscle function as measured by the ratio of Ppl during tidal inspiration to that generated by a maximal static inspiratory effort (Ppl_{max}). The Ppl/Ppl_{max} ratio improved after 2 months of treatment with theophylline compared with placebo ($p < 0.0001$). Furthermore, there was a significant correlation between the changes in the Ppl/Ppl_{max} ratio and those in the dyspnea score (using a VAS) during theophylline treatment ($r = 0.68$, $p < 0.001$). Finally, Jaeschke et al. (1991) indicated that PI_{max} increased with theophylline compared with placebo in the previously reported study by Guyatt et al. (1987b). The alleviation of dyspnea was statistically related to both bronchodilation (changes in FEV_1; $r = 0.50$, $p < 0.001$) and enhanced respiratory muscle function (changes in PL_{max}; $r = 0.40$, $p < 0.001$).

These collective results demonstrate that theophylline relieves dyspnea in patients with symptomatic COPD. The apparent mechanisms for reduction in breathlessness are modest bronchodilation and/or improvement in respiratory muscle function. Enhanced respiratory muscle performance with theophylline may be a result of the mechanical length-tension advantage associated with the decrease in lung volumes (FRC and trapped gas) and/or direct effects on muscle contractility.

Corticosteroids

The results of published studies on the effectiveness of corticosteroid therapy for treating patients with stable but symptomatic COPD are unclear. Callahan et al.

(1991) performed a meta-analysis and reported that patients with stable COPD receiving oral corticosteroid therapy have a 20% or greater improvement in baseline FEV_1 approximately 10% more often than similar patients receiving placebo. More recent investigations demonstrated both positive (Thompson et al., 1992; Kerstjens et al., 1992) and negative (Wempe et al., 1992) results for inhaled or oral corticosteroids on airway inflammation and hyperresponsiveness. However, none of these randomized, placebo-controlled studies examined dyspnea as an outcome measure.

Improvement in lung function has been considered critical for demonstrating efficacy of corticosteroid therapy in patients with COPD for two reasons: (1) the drug can affect an individual's sense of well-being and mood, causing euphoria or depression in some patients; and (2) side effects are common with prolonged use. On the other hand, it is possible that corticosteroids reduce dyspnea without necessarily causing bronchodilation, for example by prevention of bronchoconstriction (Kerstjens et al., 1992; Dompeling et al., 1993). In addition, corticosteroids could act within the central nervous system to relieve breathlessness. These examples of possible mechanisms of action illustrate the problem of focusing on lung function as an absolute criterion for evaluating corticosteroid therapy in patients with COPD. At the present time health care providers should employ a trial of corticosteroid therapy in individual patients who remain limited by dyspnea but are otherwise receiving "optimal" therapy.

F. Oxygen

Hypoxemia stimulates peripheral chemoreceptors to increase ventilation and is frequently associated with breathlessness. Breathing supplemental oxygen reduces ventilatory drive, $\dot{V}_E$, and tidal volume (Criner and Celli, 1987) and is clearly indicated for patients with resting hypoxemia (Nocturnal Oxygen Therapy Trial Group, 1980). There are six controlled studies evaluating the effects of supplemental oxygen on dyspnea in patients with COPD. Two investigations examined the benefits of oxygen in patients with hypoxemia *at rest*. Liss and Grant (1988) studied 8 patients with COPD (mean ± SD arterial oxygen pressure, Pa_{O_2}, 53 ± 7 mm Hg); no flow, air at 2 and 4 L/minute, and O_2 at 2 and 4 L/minute were given through a nasal cannula for 5 minutes before having the patient select a breathlessness rating on a VAS. The authors found that reduction in breathlessness by nasal oxygen was the result of a placebo effect, not related to either gas flow or an increase in Pa_{O_2}. However, 5 minutes may be too short a time to observe physiological and/or perceptive adaptations. Although there was considerable variability in individual responses, breathlessness was actually lower with 4 L/minute of air (39 ± 23 versus 50 ± 24). Swinburn and colleagues (1991) administered 28% oxygen or air through a face mask for 10 minutes, with each gas given twice in a randomized sequence. There was a significant decrease in dyspnea with oxygen compared with air in the VAS (30 ± 5 versus 46 ± 6) in 12 patients with hypoxemic COPD (mean ± standard error of the mean, SEM, Pa_{O_2}, 50 ± 4 mm Hg; Fig. 2). Furthermore, there was a corresponding reduction in $\dot{V}_E$ during oxygen breathing as measured by magnetometers.

There is consistent evidence for reduction in dyspnea during exertion even in patients who may have acceptable levels of oxygenation at rest. Woodcock et al. (1981) found that patients with emphysema reported significantly less breathlessness and walked farther while breathing O_2 at 4 L/minute compared with air. The degree of improvement did not correlate with lung function, arterial blood gases, or exercise capacity, and no clinical information predicted those patients who benefited most except by testing. Lane et al. (1987) reported a significant decrease in VAS scores for breathlessness with supplemental oxygen that could not be completely explained by corresponding reductions in ventilation. Davidson et al. (1988) observed a 25% decline in dyspnea ratings on a VAS during endurance cycle ergometry in 17 patients with COPD who had an SaO_2 of 94% at rest but desaturated to 88% during exercise. In addition, supplemental oxygen improved endurance cycling time and mean speed achieved during a 6 minute walking test. Finally, Dean and colleagues (1992) studied 12 patients with severe COPD who had Pa_{O_2} of 71 ± 3 mm Hg (mean ± SEM) and noted significant decreases in dyspnea scores on a VAS, $\dot{V}_E$, and heart rate while breathing 40% O_2 through a mouthpiece compared with air. Exercise duration also improved with O_2, and the increase in exercise capacity correlated with the decrease in dyspnea ratings (r = 0.66, p = 0.001).

There are various possible mechanisms whereby oxygen relieves breath-

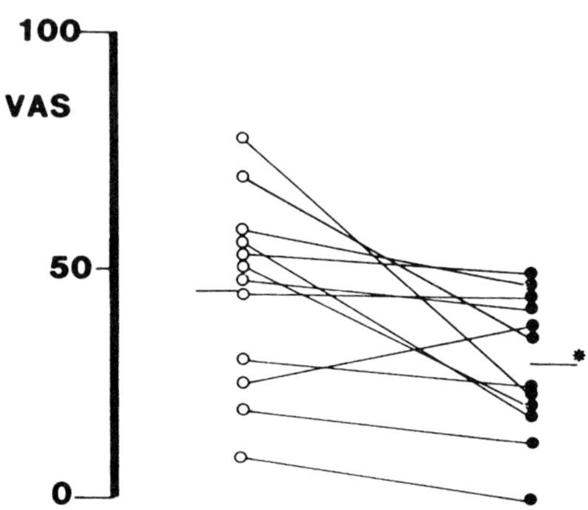

Figure 2 Effects of breathing air (open circles) and 28% oxygen (closed circles) on ratings of breathlessness using the visual analog scale (VAS) in 12 patients with hypoxemic chronic obstructive pulmonary disease. (From Swinburn et al., 1991.)

lessness. Flow-sensitive receptors in the upper airway may be stimulated by the flow of oxygen and thereby influence respiration and possibly dyspnea (McBride and Whitelaw, 1981). Supplementary oxygen may diminish dyspnea by directly decreasing peripheral chemoreceptor activity. Certainly, oxygen administration is associated with a decrease in ventilation at rest as well as with exertion (Vyas et al., 1971; Swinburn et al., 1991). In addition, oxygen may enhance respiratory muscle function. Bye et al. (1985) showed that oxygen delayed the onset of respiratory muscle fatigue, and Criner and Celli (1987) reported that O_2 altered ventilatory muscle recruitment during exercise. These changes may decrease any dyspnea signal arising from the respiratory muscles. Finally, oxygen could alter the processing and integration of respiratory discomfort in the central nervous system without necessarily affecting physiological parameters. Most likely, the benefits of oxygen on respiratory sensation are related to multiple factors rather than a single explanation in symptomatic patients.

G. Exercise Reconditioning

Effect on Dyspnea

Controlled trials have demonstrated improvements in exercise and skill performance in patients with COPD as a result of exercise reconditioning programs (Ries, 1990). Five reports describe a decrease in the intensity of breathlessness in patients with symptomatic COPD after exercise training compared with a control group who did not participate in exercise training (McGavin et al., 1977; Sinclair and Ingram, 1980; Cockcroft, et al., 1981; Strijbos et al., 1989; Goldstein et al., 1994). However, only the studies by Strijbos and colleagues (1989) and Goldstein et al. (1994) used an appropriate instrument for quantifying dyspnea. Strijbos et al. (1984) randomized patients with COPD into a treatment group (n = 30) and a control group (n = 15). After 12 weeks of exercise reconditioning, relaxation, and breathing training, the treatment group had a substantial decrease in dyspnea scores during steady-state cycle ergometry ($p < 0.001$); in contrast, the control group (who participated in the same rehabilitation program but did not exercise) exhibited no change in breathlessness ratings (Fig. 3). Goldstein et al. (1994) showed significant improvement in dyspnea ratings using the BDI/TDI and the dyspnea component of the CRQ.

Possible mechanisms for the reduction in dyspnea with exercise reconditioning include physiological adaptations as well as desensitization. Exercise training can lead to significant declines in $\dot{V}_E$ and blood lactate levels, which provide a physiological basis or explanation for diminished dyspnea (Belman and Gaesser, 1991; Casaburi et al., 1991). Also, regular exercise training can enhance a patient's tolerance of breathing distress and provide reassurance that a moderate level of breathlessness is acceptable, that is, desensitization. In fact, Belman et al. (1991) showed that ratings of dyspnea progressively decreased in patients with COPD who performed repetitive exercise tests over a 10 day period, whereas

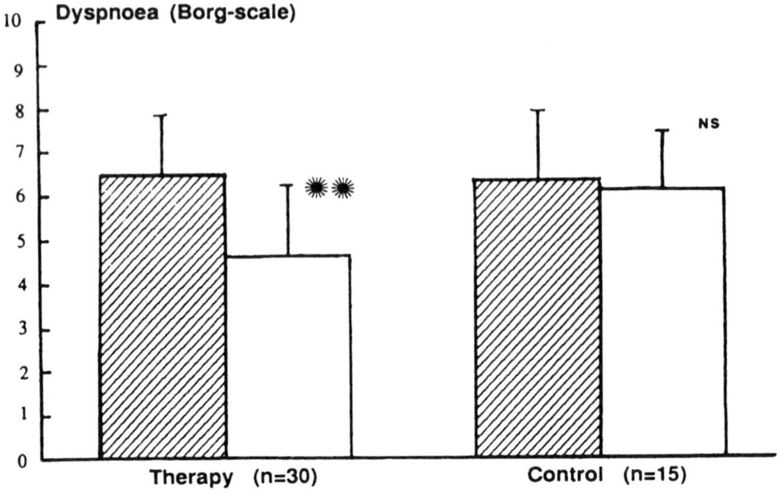

Figure 3 Scores for dyspnea on the 0–10 category ratio scale during steady-state exercise on the cycle ergometer before (matched bars) and after (open bars) a 12 week pulmonary rehabilitation program. The therapy group participated in breathing retraining, exercise reconditioning, and relaxing exercises twice a week for 2 h. The control group received breathing retraining and relaxing exercises but no exercise reconditioning. There was a significant decrease in ratings of dyspnea in the therapy group after the 12 week program ($p < 0.001$) but no change in the control group (p NS). (From Strijbos et al., 1989.)

physiological parameters stabilized after one or two tests. Additional benefits of regular exercise include enhanced sense of well-being and confidence.

Exercise Prescription

The major components of exercise prescription include type of exercise, frequency, intensity, and duration. At the present time there are no standardized guidelines for prescribing exercise training in patients with COPD. In general, recommendations established by the American College of Sports Medicine (1990) for quantity and quality of exercise for healthy adults are modified and applied to patients with chronic respiratory disease (American College of Sports Medicine, 1995).

Various types of exercise, such as, walking, cycling, and rowing, are appropriate for patients with COPD. Continuous exertion involving large muscle groups is important. Ideally, the individual patient trains the muscle groups involved in the activities that commonly provoke dyspnea. Low-impact exertion is preferred to reduce musculoskeletal injury. An indoor activity should be available when the weather conditions limit outdoor exercise.

The suggested frequency of exercise training is 3–5 days per week (American College of Sports Medicine Position Stand, 1990). An every-other-day schedule of exertion fits this recommendation and allows recovery after the training day.

There is controversy about the appropriate training intensity for patients with COPD. The recommended intensities range from a low of 50% of peak oxygen consumption ($\dot{V}O_2$) to a high of nearly maximal exercise capacity. The rationale for each of the two extreme intensities depends, in part, on the targeted outcome. There is clear evidence that a modest training intensity, approximately 50% of peak $\dot{V}O_2$, increases exercise performance in patients with COPD (Niederman et al., 1991). This training level can enhance compliance and reduce the risk of injury compared with high-intensity exercise. In contrast, Casaburi et al. (1991) suggested that patients with COPD need to train above the anaerobic threshold (AT) to achieve a physiological training response, that is, reduced $\dot{V}E$ and reduced lactic acidosis. On the other hand, Punzal et al. (1991) reported that patients with moderate to severe COPD can train at 95% of the maximal treadmill workload and that increases in exercise performance were independent of the ability to reach an AT.

I recommend an *initial* training intensity of about 50% of peak $\dot{V}O_2$, or peak power production, because many patients with severe COPD have been sedentary and may be reluctant or find it difficult to exercise at a high intensity at the start of an exercise reconditioning program. Both perceived intensity of dyspnea (Horowitz and Mahler, 1993) and a target heart rate obtained from results of a progressive incremental exercise test can be used to monitor the training sessions. This approach appears more realistic for patients who are training mostly on their own at home, whereas a higher training intensity may be feasible in a supervised exercise program in a clinic or hospital.

Both intensity and duration of training are interrelated. Low-intensity/long-duration training achieves physiological benefits comparable to those of high-intensity/short-duration exertion as long as the energy costs are equivalent. The recommended 20–60 minutes of continuous activity for healthy adults (American College of Sports Medicine, 1990) exceeds the ability of most patients with moderate to severe COPD who are deconditioned. A more reasonable target is 20–30 minutes of continuous exercise. A patient with severe COPD may initially be able to perform only 5 minutes of exercise before dyspnea or exhaustion limits further exertion. A repeated exercise-rest schedule may be required to increase endurance slowly and to promote confidence. Achievement of 20 minutes of exercise training may take weeks to months for certain patients.

Continuous Positive Airway Pressure (CPAP)

O'Donnell and colleagues (1988b) applied 4–5 cm H_2O CPAP during steady-state submaximal exercise in five patients with COPD and observed a consistent reduction in dyspnea but "harder" breathing when the CPAP was removed. Separation of the pressures into continuous positive inspiratory (CPIP) or continuous positive expiratory (CPEP) pressures revealed, in general, symptomatic relief with CPIP and worsening of dyspnea with CPEP. These investigators suggested that CPAP relieved dyspnea primarily by counterbalancing the threshold elastic load and thereby unloading the inspiratory muscles (O'Donnell et al., 1988b). In a separate study, O'Donnell et al. (1988a) showed an improvement in exercise endurance with CPAP in patients with COPD chiefly by alleviating exertional dyspnea (Fig. 4).

Petrof et al. (1990) investigated the effect of CPAP in patients with severe COPD by measuring esophageal (Pes) and gastric (Pga) pressures during cycle ergometry. Of eight patients five reported a reduction in breathlessness with 7.5–10 cm H_2O CPAP, and the amelioration of dyspnea was directly related to reductions in the pressure-time integral of Pes (reduced inspiratory muscle effort) and inversely related to increases in the pressure-time integral of Pga (increased expiratory muscle effort).

In summary, CPAP can reduce breathlessness in patients with COPD by unloading the inspiratory muscles. However, in some patients there may be substantial increases in expiratory muscle activity that could negate any relief of dyspnea experienced during inspiration (Petrof et al., 1990). Therefore, the level of CPAP must be individually titrated. Separate levels of inspiratory and expiratory pressure (BiPAP) or proportional assist ventilation (PAV) may be useful to unload the inspiratory muscles optimally and/or to avoid excessive expiratory pressure with the associated recruitment of expiratory abdominal muscles. The application of CPAP, BiPAP, or PAV may allow patients with COPD to experience less breathlessness during exercise training and thereby improve reconditioning beyond that achieved by standard exercise programs (Mahler and O'Donnell, 1991).

Upper Extremity Training

An exercise reconditioning program should include upper extremity training (American College of Sports Medicine, 1990). High-repetition and low-intensity efforts are generally recommended to develop endurance and strength of the arm and shoulder muscles. Ellis and Ries (1991) showed improvements in upper extremity exercise performance and reductions in ratings of breathlessness in an observational, uncontrolled study of 72 patients with COPD. Simpson et al. (1992) reported significant improvement in the dyspnea score of the CRQ questionnaire in 14 patients with COPD who performed resistance training (weight lifting) of upper and lower limb muscles compared with a control group.

Upper extremity exercise can include gravity resistance and proprioceptive neuromuscular facilitation (Ries et al., 1988). Gravity resistance includes low-

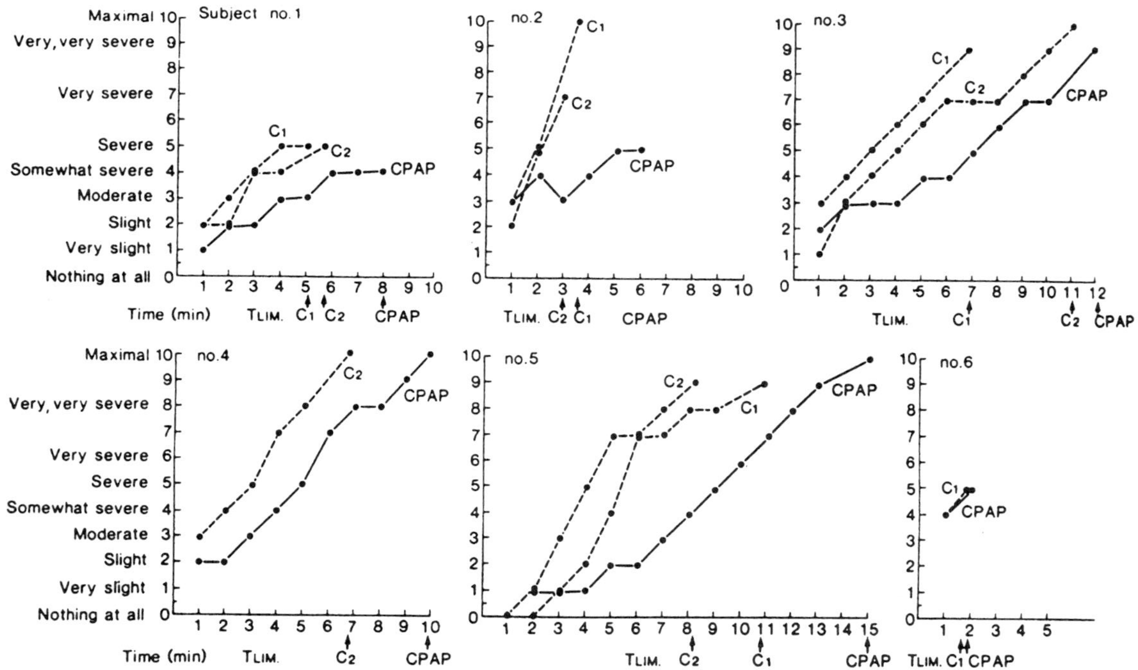

Figure 4 Breathlessness ratings plotted against time during CPAP-assisted exercise (solid lines) compared with unassisted controls, C1 and C2 (dashed lines) during submaximal, constant-load exercise on the cycle ergometer at 50% of peak oxygen consumption in six patients with chronic obstructive pulmonary disease. There were increases in exercise duration and decreases in the intensity of breathlessness with CPAP in subjects 1–5, but not in subject 6. (From O'Donnell et al., 1988.)

resistance, high-repetition activities aimed at increasing the endurance of the arm and shoulder muscles. The patient can perform one to two sets of 10 repetitions; each set includes three to five exercises with either no weight or added hand weights (0.5–2 kg). Proprioceptive neuromuscular facilitation (PNF) involves lower frequency, progressive resistance training with weights to improve both strength and endurance. Diagonal combinations of muscle movements can be used to strengthen weaker muscles by exercising functionally related muscles. Exercises are performed in three sets of 4–10 repetitions each with a weight; the initial weight can be determined by the maximal weight with which each patient could complete 6 repetitions of the first set of exercises (Ries et al., 1988). Training frequency for gravity resistance and PNF can be every other day for the first few weeks and then progress to daily exercise. Exercises should be coordinated with breathing (entrainment) so that patients exhale during exertion or lifting.

H. Resistive Inspiratory Muscle Training (RIMT)

The major objective of RIMT is to increase strength and/or endurance of the respiratory muscles, thereby allowing the patient to use a lower percentage of respiratory muscle capacity during exertional activities. This should translate into a reduction in the severity of breathlessness.

Smith and colleagues (1992) performed a metaanalysis of 17 randomized trials of both resistance and volume types of respiratory muscle training in patients with COPD. Although the collective data showed no evidence of clinical benefit, 12 of the 17 studies did not adequately ensure an appropriate training intensity. However, subgroup analysis of 5 studies that incorporated targeted intensities of training demonstrated improvement in various functional outcomes.

In one study, Harver and colleagues (1989) performed a randomized, placebo-controlled, parallel design trial of targeted RIMT over an 8 week period in patients with COPD. Patients used a resistance device modified to give visual feedback on breath-to-breath changes related to inspiratory muscle pressure. In the experimental group, 10 patients trained at six progressive levels of inspiratory resistance (range 5–35 cm (H_2O/L/s). In this group, PI_{max} at FRC increased from 47 ± 22 to 62 ± 29 cm H_2O ($p = 0.01$). The 9 patients in the control group trained at a constant, nominal level of resistance (approximately 5 cm H_2O/L/s); these patients showed a slight increase in PI_{max} from 43 ± 10 to 48 ± 23 cm H_2O (p not significant, NS), which is consistent with a learning effect. Compared with the control group, the experimental group showed a significant improvement in dyspnea, as assessed by the multidimensional BDI and TDI ($p = 0.003$). Improvements in physiological values and in dyspnea ratings were correlated.

Patients with COPD who are "limited" by dyspnea but do not have severe hyperinflation may benefit from RIMT. A clinical trial of RIMT may be warranted in symptomatic patients who have diminished respiratory muscle strength despite optimal application of the previously described therapeutic strategies for reducing breathlessness. Certainly, it is critical to achieve a target inspiratory pressure (or flow rate) and to provide a feedback signal to the patient during training (Belman et al., 1986). A threshold loading device is commercially available for RIMT; it requires that a target inspiratory pressure be achieved by the patient to overcome the selected resistance and to generate airflow. An initial intensity of training can be 25–35% of PI_{max} measured at FRC for 15–30 minutes per day. The target pressure can be adjusted every 2–3 weeks according to the training response (Mahler, 1990b). An alternative approach is to have the patient perform 10 maximal inspiratory efforts from FRC against a closed airway twice a day and sustain the effort for 5 s (Redline et al., 1991).

I. Miscellaneous

Jobst and colleagues (1986) performed a randomized, controlled trial of acupuncture in 26 patients with COPD in whom disabling breathlessness was present for at least 5 years. Subjects received traditional Chinese acupuncture on 13 occasions over 3 weeks or similar therapy except that the needles were inserted into "dead" points (control group). The acupuncture-treated group reported significant relief of breathlessness on each of three different scales for quantifying the severity of dyspnea compared with the control group, along with a greater increase in the 6 minute walking distance. The authors speculate that acupuncture releases endogenous opiates that could modify the intensity of breathlessness.

Sibuya et al. (1994) demonstrated that in-phase chest wall vibration reduced the intensity of dyspnea in patients with COPD; this suggests that afferent information from chest wall respiratory muscles may contribute to respiratory sensation.

Other strategies described in uncontrolled studies or case reports include biofeedback, hypnosis, and yoga. However, further studies of these modalities are required before such approaches can be recommended.

IV. Summary

Patients with severe COPD develop two major breathing strategies during physical exertion in an attempt to adapt to impaired ventilatory mechanics: dynamic hyperinflation and prolongation of expiration. Dynamic hyperinflation leads to an increase in end-expiratory lung volume, which increases elastic recoil (and creates a threshold elastic load during inspiration) and shortens the costal muscle fibers of the diaphragm. Prolongation of expiration forces the respiratory muscles to increase inspiratory flow to compensate for a shorter inspiratory time. These adaptations place increased demands on the respiratory muscles, especially the diaphragm, and presumably cause an increase in the effort or work of breathing reported by patients with COPD.

A careful and comprehensive history is the most important part of the clinical assessment of the patient. Particular attention should be directed toward characteristics of the patient's breathlessness, provoking activities, positional influence, and efforts that relieve the severity of breathing difficulty. Physical findings of the chest are usually normal in patients with COPD unless there is severe physiological impairment ($FEV_1 < 50\%$ of predicted). Pulmonary function testing is essential to establish a diagnosis and to determine the severity of airflow obstruction. Clinical rating instruments and/or measurement during exercise are recommended to quantify the intensity of a patient's breathlessness at an initial time and to evaluate response to therapy.

Treatment strategies for reducing the severity of breathlessness include breathing training, chest physiotherapy, coping and self-care efforts, environmental control, bronchodilator medications, supplemental oxygen, exercise reconditioning and training, and inspiratory muscle training. These options should be selected and tried based on individual considerations, especially the patient's desire and request for relief from the distress of breathlessness. Additional approaches for relieving breathlessness, such as opioid medications and psychosocial management, are presented in Chaps. 14 and 15, respectively.

References

Adams, L., Chronos, N., Lane, R., and Guz, A. (1985). The measurement of breathlessness induced in normal subjects: validity of two scaling techniques. Clin. Sci. 69:7–16.

Aitken, R.C.B. (1969). Measurement of feelings using visual analog scales. Proc. R. Soc. Med. 62:989–993.

American College of Sports Medicine (1995). Guidelines for Exercise Testing and Prescription, 5th ed. Lea & Febger, Philadelphia.

American College of Sports Medicine Position Stand (1990). The recommended quantity and quality of exercise for developing and maintaining cardiorespiratory and muscular fitness in healthy adults. Med. Sci. Sports. Exerc. 22:265–274.

Anthonisen, N.R., Wright, E.C., and the IPPB Trial Group (1986). Bronchodilator response in chronic obstructive pulmonary disease. Am. Rev. Respir. Dis. 133:814–819.

Belman, M.J., and Gaesser, G.A. (1991). Exercise training below and above the lactate threshold in the elderly. Med. Sci. Sports Exerc. 23:562–568.

Belman, M.J., Thomas, S.G., and Lewis, M.I. (1986). Resistive breathing training in patients with chronic obstructive pulmonary disease. Chest 90:662–669.

Belman, M.J., Brooks, L.R., Ross, D.J., and Mohsenifar, Z. (1991). Variability of breathlessness measurement in patients with chronic obstructive pulmonary disease. Chest 99:566–571.

Berger, R., and Smith, D. (1988). Effort of inhaled mataproterenol on exercise performance in patients with stable "fixed" airway obstruction. Am. Rev. Respir. Dis. 138:624–629.

Bernstein, D.A., and Borkovec, T.D. (1973). Progressive Relaxation Training. A Manual for the Helping Professions. Research Press, Champaign, IL.

Bohadana, A.B., Peslin, R., and Uffholtz, H. (1978). Breath sounds in the clinical assessment of airflow obstruction. Thorax 33:345–351.

Borg, G.A.V. (1982). Psychophysical bases of perceived exertion. Med. Sci. Sports Exerc. 14:377–381.

Breslin, E.H. (1992). The pattern of respiratory muscle recruitment during pursed-lip breathing. Chest 101:75–78.

Burrows, B., and Earle, R.H. (1969). Course and prognosis of chronic obstructive lung disease. A prospective study of 200 patients. N. Engl. J. Med. 280:397–404.

Bye, P.T.P., Esau, S.A., and Levy, R.D. (1985). Ventilatory muscle function during exercise in air and oxygen in patients with chronic air-flow limitation. Am. Rev. Respir. Dis. 132:236–240.

Callahan, C.M., Dittus, R.S., and Katz, B.P. (1991). Oral corticosteroid therapy for patients with stable chronic obstructive pulmonary disease: a meta-analysis. Ann. Intern. Med. 114:216–223.

Casaburi, R., Patessio, A., Ioli, F., Zanaboni, S., Donner, C.F., and Wasserman, K. (1991). Reductions in exercise lactate acidosis and ventilation as a result of exercise training in patients with obstructive lung disease. Am. Rev. Respir. Dis. 143:9–18.

Celli, B.R., Rassulo, J., and Make, B.J. (1986). Dyssynchronous breathing during arm but not leg exercise in patients with chronic airflow obstruction. N. Engl. J. Med. 314:1485–1490.

Chrystyn, H., Mulley, B.A., and Peake, M.D. (1988). Dose response relation to oral theophylline in severe chronic obstructive airways disease. B. M. J. 297:1506–1510.

Cockcroft, A.E., Saunders, M.J., and Berry, G. (1981). Randomized controlled trial of rehabilitation in chronic respiratory disability. Thorax 36:200–203.

Criner, G.J., and Celli, B.R. (1987). Ventilatory muscle recruitment in exercise with O_2 in obstructed patients with mild hypoxemia. J. Appl. Physiol. 63:195–200.

Davidson, A.C., Leach, R., George, R.J.D., and Geddes, D.M. (1988). Supplemental oxygen and exercise ability in chronic obstructive airways disease. Thorax 43: 965–971.

Dean, N.C., Brown, J.K., Himelman, R.B., Doherty, J.J., Gold, W.M., and Stulbarg, M.S. (1992). Oxygen may improve dyspnea and endurance in chronic obstructive pulmonary disease patients with only mild hypoxemia. Am. Rev. Respir. Dis. 146: 941–945.

Dompeling, E., van Schayck, C.P., van Grunsven, P.M., van Herwaarden, C.L.A., Akkermans, R., Molemia, J., Folgering, H., and van Weel, C. (1993). Slowing the deterioration of asthma and chronic obstructive pulmonary disease observed during bronchodilator therapy by adding inhaled corticosteroids. Ann. Intern. Med. 118: 770–778.

Drazen, J.M., and Gerard, C. (1989). Reversing the irreversible (editorial). N. Engl. J. Med. 320:1555–1556.

Dull, W.L., and Alexander, M.R. (1984). Theophylline in stable chronic airflow obstruction: a reappraisal. Arch. Intern. Med. 144:2399–2401.

Dullinger, D., Kronenberg, R., and Niewoehner, D.E. (1986). Efficacy of inhaled metaproteronol and orally-administered theophylline in patients with chronic airflow obstruction. Chest 89:171–173.

Eaton, M.L., MacDonald, F.M., Church, T.R., and Niewoehner, D.E. (1982). Effects of theophylline on breathlessness and exercise tolerance in patients with chronic air-flow obstruction. Chest 82:538–542.

Elliott, M.W., Adams, L., Cockcroft, A., Macrea, K.D., Murphy, K., and Guz, A. (1991). The language of breathlessness. Am. Rev. Respir. Dis. 144:826–832.

Ellis, B., and Ries, A.L. (1991). Upper extremity exercise training in pulmonary rehabilitation. J. Cardiopulm. Rehab. 11:227–231.

Goldstein, R.S., Gort, E.H., Stubbing, D., Avendano, M.A. Guyatt, G.H. (1994). Randomised controlled trial of respiratory rehabilitation. Lancet 344:1394–1397.

Guyatt, G.H., Berman, L.B., Townsend, M., Pugsley, S.O., and Chambers, L.W. (1987a). A measure of quality of life for clinical trials in chronic lung disease. Thorax 42: 773–778.

Guyatt, G.H., Townsend, M., Pugsley, S.O., Keller, J.L., Short, H.D., Taylor, D.W., and Newhouse, M.T. (1987b). Bronchodilators in chronic air-flow limitation: effects of airway function, exercise capacity, and quality of life. Am. Rev. Respir. Dis. 135: 1069–1074.

Guyatt, G.H., Townsend, M., Nogradi, S., Pugsley, S.O., Keller, J.L., and Newhouse, M.T. (1988). Acute response to bronchodilator: an imperfect guide for bronchodilator therapy in chronic airflow limitation. Arch. Intern. Med. 148:1949–1952.

Harver, A., Mahler, D.A., and Daubenspeck, J.A. (1989). Targeted inspiratory muscle training improves respiratory muscle function and reduces dyspnea in patients with chronic obstructive pulmonary disease. Ann. Intern. Med. 111:117–124.

Hay, J.G., Stone, P., Carter, J., Church, S., Eyre-Brook, A., Pearson, M.G., Woodcock, A.A., and Calverly, P.M.A. (1992). Bronchodilator reversibility, exercise performance, and breathlessness in stable chronic obstructive pulmonary disease. Eur. Respir. J. 5:659–664.

Hill, N.S. (1987). The cardiac exam in lung disease. Clin. Chest. Med. 8:273–285.

Horowitz, M.B., and Mahler, D.A. (1993). The validity of using dyspnea ratings for exercise prescription in patients with COPD (abstract). Am. Rev. Respir. Dis. (Suppl.) 147:A744.

Jaeschke, R., Guyatt, G.H., Singer, J., Keller, J., and Newhouse, M.T. (1991). Mechanism of bronchodilator effect in chronic airflow limitation. Can. Med. Assoc. J. 144:35–39.

Jobst, K., Chen, J.H., McPherson, K., Arrowsmith, J., Brown, V., Efthimiou, J., Fletcher, H.J., Maciocia, G., Mole, P., Shifrin, K., and Lane, D.J. (1986). Controlled trial of acupuncture for disabling breathlessness. Lancet 2:1416–1419.

Kerstjens, H.A.M., Brand, P.L.P., Hughes, M.D., Robinson, N.J., Postma, D.S., Sluiter, H.J., Bleecker, E.R., Dekhuijzen, P.N.R., de Jong, P.M., Mengelers, H.J.J., Overbeek, S.E., and Schoonbroad, D.F.M.E. (1992). A comparison of bronchodilator therapy with or without inhaled corticosteroid therapy for obstructive airways disease. N. Engl. J. Med. 327:1413–1419.

Killian, K.J., Leblanc, P., Martin, D.H., Summers, E., Jones, N.L., and Moran, E.J.M. (1992). Exercise capacity and ventilatory, circulatory, and symptom limitation in patients with chronic airflow limitation. Am. Rev. Respir. Dis. 146:935–940.

Kohlman-Carrieri, C., and Janson-Bjerklie, S. (1990). Coping and self-care strategies.

In: Dyspnea. Edited by D.A. Mahler. Futura Publishing, Mount Kisco, NY, pp. 201–230.

Lane, R., Cockcroft, A., Adams, L., and Guz, A. (1987). Arterial oxygen saturation and breathlessness in patients with chronic obstructive airways disease. Clin. Sci. 72:693–698.

LeBlanc, D.M., Bowie, D.M., Summers, E., Jones, N.L., and Killian, K.J. (1986). Breathlessness and exercise in patients with cardiorespiratory disease. Am. Rev. Respir. Dis. 133:21–25.

Liss, H.P., and Grant, B.J.B. (1988). The effect of nasal flow on breathlessness in patients with chronic obstructive pulmonary disease. Am. Rev. Respir. Dis. 137:1285–1288.

Mador, M.J., and Kufel, T.J. (1992). Reproducibility of visual analog scale measurements of dyspnea in patients with chronic obstructive pulmonary disease. Am. Rev. Respir. Dis. 146:82–87.

Mahler, D.A. (1990a). Positional dyspnea. In: Dyspnea. Edited by D.A. Mahler. Futura Publishing, Mount Kisco, NY, pp. 145–164.

Mahler, D.A. (1990b). Therapeutic strategies. In: Dyspnea. Edited by D.A. Mahler. Futura Publishing, Mount Kisco, NY, pp. 231–263.

Mahler, D.A. (1992). The measurement of dyspnea during exercise in patients with lung disease. Chest (Suppl.) 101:242S–247S.

Mahler, D.A., and Harver, A. (1988). Prediction of peak oxygen consumption in obstructive airway disease. Med. Sci. Sports Exerc. 20:574–578.

Mahler, D.A., and Harver, A. (1990). Clinical measurement of dyspnea. In: Dyspnea. Edited by D.A. Mahler. Futura Publishing, Mount Kisco, NY, pp. 75–126.

Mahler, D.A., and Harver, A. (1992). A factor analysis of dyspnea ratings, respiratory muscle strength, and lung function in patients with chronic obstructive pulmonary disease. Am. Rev. Respir. Dis. 145:467–470.

Mahler, D.A., and O'Donnell, D.E. (1991). Alternative modes of exercise training for pulmonary patients. J. Cardiopulm. Rehab. 11:58–63.

Mahler, D.A., and Wells, C.K. (1988). Evaluation of clinical methods for rating dyspnea. Chest 93:580–586.

Mahler, D.A., Weinberg, D.H., Wells, C.K., and Feinstein, A.R. (1984). The measurement of dyspnea: contents, interobserver agreement, and physiologic correlates of two new clinical indexes. Chest 85:751–758.

Mahler, D.A., Matthay, R.A., Snyder, R.E., Wells, C.K., and Loke, J. (1985). Sustained-release theophylline reduces dyspnea in nonreversible obstructive airway disease. Am. Rev. Respir. Dis. 131:22–25.

Mahler, D.A., Rosiello, R.A., Harver, A., Lentine, T., McGovern, J.F., and Daubenspeck, J.A. (1987). Comparison of clinical dyspnea ratings and psychophysical measurements of respiratory sensation in obstructive airway disease. Am. Rev. Respir. Dis. 135:1229–1233.

Mahler, D.A., Faryniarz, K., Lentine, T., Ward, J., Olmstead, E.M., and O'Connor, G.T. (1991). Measurement of breathlessness during exercise in asthmatics: predictor variables, reliability, and responsiveness. Am. Rev. Respir. Dis. 144:39–44.

Mahler, D.A., Faryniarz, K., Tomlinson, D., Colice, G.L., Robins, A.G., Olmstead, E.M., and O'Connor, G.T. (1992). The impact of dyspnea and physiologic function on general health status in patients with chronic obstructive pulmonary disease. Chest 102:395–401.

Manning, H.L., Harver, A., and Mahler, D.A. (1993). Dyspnea in the elderly. In: Pulmonary Disease in the Elderly Patient. Edited by D.A. Mahler. Marcel Dekker, New York, pp. 81–112.

Martinez, F.J., Couser, J.I., and Celli, B.R. (1990). Factors influencing ventilatory muscle recruitment in patients with chronic airflow obstruction. Am. Rev. Respir. Dis. 142:276–282.

McBride, B., and Whitelaw, W.A. (1981). A physiological stimulus to upper airway receptors in humans. J. Appl. Physiol. 51:1189–1197.

McGavin, C.R., Gupta, S.P., Lloyd, E.L., and McHardy, G.J.R. (1977). Physical rehabilitation for the chronic bronchitic: results of a controlled trial of exercises in the home. Thorax 32:307–311.

Medical Section of the American Lung Association (1987). Standards for the diagnosis and care of patients with chronic obstructive pulmonary disease (COPD) and asthma. Am. Rev. Respir. Dis. 136:225–244.

Medical Section of the American Lung Association (1991). Lung function testing: selection of reference values and interpretative strategies. Am. Rev. Respir. Dis. 144:1202–1218.

Mendella, L.A., Manfreda, J., Warren, C.P.W., and Anthonisen, N.R. (1982). Steroid response in stable chronic obstructive pulmonary disease. Ann. Intern. Med. 96: 17–21.

Morrison, J.F.J., Jones, P.C., and Muers, M.F. (1992). Assessing physiological benefit from domiciliary nebulized bronchodilators in severe airflow limitation. Eur. Respir. J. 5:424–429.

Mueller, R.E., Petty, T.L., and Filley, G.F. (1970). Ventilation and arterial blood gas changes induced by pursed lips breathing. J. Appl. Physiol. 28:784–789.

Murciano, D., Auclair, M.H., Pariente, R., and Aubier, M. (1989). A randomized, controlled trial of theophylline in patients with severe chronic obstructive pulmonary disease. N. Engl. J. Med. 320:1521–1525.

Muza, S.R., Silverman, M.T., Gilmore, G.C., Hellerstein, H.K., and Kelsen, S.G. (1990). Comparison of scales used to quantitate the sense of effort to breathe in patients with chronic obstructive pulmonary disease. Am. Rev. Respir. Dis. 141:909–913.

Nath, A.R., and Capel, L.H. (1974). Inspiratory crackles: early and late. Thorax 29: 223–227.

Niederman, M.S., Clemente, P.H., Fein, A.M., Feinsilver, S.H., Robinson, D.A., Ilowite, J.S., and Bernstein, M.G. (1991). Benefits of a multidisciplinary pulmonary rehabilitation program improvements are independent of lung function. Chest 99: 798–804.

Nocturnal Oxygen Therapy Trial Group (1980). Continuous or nocturnal oxygen therapy in hypoxemic chronic obstructive lung disease: a clinical trial. Ann. Intern. Med. 93:391–398.

O'Connell, J.M., and Campbell, A.H. (1976). Respiratory mechanics in airways obstruction associated with inspiratory dyspnoea. Thorax 31:669–677.

O'Donnell, D.E., and Webb, K.A. (1993). Exertional breathlessness in patients with chronic airflow limitation: the role of lung hyperinflation. Am. Rev. Respir. Dis. 148:1351–1357.

O'Donnell, D.E., Sanii, R., and Younes, M. (1988a). Improvement in exercise endurance in patients with chronic airflow obstruction using continuous positive airway pressure. Am. Rev. Respir. Dis. 138:1510–1514.

O'Donnell, D.E., Sanii, R., Giesbrecht, G., and Younes, M. (1988b). Effect of continuous positive airway pressure on respiratory sensation in patients with chronic obstructive pulmonary disease during submaximal exercise. Am. Rev. Respir. Dis. 138:1185–1191.

Petrof, B.J., Calderini, E., and Gottfried, S.B. (1990). Effect of CPAP on respiratory effort and dyspnea during exercise in severe COPD. J. Appl. Physiol. 69:179–188.

Pratter, M.R., and Irwin, R.S. (1988). Predicting response to bronchodilator therapy in chronic obstructive pulmonary disease. Arch. Intern. Med. 148:1909–1910.

Pratter, M.R., Curley, F.J., Dubois, J., and Irwin, R.S. (1989). Cause and evaluation of chronic dyspnea in a pulmonary disease clinic. Arch. Intern. Med. 149:2277–2282.

Punzal, P.A., Ries, A.L., Kaplan, R.M., and Prewitt, L.M. (1991). Maximum intensity exercise training in patients with chronic obstructive pulmonary disease. Chest 100:618–623.

Redline, S., Gottfried, S.B., and Altose, M.D. (1991). Effects of changes in inspiratory muscle strength on the sensation of respiratory force. J. Appl. Physiol. 70:240–245.

Renfroe, K.L. (1988). Effect of progressive relaxation on dyspnea and state anxiety in patients with chronic obstructive pulmonary disease. Heart Lung 17:408–413.

Ries, A.L. (1990). Scientific basis of pulmonary rehabilitation: position paper of the American Association of Cardiovascular and Pulmonary Rehabilitation. J. Cardiopulm. Rehab. 10:418–441.

Ries, A.L., Ellis, B., and Hawkins, R.W. (1988). Upper extremity exercise training in chronic obstructive pulmonary disease. Chest 93: 688–692.

Rochester, D.F. (1991). Effects of COPD on the respiratory muscles. In: Chronic Obstructive Pulmonary Disease. Edited by N.S. Cherniack. W.B. Saunders, Philadelphia, pp. 134–157.

Schneider, I.C., and Anderson, A.E. (1965). Correlation of clinical signs with ventilatory function in obstructive lung disease. Ann. Intern. Med. 62:477–485.

Schwartzstein, R.M., Lahive, K., Pope A., Weinberger, S.E., and Weiss, J.W. (1987). Cold facial stimulation reduces breathlessness induced in normal subjects. Am. Rev. Respir. Dis. 136:58–61.

Sexton, D.L. (1987). Relaxation techniques and biofeedback. In: Chronic Obstructive Pulmonary Disease: Current Concepts. Edited by J.E. Hodgkin and T.L. Petty. W.B. Saunders, Philadelphia, pp. 99–112.

Sharp, J.T., Drutz, W.S., Moisan, R., Foster, J., and Machnach, W. (1980). Postural relief of dyspnea in severe chronic obstructive pulmonary disease. Am. Rev. Respir. Dis. 122: 201–211.

Sibuya, M., Yamada, M., Kanamaru, A., Tanaka, K., Suzuki, H., Noguchi, E., Altose, M.D., and Homma, I. (1994). Effect of chest wall vibration on dyspnea in patients with chronic respiratory disease. Am. J. Respir. Crit. Care Med. 149:1235–1240.

Simon, P.M., Schwartzstein, R.M., Weiss, J.W., Lahive, F., Fencl, V., Teghtsoonian, M., and Weinberger, S.E. (1989). Distinguishable sensations of breathlessness induced in normal volunteers. Am. Rev. Respir. Dis. 140:1021–1027.

Simon, P.M., Schwartzstein, R.M., Weiss, J.W., Fencl, V., Teghtsoonian, M., and Weinberger, S.E. (1990). Distinguishable types of dyspnea in patients with shortness of breath. Am. Rev. Respir. Dis. 142:1009–1014.

Simon, P.M., Basner, R.C., Weinberger, S.E., Fencl, V., Weiss, J.W., and Schwartzstein, R.M. (1991). Oral mucosal stimulation modulates the intensity of breathlessness induced in normal subjects. Am. Rev. Respir. Dis. 144:419–422.

Similowski, T., Yan, S., Gauthier, A.P., Macklem, P.T., and Bellamare, F. (1991). Contractile properties of the human diaphragm during chronic hyperinflation. N. Engl. J. Med. 325:917–923.

Simpson, K., Killian, K., McCartney, N., Stubbing, D.G., and Jones, N.L. (1992). Randomized controlled trial of weight lifting exercise in patients with chronic airflow limitation. Thorax 47:70–75.

Sinclair, D.J.M., and Ingram, C.G. (1980). Controlled trial of supervised exercise training in chronic bronchitis. B. M. J. 280:519–521.

Smith, K., Cook, D., Guyatt, G.H., Madhaven, J., and Oxman, A.D. (1992). Respiratory muscle training in chronic airflow limitation: a meta-analysis. Am. Rev. Respir. Dis. 145:533–539.

Spence, D.P.S., Graham, D.R., Ahmed, J., Rees, K., Pearson, M.G., and Calverley, P.M.A. (1993). Does cold air affect exercise capacity and dyspnea in stable chronic obstructive pulmonary disease? Chest 103:693–696.

Strijbos, J.H., Sluiter, H.J., and Postma, D.S. (1989). Objective and subjective performance indicators in COPD. Eur. Respir. J. 2:666–669.

Stubbing, D.G., Mathur, P.N., Roberts, R.S., and Campbell, E.J.M. (1982). Some physical signs in patients with chronic airflow obstruction. Am. Rev. Respir. Dis. 125:549–552.

Suero, J.T., and Woolf, C.R. (1970). Alterations in the mechanical properties of the lung during dyspnea in chronic obstructive pulmonary disease. J. Clin. Invest. 49:747–751.

Swinburn, C.R., Mould, H., Stone, T.N., Corris, P.A., and Gibson, G.J. (1991). Symptomatic benefit of supplemental oxygen in hypoxemic patients with chronic lung disease. Am. Rev. Respir. Dis. 143:913–915.

Thompson, A.B., Mueller, M.B., Heires, A.J., Bohling, T.L., Daughton, D., Yancey, S.W., et al. (1992). Aerosolized beclomethasone in chronic bronchitis. Am. Rev. Respir. Dis. 146:388–395.

Tiep, B.L., Burns, M., Kao, D., Madison, R., and Herrara, J. (1986). Pursed lips breathing training using ear oximetry. Chest 90:218–221.

Vyas, M.N., Banister, E.W., Morton, J.W., and Grzybowski, S. (1971). Response to exercise in patients with chronic airway obstruction. II. Effects of breathing 40 percent oxygen. Am. Rev. Respir. Dis. 103:401–412.

Wempe, J.B., Postma, D.S., Breederveld, N., Kort, E., van der Mark, T.W., and Koeter, G.H. (1992). Effects of cortocosteroids on bronchodilator action in chronic obstructive lung disease. Thorax 47:616–621.

Wilson, R.C., and Jones, P.W. (1989). A comparison of the visual analogue sale and modified Borg scale for the measurement of dyspnoea during exercise. Clin. Sci. 76:277–282.

Woodcock, A.A., Gross, E.R., and Geddes, D.M. (1981). Oxygen relieves breathlessness in "pink puffers." Lancet 1:907–909.

11

Breathlessness in Heart Disease

ANDREW CLARK and PHILIP POOLE-WILSON

National Heart and Lung Institute
London, England

I. Introduction

The sensation of breathlessness is one of the most common presenting complaints of patients with heart disease, but it may arise in many different clinical settings (Braunwald, 1988). Differentiating the underlying clinical syndrome responsible for breathlessness in patients with heart disease and understanding the pathophysiological mechanisms are important to establish the most appropriate management of the patient.

When obtaining a history from a patient complaining of breathlessness, physicians often have difficulty determining just what the patient is describing. Tiredness and fatigue can be confused with breathlessness, and on occasion, chest pain may masquerade as shortness of breath. It is of great importance to obtain a detailed description from the patient. A working definition of *breathlessness* is an abnormally uncomfortable awareness of breathing, and there are three main cardiac syndromes in which breathlessness may occur: acute ischemia ("angina equivalent"), acute heart failure, and chronic heart failure. Breathlessness is caused by other conditions, but these are much less common.

The pathophysiology and mechanisms underlying the sensation of breathlessness in heart disease have not been clearly delineated, and little, if any, formal work has been conducted into the sensation of dyspnea. Breathlessness may rise from a variety of pathological changes occurring under different clinical circumstances, but it is important to recognize before further discussion that "breathlessness" as a symptom is mutable. Patients with chronic heart failure may be limited during different forms of exercise, with either breathlessness or fatigue as their predominant symptom despite identical hemodynamics and ventilatory responses (Lipkin et al., 1986b). Furthermore, although to the patient symptomatology is of central importance, breathlessness is of little relevance in predicting outcome (Bittner et al., 1993). Study of the causes of exercise limitation in heart disease may be more profitable than elucidation of the nature of symptoms at peak exercise. In this chapter, we focus the discussion on the nature of the increased ventilatory response to exercise in patients with heart disease rather than on the symptom of breathlessness per se, because breathlessness in heart disease is likely to arise from abnormal ventilatory activation.

II. Acute Ischemia

Ischemic heart disease is commonly manifested as angina pectoris, myocardial infarction, or sudden death. During an attack of ischemia, a segment of myocardium is deprived of its blood supply as a result of atheromatous obstructive disease in an epicardial vessel. This usually causes typical chest pain—central, crushing, related to exertion, and radiating to the arms and neck—but it has long been recognized that ischemia can cause a sensation of breathlessness in the absence of pain (Gallavardin, 1933). As a symptom of coronary artery disease, breathlessness on exertion may precede the development of chest pain (Hagman and Wilhelmsen, 1981; Cook and Shaper, 1989) and can cause considerable difficulty in reaching a diagnosis (Rose, 1962). The British Regional Heart Study, looking at a random sample of men aged 40–59, found a strong relationship between breathlessness and the development of angina and myocardial infarction; at 5 year follow-up, 37.2% of mean with severe breathlessness but no evidence of coronary artery disease had had a heart attack compared with only 8.1% of men without breathlessness (Cook and Shaper, 1988, 1989). The breathlessness was independent of the smoking history of the individual (Cook and Shaper, 1989).

The mechanism by which myocardial ischemia produces the sensation of breathlessness is similar to that of transient left ventricular dysfunction (Hagman and Wilhelmsen, 1981; Taki et al., 1992; Kléber and Oetliker, 1992).

III. Heart Failure

Heart failure is a clinical syndrome rather than a diagnosis in itself (Poole-Wilson, 1985). Many definitions have been used over the years. A good theoretical definition has some attractions—"a pathophysiological state in which an abnormality of cardiac function is responsible for the failure of the heart to pump blood at a rate commensurate with the requirements of the metabolizing tissues" (Braunwald, 1988)—but lacks precision and applicability at the bedside. A working definition is more useful: a clinical syndrome caused by an abnormality of the heart and recognized by a characteristic pattern of hemodynamic, renal, neural, and hormonal responses. A simpler definition is ventricular dysfunction with symptoms (Poole-Wilson, 1985, 1989). Older descriptions of heart failure, such as forward and backward failure, right and left heart failure, and congestive heart failure, are often not helpful in understanding the physiology but can be useful shorthand for the transmission of clinical details between doctors. In practical terms, acute heart failure, circulatory collapse, and chronic heart failure are sufficient to describe most clinical conditions.

A. Acute Heart Failure

Physiology

In a normal person, the left ventricle accepts blood returning from the lungs via the pulmonary veins. The force with which the left ventricle ejects the blood is a function of the end-diastolic pressure in the ventricle, the well-known Frank-Starling mechanism, the blood pressure, and the inotropic state of the myocardium. If the left ventricle fails, the left ventricular filling pressure rises and contributes to the maintenance of the forward flow of blood. An increase in stiffness of the failing left ventricle has similar consequences. As has been recognized for many years, acute heart failure is characterized par excellence by breathlessness (Lewis, 1933). The sensation of breathlessness arises from an increase in left ventricular filling pressure, with the result that the hydrostatic pressure in the pulmonary veins exceeds the osmotic pressure. Fluid is thus lost from the circulation and enters the tissues at a rate dependent upon the size of the pressure gradient, the oncotic pressure (Guyton and Lindsey, 1959), and the functional capacity of the lymphatics to remove accumulating fluid (Cross et al., 1970). Acute heart failure is synonymous with acute pulmonary edema. Orthopnea can be considered a variant of acute heart failure; in the recumbent posture, there is pooling of the blood within the thorax, resulting in increased venous return, or preload. In turn, this leads to a further rise in left ventricular filling pressure. In addition, as the effects of gravity pulling down on the thoracic viscera are lost, the diaphragm is raised and vital capacity is reduced (Braunwald, 1988).

From Pulmonary Edema to Breathlessness

The breathlessness seen in patients with acute heart failure correlates with left ventricular end-diastolic pressure, suggesting that the sensation is dependent upon the head of pressure tending to force fluid into the lung tissues. The strongest evidence for this is that breathlessness is relieved immediately by acute lowering of the end-diastolic pressure regardless of the means, such as nitrates, bleeding, diuretics, or opiates (Dikshit et al., 1973; Pouleur et al., 1980). A number of possible mechanisms may be responsible for translating the pulmonary fluid accumulation into breathlessness.

Pulmonary Mechanical Changes

As fluid accumulates the lungs become stiffer, and in consequence there is early closure of airways with air trapping (Collins et al., 1975). With increased stiffness and decreased lung compliance the work required by the respiratory muscles to reduce intrathoracic pressure during inspiration rises (Marshall et al., 1954; White et al., 1958; Depeursinge et al., 1986). Accumulation of fluid in the airways results in an increase in resistance to airflow (Hogg et al., 1972) and reflex bronchoconstriction (Murray, 1985). Receptors in the alveolar wall (J receptors) (Paintal, 1973) may be stimulated by the accumulation of interstitial fluid, resulting in the sensation of dyspnea (Paintal, 1969; Guyton, 1991).

Cardiac Asthma

In the normal lung, the proximal bronchial veins drain into the systemic circulation and the more distal into the pulmonary veins (Schoenmackers, 1960; Deffebach et al., 1987). Patients with acute heart failure may have respiratory function tests indicative of bronchospasm that improves on treatment (Light and George, 1983; Petermann et al., 1987). This can be a result of the formation of edema in the bronchial walls, causing narrowing of the airways. In addition, stimulation of bronchial receptors may result in parasympathetic activation and bronchospasm (Lloyd, 1980).

Cabanes et al. (1989) have found that there is indeed increased bronchial reactivity in patients with heart failure compared with controls using the cholinergic agent methacholine. Furthermore, this effect is partially reversed by the administration of the β-adrenergic stimulant albuterol. Cabanes et al. suggested that patients with heart failure develop raised pressure in the bronchial veins on exercise (because these drain into the left atrium) and that this results in vasodilation, extravasation of plasma in the small airways, and hence bronchospasm. In support of this hypothesis is the observation that inhaled methoxamine, a vasoconstrictor, results in a greatly improved exercise time at constant workload (Cabanes et al., 1992). The methoxamine could only have reached the bronchial vessels, because there was no hemodynamic evidence of a systemic effect.

Systemic Changes

The accumulation of alveolar fluid results in impairment of metabolic gas exchange; as the pulmonary capillary pressure rises, hypoxemia worsens (Fillmore et al., 1972). Metabolic acidosis develops as a result of reduced tissue perfusion and the accumulation of lactate (Weil and Afifi, 1970). Less commonly, carbon dioxide retention occurs (Aberman and Fulop, 1972). Respiratory or metabolic acidosis increases the ventilatory drive.

Respiratory Muscles

As the work of breathing increases, so respiratory muscles must expend more energy. The respiratory muscles may be less well perfused, leading to fatigue (Macklem, 1980; Aubier et al., 1981), possibly stimulating breathlessness (Gandevia et al., 1981). An intriguing theory is that the work required for a given inspiratory volume is increased, resulting in a change to the length-tension relationships in the respiratory muscles, perhaps resulting in a sensation of breathlessness (Campbell and Howell, 1963; Campbell et al., 1970).

Summary

To summarize, in acute heart failure, the central event is a rise in the left ventricular filling pressure resulting in a rise in pulmonary venous pressure. Accumulation of fluid in the alveoli results in impaired gas exchange and in the interstitium results in increased lung stiffness. In the bronchial walls, fluid accumulation may result in bronchospasm and increased airflow resistance. There is decreased perfusion of the tissues generally, resulting in metabolic acidosis and, more specifically, decreased perfusion of the respiratory muscles.

All these factors combine to increase both the ventilatory drive and the metabolic cost of breathing. The final common pathway by which these abnormalities generate the signals leading to the sensation of dyspnea remains unclear.

B. Chronic Heart Failure

This group of patients have impaired left ventricular function and between episodes of acute heart failure do not have fluid retention because of treatment with diuretics, vasodilators, and angiotensin converting enzyme inhibitors (Anand et al., 1989). Although it is easy to appreciate why patients with an increase in lung water feel breathless, if only because of the reduction in available gas exchange area, understanding breathlessness and exercise limitation in chronic heart failure is more challenging.

Assessment of Exercise Limitation

Patients with chronic heart failure complain of exercise limitation. This is usually associated with such symptoms as breathlessness or fatigue on exertion; to assess the severity of possible heart disease, the symptoms must be considered against the background of the patient's normal activities. A range of different methods for assessing exercise function has been described, from treadmill and cycle exercise protocols to measurements of everyday activity, such as a 6 minute walking test (Lipkin et al., 1986a; Cowley et al., 1990, 1991; Cohen-Solal et al., 1991).

The most widely used objective measure of exercise limitation in chronic heart failure is an exercise test with metabolic gas exchange analysis to measure peak oxygen consumption (peak $\dot{V}O_2$) (Weber et al., 1984; Lipkin et al., 1985). Chronic heart failure results in a reduction in peak exercise oxygen consumption, and exercise is usually terminated by either breathlessness or fatigue. Which symptom dominates is a function of the type of exercise performed. Cycle exercise is more often stopped because of fatigue rather than breathlessness (Fink et al., 1986). Lipkin et al. (1986b) showed that *in the same subjects* using a rapidly incremental treadmill protocol exercise was limited by breathlessness but, using a slowly incremental test, resulted in exercise being stopped by fatigue. More importantly, there are no objective differences in exercise capacity and ventilatory response to exercise between those patients stopping because of fatigue and those stopping because of breathlessness (Clark et al., 1995a). Unlike symptomatology in chronic heart failure, peak $\dot{V}O_2$ is a highly reproducible variable (Weber et al., 1984; Hansen et al., 1987; Sullivan and Cobb, 1990).

It therefore appears that the symptoms of shortness of breath and fatigue are closely linked and, in turn, closely allied with exercise limitation in chronic heart failure. Little formal work has been conducted into the sensation of dyspnea in patients with chronic heart failure. Nevertheless, there has been much interest in the objective ventilatory response to exercise in this group of patients; at any stage of exercise, ventilation is increased compared with controls (Sullivan et al., 1988; Rubin and Brown, 1984; Higginbotham et al., 1983). This has been characterized as an alteration in the slope of the relationship between minute ventilation and carbon dioxide production (or $\dot{V}E/\dot{V}CO_2$ slope). This is described by a linear regression equation with a coefficient of more than 0.9 in most cases, as in normal individuals. The slope is steeper in heart failure. Per unit CO_2 production, the ventilatory response is greater in heart failure, and the more severe the exercise limitation, the steeper is the $\dot{V}E/\dot{V}CO_2$ slope (see later) (Buller and Poole-Wilson, 1990; Davies et al., 1991). Much of this discussion therefore centers on the mechanisms underlying exercise limitation and the increased ventilatory response in heart failure, because the possible mechanisms have implications for the understanding of exercise limitation and dyspnea in other fields.

Central Hemodynamics

An initial and a priori thought is that exercise capacity and peak oxygen consumption should be a function of left ventricular function. It is now very clear, however, that this is not the case, although this point is still often not fully appreciated. There is poor correlation between exercise capacity and left ventricular ejection fraction and velocity of fiber shortening (Franciosa et al., 1981) and cardiac index and left ventricular filling pressure (Weber et al., 1984; Lipkin and Poole-Wilson, 1986). Acute reduction in left ventricular filling pressure with dobutamine or prazosin does not affect peak $\dot{V}O_2$ (Fink et al., 1986).

Some observers have found a correlation between peak $\dot{V}O_2$ and *right* ventricular ejection fraction (Baker et al., 1984), but this has not been confirmed by other workers in the context of acute myocardial infarction (Gadsboll et al., 1991). We recently studied patients who had undergone Fontan's procedure for congenital heart disease. In this group of patients, the systemic venous return is routed directly into the pulmonary arterial system, and thus there is no right ventricular contribution. Many of the Fontan patients had normal exercise capacity and ventilatory response to exercise, and we found no relationship between right ventricular ejection fraction and either exercise capacity or the ventilatory response to exercise in patients with chronic heart failure (Clark et al, 1994a). Interestingly, there appears to be a correlation between exercise capacity and indices reflecting resting right heart function, such as pulmonary arterial pressure and pulmonary vascular resistance (Franciosa et al., 1985), and pulmonary capillary wedge pressure (Szlachcic et al., 1985). A more comprehensive study of the influence of pulmonary artery pressure using ambulatory pulmonary artery pressure monitoring has shown wide variations in pressure and no correlation with exercise tolerance (Gibbs et al., 1990). Nevertheless, some of these findings have led some authorities to suggest that left ventricular diastolic function is the key abnormality (Packer, 1990).

There are major reservations to the idea that any aspect of left ventricular function is the central determinant of exercise limitation and breathlessness in chronic heart failure. If this were the case, then improvements in left ventricular function ought to result in acute improvements in exercise performance. This is not seen with pharmacological intervention (Massie et al., 1981; Maskin et al., 1983). Indeed, there is no acute improvement following repair of valvular stenosis (Marzo et al., 1991) or even cardiac transplantation (Sinoway et al., 1988; Marzo et al., 1992). However, delayed improvements are seen following transplantation (Banner et al., 1989) and after treatment with angiotensin converting enzyme inhibitors (Drexler et al., 1989). These findings have important implications for understanding breathlessness in heart failure; it seems likely that a dominant role is played by a peripheral factor that takes some months to recover following correction of left ventricular function. This factor is possibly the resistance to blood flow in the arterioles of exercising skeletal muscle.

Metabolic Gas Exchange

A possible contributor to breathlessness on exertion is derangement of metabolic gas exchange, which at least partially contributes to the syndrome of acute heart failure (Fillmore et al., 1972). However, there appears to be no alteration in arterial blood gas tensions during exercise in chronic heart failure (Ruin et al., 1982; Franciosa et al., 1984). Indeed, there is even a small fall in arterial carbon dioxide tension at peak exercise, suggesting that there is hyperventilation relative to arterial gases (Sullivan et al., 1988; Rajfer et al., 1987; Moore et al., 1989), and although there is a widening of the arterial-mixed venous CO_2 difference, this appears to be caused solely by a reduction in arterial CO_2 content than a rise in mixed venous CO_2 (Hachamovitch et al., 1991). These findings make it extremely unlikely that carbon dioxide production of itself is a major stimulant either to ventilation or to the symptom of dyspnea under physiological conditions.

There appears to be an increase in the oxygen-carrying capacity of the blood in chronic heart failure (Herrlin and Sylvén, 1991), and increasing the inspired oxygen concentration during exercise results in a decrease in the respiratory response (Moore et al., 1992). These findings suggest that there may be occult hypoxia, not appearing clinically significant, resulting in a mild polycythemia. Nevertheless, there are no observed falls in oxygen tension during exercise, and this is unlikely to be responsible for dyspnea. We have found that, on the contrary, oxygen saturation and arterial tension rise slightly during exercise and more markedly during the recovery phase at the same time the arterial carbon dioxide tension is falling (Clark and Coats, 1994). Again, hyperventilation is present with respect to blood gas transport.

Ventilation-Perfusion Matching

Despite the normal arterial blood gas tensions, there is an objective increase in ventilation during exercise relative to normal subjects in patients with chronic heart failure (Rubin and Brown, 1984; Sullivan et al., 1988; Buller and Poole-Wilson, 1990). The slope of the ventilation to carbon dioxide production relationship is described by a linear correlation with a coefficient greater than 0.9, but the increased ventilation results in an increase in the slope of the relationship ($\dot{V}_E/\dot{V}_{CO_2}$ slope) (Buller and Poole-Wilson, 1990; Davies et al., 1991). An analysis of the alveolar ventilation equation

$$\dot{V}_E = \dot{V}_{CO_2} \times \frac{863}{P_{A_{CO_2}}} \left(1 - \frac{V_D}{V_T}\right) \qquad (1)$$

(where V_D/V_T describes dead space ventilation as a proportion of tidal ventilation, Pa_{CO_2} is the arterial partial pressure of carbon dioxide, and 863 is a constant to standardize gas measurements to body temperature, pressure, and saturation) in the face of nearly normal arterial carbon dioxide tensions leads to the conclusion that the cause of the increase slope is ventilation-perfusion matching and, specifically, an increase in dead space ventilation (Sullivan et al. 1988; Metra et al., 1992).

However, the alveolar ventilation equation is strictly applicable only in steady-state situations (Whipp, 1983), not in the relatively rapidly incremental protocols used in cardiopulmonary exercise testing (Clark et al., 1993). Nevertheless, the increase in $\dot{V}E/\dot{V}CO_2$ slope correlates with the reduction in peak $\dot{V}O_2$ (Buller and Poole-Wilson, 1990; Davies et al., 1991). This raises the question of what may constitute the dead space. Some observers have suggested that it lies in an increase in anatomical dead space ventilation as a result of an altered respiratory pattern; if minute ventilation is constant but respiratory rate increases, then the contribution of anatomical dead space increases (Weber et al., 1982). However, we have shown that in normal subjects altered respiratory rate at a given minute ventilation does not increase the $\dot{V}E/\dot{V}CO_2$ slope (Clark and Coats, 1993).

The alternative possibility is that perfusion to underventilated areas or a relative shunt must also be considered. Should significant shunting occur, then there should be an increase in the alveolar-arterial oxygen difference. Some observers have shown such an increase but with an overall fall in the contribution of shunt (Rubin et al., 1982). Others have found the alveolar-arterial oxygen difference to be unchanged (Rajfer et al., 1987), and it has been shown that perfusion to the apices of the lungs is increased at rest in patients with heart failure and that perfusion does not increase further with exercise, suggesting uniform perfusion, at least at an observable level (Mohsenifar et al., 1989). A study using radioisotope techniques has shown improvement in ventilation-perfusion matching during exercise (Uren et al., 1993). If ventilation-perfusion mismatch is occurring to a significant degree in chronic heart failure, then this begs the question of how the body senses an increase in dead space causing the sensation of breathlessness and the increased ventilation.

Control of Ventilation in Chronic Heart Failure

The nature of the "straight-line" relationship between ventilation and carbon dioxide production has led many cardiologists to assume that ventilation is controlled by $\dot{V}CO_2$. This does not sit easily with the small fall in arterial carbon dioxide tension seen during exercise (Sullivan et al., 1988; Rajfer et al., 1987; Moore et al., 1989; Clark and Coats, 1994). Some investigators have attempted to dissociate ventilation from carbon dioxide production. Using bouts of heavy exercise to deplete muscle glycogen forces muscle to use an alternative substrate during subsequent exercise. At a given load, carbon dioxide production thus falls, and if it is coupled to ventilation, then ventilation at a given load should fall. This has been found not to occur, suggesting that the two are not causally linked (Hughes et al., 1982; Heigenhauser et al., 1983). In these experiments, however, dead space fraction and arterial carbon dioxide are assumed to remain constant, neither of which may be the case. Caiozzo et al. (1987) have found a decrease in arterial carbon dioxide tension during exercise following glycogen depletion, which would accord with the hypothesis that something other than carbon dioxide production is the principal respiratory stimulant. We have shown that the ventilation to carbon dioxide production ratio during exercise is not constant in patients with heart failure and that the ratio rises toward peak exercise: the higher the ratio at peak exercise, the worse the heart failure (Clark et al., 1992). These findings suggest that a factor other than carbon dioxide production drives ventilation and that the degree to which this factor is present is a function of the severity of heart failure.

Contribution of Skeletal Muscle

In chronic heart failure, skeletal muscle becomes both qualitatively and quantitatively altered. The histology of muscle is altered with an increase in fast-twitch fibers, which are smaller than normal, at the expense of slow-twitch muscles (Lipkin et al., 1988; Sullivan et al., 1990). There is generalized wasting of muscle (McMurray et al., 1991; Mancini et al., 1992a). The muscle is metabolically abnormal, with a reduction in enzymes of the Krebs cycle (Sullivan et al., 1991) and a decrease in cytochrome oxidase activity (Drexler et al., 1991), indicating reduced oxidative capacity. There is early acidosis during exercise and a reduction in endurance with early fatigue (Minotti et al., 1991, 1992).

There are many ways in which these changes could result in breathlessness and increased ventilation. Respiratory muscle itself is abnormal in heart failure, with reduced respiratory muscle strength (Hammond et al., 1990; Mancini et al., 1992b; McParland et al., 1992) and early deoxygenation (Mancini et al., 1991). This could certainly contribute to a feeling of breathlessness. Metabolically abnormal exercising skeletal muscle itself could be the origin of an abnormal signal resulting in an increased ventilatory drive.

Lactate

Acidosis from skeletal muscle is observed early during exercise in heart failure (Massie et al., 1987). Reddy et al. (1988) have demonstrated a prolonged rise in blood lactate levels in patients following light exercise. The anaerobic threshold, a point during exercise when there is a rise in the ventilation to oxygen consumption ratio while the ventilation to carbon dioxide production remains unaltered, is thought to be caused by a blood lactate threshold and occurs earlier in patients with heart failure than in normal subjects (Sullivan and Cobb, 1990; Metra et al., 1990). Analysis of venous and arterial blood lactate fails to show a distinct threshold (Yeh et al., 1983), and patients with McArdle's syndrome, although not being metabolically able to generate lactate, display a ventilatory threshold similar to that seen in normal individuals (Paterson et al., 1990). If patients with heart failure are infused with dichloroacetate, which reduces blood lactate, exercise performance and ventilation are unchanged (Wilson et al., 1988). Finally, the time course of the rise in blood lactate during exercise does not parallel the rise in ventilation (Paterson et al., 1989). This combination of findings makes lactate an unlikely candidate for a role as physiological respiratory stimulant.

Potassium

During exercise, potassium is released from within cells (Kilburn, 1965) and arterial potassium rises. The rise in potassium closely parallels the rise in ventilation (Tibes et al., 1977; Paterson et al., 1989) and thus could be a respiratory stimulant. Some investigators have found a greater rise in arterial potassium at matched work rates in heart failure patients that is reduced by a training regimen (Barlow et al., 1994). However, in patients taking β blockers, which cause a greater rise in potassium during exercise, there is no increase in ventilation (Lim et al., 1981). Studies at our institute have also suggested that although the time course of the rise in potassium is similar to that of the rise in ventilation, potassium is more likely to reflect the duration and intensity of exercise rather than to act as the prime stimulus to the excessive ventilatory response of chronic heart failure (Clark et al., 1995b).

Muscle Bulk

Many of the features of chronic heart failure are similar to those seen after detraining, and it may be that in heart failure muscle bulk is a determinant of exercise capacity. Muscle wasting occurs in even mildly affected patients (Mancini et al., 1992a) and correlates modestly with exercise capacity. We recently showed a correlation between exercise performance and both muscle bulk and muscle strength (Volterrani et al., 1994). Decreased muscle bulk may also be responsible for the increased peripheral vascular resistance and a reduction in leg muscle blood flow.

Neural Signaling

The abnormal skeletal muscle of patients with chronic heart failure may be the origin of neural signals stimulating an excessive ventilatory response. Occluding the circulation to exercising muscle results in an increased ventilatory response that can only be neural in origin (Asmussen and Nielsen, 1964). In animal experiments, this stimulus is mimicked by infusing muscle with potassium and abolished by blocking small unmyelinated fibers (McCloskey and Mitchell, 1972). These workload receptors have been described as "ergoreceptors" (Iaria et al., 1959) or mechanoreceptors (Rowell and O'Learly, 1990). The receptors respond to work performed and stimulate ventilation. The accumulation of metabolites in the active muscle results in an enhanced ergoreceptor response (Tallarida et al., 1985; Rowell, 1986).

Skeletal muscle in heart failure fatigues early and is metabolically abnormal. The abnormalities may result in an abnormal ergoreflex signal stimulating increased ventilation. This hypothesis would unite the two common symptoms of heart failure, fatigue and breathlessness (Clark and Coats, 1992).

Effects of Training

Evidence for the dominant role of skeletal muscle is provided by controlled experiments on the effects of a training program in patients with heart failure. Exercise performance is improved (Coats et al., 1990, 1992), and the $\dot{V}E/\dot{V}CO_2$ slope is reduced (Davey et al., 1992). Following heart transplantation, despite immediate improvement in central hemodynamics, exercise capacity improves slowly (Sinoway et al., 1988; Marzo et al., 1992), and the improvement is accelerated by following a training program (Kavanagh et al., 1988; Keteyian et al., 1991). These findings are consistent with the idea that skeletal muscle changes are the determinant of exercise intolerance and breathlessness in chronic heart failure.

Respiratory Sensation

Some attention has been given to the possible mechanisms underlying the sensation of dyspnea. It may be thought that the sensation of breathlessness arises from excessive stimulation of J receptors (Paintal, 1969), perhaps because of excessive intrapulmonary collection of fluid. However, aerosol administration of lignocaine resulted in no change in the sensation of breathlessness, despite abolishing the cough response to capsaicin (Davies et al., 1990b). Exercise capacity and the ventilatory response to exercise were also unaltered. In contrast, inhaled diacetylmorphine immediately before exercise resulted in an increase in peak $\dot{V}O_2$ (Uren et al., 1991). Although exercise time was also increased, there was no change in the $\dot{V}E/\dot{V}CO_2$ slope and no change in the sensation of dyspnea on a visual analog scale either at peak exercise or at the same submaximal exercise level. Davies et al. (1990a) also found a decrease in dyspnea at a standard workload in patients given dihydrocodeine orally.

It is difficult to be certain from these experiments whether opiates are acting centrally or peripherally in the lungs, although the effect of dihydrocodeine suggests that central action is more important. That the $\dot{V}E/\dot{V}CO_2$ slope was unaltered although exercise time improved suggests that there is a central perception of the tolerability of discomfort that is modulated by opiates.

In contrast to the effects of opiates, Moore et al. (1992) found that increasing the fraction of inspired oxygen to 50% resulted in an improvement in exercise time and a reduction in the sensation of dyspnea at each stage of exercise. Others have found that in endurance walk testing and 6 minute walking tests, there was no effect of oxygen at flow rates up to 5 L/minute on either exercise capacity or breathlessness (Restrick et al., 1992). The difference between the two studies may be related to the difference in exercise protocols, Moore using maximal exercise testing and Restrick using patient-determined levels of exercise. As discussed, it seems unlikely that hypoxia is an important contributing factor to breathlessness in chronic heart failure, and it may be that additional oxygen works as in normal subjects (Bannister and Cunningham, 1954), perhaps by suppressing chemoreceptor activity.

IV. Summary

Breathlessness is one of the cardinal manifestations of cardiac disease. The common underlying phenomenon causing breathlessness is left ventricular dysfunction; when this happens acutely, the breathlessness appears to be directly related to an increase in left ventricular filling pressures resulting in fluid accumulation within the lung tissues. The consequences are an increase in the work of breathing and derangement of metabolic gas exchange with the resulting sensation of breathlessness.

In chronic heart failure, the situation is more complex. The symptom of shortness of breath is tied to the sensation of fatigue and with the causes of exercise limitation. The symptom of breathlessness is inconsistent and, although subjectively important for the patient, does not seem readily to have important objective correlates. There is an increase in the ventilatory response to exercise that increases further with worsening exercise limitation. There are widespread changes in the body, and neural and metabolic signals from skeletal muscle are a major factor in determining the ventilatory response to exercise.

References

Aberman, A., and Fulop, M. (1972). The metabolic and respiratory acidosis of acute pulmonary edema. Ann. Intern. Med. 76:173–184.

Anand, A.S., Veall, N., Kabra, G.S., Ferrari, R., Sutton, G., Lipkin, D., Harris, P., and Poole-Wilson, P.A. (1989). Treatment of heart failure with diuretics: body compartments, renal function and plasma hormones. Eur. Heart J. 10:455–450.

Asmussen, E., and Nielsen, M. (1964). Experiments on nervous factors controlling respiration and circulation during exercise employing blocking of the blood flow. Acta Physiol. Scand. 60:103–111.

Aubier, M., Trippenbach, T., and Roussos, C. (1981). Respiratory muscle fatigue during cardiogenic shock. J. Appl. Physiol. 51:449–508.

Baker, B.J., Wilen, M.M., Boyd, C.M., Dinh, H.A., and Franciosa, J.A. (1984). Relation of right ventricular ejection fraction to exercise capacity in chronic left ventricular failure. Am. J. Cardiol. 54:596–599.

Banner, N.R., Lloyd, M.H., Hamilton, R.D., Innes, J.A., Guz, A., and Yacoub, M.H. (1989). Cardiopulmonary response to dynamic exercise after heart and combined heart-lung transplantation. Br. Heart J. 61:215–223.

Bannister, R.G., and Cunningham, D.J. (1954). The effects on the respiration and performance during exercise of adding oxygen to the inspired air. J. Physiol. (Lond.) 125:118–137.

Barlow, C.W., Qayyum, M.S., Davey, P.P., Conway, J., Paterson, D.J., and Robbins, P.A. (1994). Effect of physical training on exercise-induced hyperkalemia in chronic heart failure: relation with ventilation and catecholamines. Circulation 89:1144–1152.

Bittner, V., Weiner, D.H., Yusuf, S., Rogers, W.J., McIntyre, K.M., Bangdiwala, S.I., Kronenberg, M.W., Kostis, J.B., Kohn, R.M., Guillotte, M., Greenberg, B., Woods, P.A., and Bourassa, M.G., for the SOLVD investigators (1993). Prediction of mortality and morbidity with a 6-minute walk test in patients with left ventricular dysfunction. JAMA 270:1702–1707.

Braunwald, E. (1988). Heart Disease: A Textbook of Cardiovascular Medicine, 3rd ed. Harcourt Brace Jovanovich, Philadelphia.

Buller, N.P., and Poole-Wilson, P.A. (1990). Mechanism of the increased ventilatory response to exercise in patients with chronic heart failure. Br. Heart J. 63:281–283.

Cabanes, L.R., Weber, S.N., Matran, R., Regnard, J., Richard M.O., Degeorges, M.F., and Lockhart, A. (1989). Bronchial hyperresponsiveness to methacholine in patients with impaired left ventricular function. N. Engl. J. Med. 320:1317–1322.

Cabanes, L., Costes, F., Weber, S., Regnard, J., Benvenuti, C., Castaigne, A., Guerin, F., and Lockhart, A. (1992). Improvement in exercise performance by inhalation of methoxamine in patients with impaired left ventricular function. N. Engl. J. Med. 326:1661–1665.

Caiozzo, V.J., Davis, J.A., Berriman, D.J., Vandagriff, R.B., and Prietto, C.A. (1987). Effects of high intensity exercise on the $\dot{V}E/\dot{V}CO_2$ relationship. J. Appl. Physiol. 62:1460–1464.

Campbell, E.M., and Howell, J.B.L. (1963). The sensation of breathlessness. Br. Med. Bull. 19:36–40.

Campbell, E.J.M., Agostoni, E., and Newsom, Davis, J. (1970). The Respiratory Muscles: Mechanisms and Neural Control, 2nd ed. W.B. Saunders, Philadelphia.

Clark, A.L., and Coats, A.J.S. (1992). The mechanisms underlying the increased ventilatory response to exercise in chronic stable heart failure. Eur. Heart J. 13:1698–1708.

Clark, A.L., and Coats, A.J.S. (1993). Effects of induced changes in anatomical dead space ventilation on the relationship between ventilation and carbon dioxide production in normal man. Eur. J. Clin. Invest. 27:428–432.

Clark, A.L., and Coats, A.J.S. (1994). Usefulness of arterial blood gas estimations during exercise in patients with chronic heart failure. Br. Heart J. 71:528–530.

Clark, A.L., Poole-Wilson, P.A., and Coats, A.J.S. (1992). The relationship between ventilation and carbon dioxide production in patients with chronic heart failure. J. Am. Coll. Cardiol. 20:1326–1332.

Clark, A.L., Volterrani, M., Piepoli, M., Poole-Wilson, P.A., and Coats, A.J.S. (1993). The influence of stage duration during incremental treadmill exercise on metabolic gas exchange measurements. Eur. Heart J. (Suppl.) 14:417.

Clark, A.L., Sparrow, J.L., and Coats, A.J.S. (1995a). Muscle fatigue and dyspnoea in chronic heart failure: two sides of the same coin? Eur. Heart J. 16:49–52.

Clark, A.L., Swan, J.W., Laney, R., Connelly, M., Somerville, J., and Coats, A.J.S. (1994a). The role of right and left ventricular function in the ventilatory response to exercise in chronic heart failure. Circulation 89:2062–2069.

Clark, A.L., Volterrani, M., Cerquetani, E., Ludman, P.F., Swan, J.W., Poole-Wilson, P.A., and Coats, A.J.S. (1995b). The relationship between arterial potassium and ventilation during exercise in patients whit chronic heart failure. J. Cardiac Failure: in press.

Coats, A.J.S., Adamopoulos, S., Meyer, T.E., Conway, J., and Sleight, P. (1990). Effects of physical training in chronic heart failure. Lancet 335:63–66.

Coats, A.J.S., Adamopoulos, S., Radaelli, A., McCance, A., Meyer, T.E., Bernardi, L., Solda, P.L., Davey, P., Ormerod, O., Forfar, C., Conway, J., and Sleight, P. (1992). Controlled trial of physical training in chronic heart failure: exercise performance, hemodynamics, ventilation, and autonomic function. Circulation 85:2119–2131.

Cohen-Solal, A., Zannad, F., Kayanakis, J.-G., Gueret, P., Aupetit, J.F., and Kolsky, H. (1991). Multicentre study of the determination of peak oxygen uptake and ventilatory threshold during bicycle exercise in chronic heart failure. Eur. Heart J. 12:1055–1063.

Collins, J.V., Clark, T.J.H., and Brown, D.J. (1975). Airway function in healthy subjects and in patients with left heart disease. Clin. Sci. Mol. Med. 49:217–228.

Cook, D.G., and Shaper, A.G. (1988). Breathlessness, lung function and risk of heart attack. Eur. Heart J. 9:1215–1222.

Cook, D.G., and Shaper, A.G. (1989). Breathlessness, angina pectoris and coronary artery disease. Am. J. Cardiol. 63:921–924.

Cowley, A.J., Fullwood, L., Stainer, K., and Hampton, J.R. (1990). Exercise tolerance in patients with heart failure—how should it be measured? Eur. Heart J. 12:50–54.

Cowley, A.J., Fullwood, L.J., Muller, A.F., Stainer, K., Skene, A.M., and Hampton, J.R. (1991). Exercise capability in heart failure: is cardiac output important after all? Lancet 337:771–773.

Cross, C.E., Shaver, J.A., Wilson, R.J., and Robin, E.D. (1970). Mitral stenosis and pulmonary fibrosis: special reference to pulmonary edema and lung lymphatic function. Arch. Intern. Med. 125:248–254.

Davey, P., Meyer, T., Coats, A., Adamopoulos, S., Casadei, B., Cownay, J., and Sleight, P. (1992). Ventilation in chronic heart failure: effects of physical training. Br. Heart J. 68:473–477.

Davies, S.W., Jordan, S.L., and Lipkin, D.P. (1990a). Central modulation of dyspnoea in chronic heart failure related to opiod axis. Br. Heart J. 64:58P.

Davies, S.W., Jordan, S.L., Newman, S., Agnew, J., and Lipkin, D.P. (1990b). Lignocaine aerosol anaesthesia and dyspnoea in chronic left heart failure. Br. Heart J. 64:59P.

Davies, S.W., Emery, T.M., Watling, M.I.L., Wannamethee, G., and Lipkin, D.P. (1991). A critical threshold of exercise capacity in the ventilatory response to exercise in heart failure. Br. Heart J. 65:179–183.

Deffebach, M.E., Charan, N.B., Lakshminarayam, S., and Butler, J. (1987). The bronchial circulation: small but a vital attribute of the lung. Am. Rev. Respir. Dis. 135: 463–481.

Depeursinge, F.B., Depeursinge, C.D., Boutaleb, A.K., Feihl, F., and Perret, C.H. (1986). Respiratory system impedance in patients with acute left ventricular failure: pathophysiology and clinical interest. Circulation 73:386–395.

Dikshit, K., Vyden, J.K., Forrester, J.S., Chatterjee, K., Prakosh, R., and Swan, H.J.C. (1973). Renal and extrarenal hemodynamic effects of furosemide in congestive heart failure after acute myocardial infarction. N. Engl. J. Med. 288:1087–1090.
Drexler, H., Banhardt, U., Meinertz, T., Wollschläger, H., Lehmann, M., and Just, H. (1989). Contrasting peripheral short-term and long-term effects of converting enzyme inhibition in patients with congestive heart failure. A double-blind, placebo-controlled trial. Circulation 79:491–502.
Drexler, H., Funke, E., and Riede, U. (1991). The oxidative enzyme activity decreases in all fibre types in skeletal muscle of patients with chronic heart failure. Circulation 84 (Suppl. II):II-74.
Fillmore, S.J., Giumaraes, A.C., Scheidt, S.S., and Killip, T. (1972). Blood gas changes and pulmonary hemodynamics following acute myocardial infarction. Circulation 45: 583–591.
Fink, L.I., Wilson, J.R., and Ferraro, N. (1986). Exercise ventilation and pulmonary artery wedge pressure in chronic stable congestive heart failure. Am. J. Cardiol. 57: 249–253.
Franciosa, J.A., Park, M, and Levine, T.B. (1981). Lack of correlation between exercise capacity and indexes of resting left ventricular performance in heart failure. Am. J. Cardiol. 47:33–39.
Franciosa, J.A., Leddy, C.L., Wilen, M., and Schwartz, D.E. (1984). Relation between haemodynamic and ventilatory responses in determining exercise capacity in severe congestive heart failure. Am. J. Cardiol. 53:127–134.
Franciosa, J.A., Baker, B.J., and Seth, L. (1985) Pulmonary versus systemic hemodynamics in determining exercise capacity of patients with chronic left ventricular failure. Am. Heart J. 110:807–813.
Gadsboll, N., Hoiland-Carlson, P.F., and Badsberg, J.H. (1991). Cardiac function and maximal exercise capacity early after acute myocardial infarction. Eur. Heart J. 12: 1189–1194.
Gallavardin, L. (1933). Les syndromes d'effort dans les affections cardioaortiques. J. Med. Lyon 14:539–558.
Gandevia, S.C., Killian, K.J., and Campbell, E.J.M. (1981). The effect of respiratory muscle fatigue on respiratory sensations. Clin. Sci. 60:463–466.
Gibbs, J.S.R., Keegan, J., Wright, C., Fox, K.M., and Poole-Wilson, P.A. (1990). Pulmonary artery pressure changes during exercise and daily activities in chronic heart failure. J. Am. Coll. Cardiol. 15:52–61.
Guyton, A.C. (1991). Textbook of Medical Physiology, 8th ed. W.B. Saunders, Philadelphia, p. 452.
Guyton, A.C., and Lindsey, A.W. (1959). Effect of elevated left atrial pressure and decreased plasma protein concentration on the development of pulmonary edema. Circ. Res. 7:649–657.
Hachamovitch, R., Brown, H.V., and Rubin, S.A. (1991). Respiratory and circulatory analysis of CO_2 output during exercise in chronic heart failure. Circulation 84: 605–612.
Hagman, M., and Wilhelmsen, L. (1981). Relationship between dyspnea and chest pain in ischaemic heart disease. Acta Med. Scand. (Suppl.) 644:16–18.

Hammond, M.D., Bauer, K.A., Sharp, J.T., and Rocha, R.D. (1990). Respiratory muscle strength in congestive heart failure. Chest 98:1091–1094.

Hansen, J.E., Sue, D.Y., Oren, A., and Wasserman, K. (1987). Relation of oxygen uptake to work rate in normal men and men with circulatory disorders. Am. J. Cardiol. 59: 669–674.

Heigenhauser, G.J.F., Sutton, J.R. and Jones, N.L. (1983). Effect of glycogen depletion on the ventilatory response to exercise. J. Appl. Physiol. 54:470–474.

Herrlin, B., and Sylvén, C. (1991). Increased arterial oxygen content—an important compensatory mechanism in chronic moderate heart failure. Cardiovasc. Res. 25: 384–390.

Higginbotham, M.B., Morris, K.G., Conn, E.H., Coleman, R.E., and Cobb, F.R. (1983). Determinants of variable exercise performance among patients with severe left ventricular dysfunction. Am. J. Cardiol. 51:52–60.

Hogg, J.C., Agarawal, J.B., Gardiner, A.J.S., Palmer, W.H., and Macklem, P.T. (1972). Distribution of airways resistance with developing pulmonary edema in dogs. J. Appl. Physiol. 32:20–24.

Hughes, E.F., Turner, S.C., and Brooks, G.A. (1982). Effects of glycogen depletion and pedalling speed on "anaerobic threshold." J. Appl. Physiol. 52:1598–1607.

Iaria, C.T., Jalar, U.H., and Kao, F.F. (1959). The peripheral neural mechanism of exercise hyperpnoea. J. Physiol. (Lond.) 148:49P–50P.

Kavanagh, T., Yacoub, M.H., Mertens, J., Kennedy, J., Campbell, R.B., and Sawyer, P. (1988). Cardiorespiratory responses to exercise training after orthotopic cardiac transplantation. Circulation 77:162–171.

Keteyian, S., Shepard, R., Ehrman, J., Fedel, F., Glick, C., Rhoads, K., and Levine, T.B. (1991). Cardiovascular responses of heart transplant patients to exercise training. J. Appl. Physiol. 70:2627–2631.

Kilburn, K.H. (1965). Muscular origin of elevated plasma potassium during exercise. J. Appl. Physiol. 21:675–678.

Kléber, A.G., and Oetliker, H. (1992). Early contractile failure in ischaemia. In: The Heart and Cardiovascular System, 2nd ed. Edited by H.A. Fozzard, E. Haber, R.B. Jennings, A.M. Katz, and H.E. Morgan. Raven Press, New York, pp. 1975–1996.

Lewis, T. (1933). Diseases of the Heart. Macmillan, London, pp. 1–2.

Light, R.M., and George, R.B. (1983). Serial pulmonary function in patients with acute heart failure. Arch. Intern. Med. 143:429–433.

Lim, M., Linton, R.A.F., Wolff, C.B., and Band, D.M. (1981). Propranolol, exercise and arterial plasma potassium. Lancet 2:591.

Lipkin, D.P., and Poole-Wilson, P.A., (1986). Symptoms limiting exercise capacity in chronic heart failure. B. M. J. 292:653–655.

Lipkin, D.P., Perrins, J., and Poole-Wilson, P.A. (1985). Respiratory gas exchange in the assessment of patients with impaired ventricular function. Br. Heart J. 54:321–328.

Lipkin, D.P., Scriven, A.J., Crake, T., and Poole-Wilson, P.A. (1986a). Six minute walking test for assessing exercise capacity in chronic heart failure. B. M. J. 292:653–655.

Lipkin, D.P., Canepa-Anson, R., Stephens, M.R., and Poole-Wilson, P.A. (1986b). Factors determining symptoms in heart failure: comparison of fast and slow exercise tests. Br. Heart J. 55:439–445.

Lipkin, D.P., Jones, D.A., Round, J.M., and Poole-Wilson, P.A. (1988). Abnormalities of skeletal muscle in patients with chronic heart failure. Int. J. Cardiol. 18:187–195.
Lloyd, T.C., Jr. (1980). Reflex effects of left heart and pulmonary vascular distension on airways of dogs. J. Appl. Physiol. 49:620–626.
Macklem, P.T. (1980). Respiratory muscles: the vital pump: Chest 78:753–758.
Mancini, D.M., Ferraro, N., Nazzaro, D., Chance, B., and Wilson, J.R. (1991). Respiratory muscle deoxygenation during exercise in patients with heart failure demonstrated with near-infrared spectroscopy. J. Am. Coll. Cardiol. 18:492–498.
Mancini, D.M., Walter, G., Reichnek, N., Lenkinski, R., McCully, K.K., Mullen, J.L., and Wilson, J.R. (1992a). Contribution of skeletal muscle atrophy to exercise intolerance and altered muscle metabolism in heart failure. Circulation 85:1364–1373.
Mancini, D.M., Henson, D., LaManca, J., and Levine, S. (1992b). Respiratory muscle function and dyspnea in patients with chronic congestive heart failure. Circulation 86:909–919.
Marshall, R., McIroy, M.B., and Christie, R.V. (1954). The work of breathing in mitral stenosis. Clin. Sci. 13:137–146.
Marzo, K., Herrmann, H.A., Rein, A., and Mancini, D. (1991). Acute effect of balloon mitral valvuloplasty on exercise capacity ventilation and skeletal muscle oxygenation. Circulation 84 (Suppl. II):II-72.
Marzo, K.P., Wilson, J.R., and Mancini, D.M. (1992). Effects of cardiac transplantation on ventilatory response to exercise. Am. J. Cardiol. 69:547–553.
Maskin, C.S., Forman, R., Sonnenblick, E.H., Frishman, W.H., and LeJemtel, T.H. (1983). Failure of dobutamine to increase exercise capacity despite haemodynamic improvement in severe chronic heart failure. Am. J. Cardiol. 51:177–182.
Massie, B.M., Kramer, B., and Haughom, F. (1981). Acute and long-term effects of vasodilator therapy on resting and exercise hemodynamics and exercise tolerance. Circulation 64:1218–1226.
Massie, B.M., Conway, M., Yonge, R., Frostick, S., Ledingham, J., Sleight, P., Radda, G., and Rajagopalan, B. (1987). Skeletal muscle metabolism in patients with congestive heart failure: relation to clinical severity and blood flow. Circulation 76:1009–1019.
McCloskey, D.I., and Mitchell, J.H. (1972). Reflex cardiovascular and respiratory responses originating in exercising muscle. J. Physiol. (Lond.) 224:173–187.
McMurray, J., Abdullah, I., Dargie, H.J., and Shapiro, D. (1991). Increased concentrations of tumour necrosis factor in "cachectic" patients with severe chronic heart failure. Br. Heart J. 66:356–358.
McParland, C., Krishnan, B., Wang, Y., and Gallagher, C.G. (1992). Inspiratory muscle weakness and dyspnea in chronic heart failure. Am. Rev. Respir. Dis. 146:467–472.
Metra, M., Raddino, R., Dei Cas, L., and Visioli, O. (1990). Assessment of peak oxygen consumption, lactate and ventilatory thresholds and correlation with resting and exercise haemodynamic data in chronic congestive heart failure. Am. J. Cardiol. 65:1127–1133.
Metra, M., Dei Cas, L., Panina, G., and Visioli, O. (1992). Exercise hyperventilation chronic congestive heart failure and its relation to functional capacity and hemodynamics. Am. J. Cardiol. 70:622–628.
Minotti, J.R., Christoph, I., Oka, R., Weiner, M.W., Wells, L., and Massie, B.M. (1991).

Impaired skeletal muscle function in patients with congestive heart failure. Relationship to systemic exercise performance. J. Clin. Invest. 88:2077–2082.
Minotti, J.R., Pillay, P., Chang, L., Wells, L., and Massie, B.M. (1992). Neurophysiological assessment of skeletal muscle fatigue in patients with congestive heart failure. Circulation 86:903–908.
Mohsenifar, Z., Amin, D.K., and Shah, P.K. (1989). Regional distribution of lung perfusion and ventilation in patients with chronic congestive heart failure and its relationship to cardiopulmonary hemodynamics. Am. Heart J. 117:887–891.
Moore, D.P., Gilligan, D., and Oakley, C.M. (1989). Hypocapnia during exercise testing in dilated cardiomyopathy and hypertrophic cardiomyopathy: objective assessment by respiratory gas analysis. Br. Heart J. 61:435.
Moore, D.P., Weston, A.R., Hughes, J.M.B., Oakley, C.M., and Cleland, J.G.F. (1992). Effects of increased inspired oxygen concentrations on exercise performance in chronic heart failure. Lancet 339:850–853.
Murray, J.F. (1985). The lungs and heart failure. Hosp. Pract. [off.] 20:55–66.
Packer, M. (1990). Abnormalities of diastolic function as a potential cause of exercise intolerance in chronic heart failure. Circulation 81 (Suppl. III):III-78–III-86.
Paintal, A.S. (1969). Mechanism of stimulation of type J pulmonary receptors. J. Physiol. (Lond.) 203:511–532.
Paintal, A.S. (1973). Vagal sensory receptors and their reflex effects. Physiol. Rev. 53: 159–227.
Paterson, D.J., Robbins, P.A., and Conway, J. (1989). Changes in arterial plasma potassium and ventilation during exercise in man. Respir. Physiol. 78:323–330.
Paterson, D.J., Friedland, J.S., Bascom, D.A., Clement, I.D., Cunningham, D.A., Painter, R., and Robbins, P.A. (1990). Changes in arterial K^+ and ventilation during exercise in normal subjects and patients with McArdle's syndrome. J. Physiol. (Lond.) 429: 339–348.
Petermann, W., Barth, J., and Entzian, P. (1987). Heart failure and airways obstruction. Int. J. Cardiol. 17:207–209.
Poole-Wilson, P.A. (1985). Heart failure. Med. Int. 2:866–871.
Poole-Wilson, P.A. (1989). Chronic heart failure: causes, pathophysiology, prognosis, clinical manifestations, investigations. In: Diseases of the Heart. Edited by D.G. Julian, A.J. Camm, K.M. Fox, R.J.C. Hall, and P.A. Poole-Wilson. Bailliére-Tindall, London. p. 48 for quoted definition; pp. 48–57 for entire chapter.
Pouleur, H., Covell, J.W., and Ross, J., Jr. (1980). Effects of nitroprusside and central blood volume in the absence and presence of acute heart failure. Circulation 61:328–337.
Rajfer, S.A., Nemanich, J.W., Shurman, A.J., and Rossen, J.D. (1987). Metabolic responses to exercise in patients with heart failure. Circulation 76 (Suppl. VI):VI46–VI53.
Reddy, H.K., Weber, K.T., Janicki, J.S., and McElroy, P.A. (1988). Hemodynamic, ventilatory and metabolic effects of light isometric exercise in patients with chronic heart failure. J. Am. Coll. Cardiol. 12:53–58.
Restrick, L.J., Davies, S.W., Noone, L., and Wedzicha, J.A. (1992). Ambulatory oxygen in chronic heart failure. Lancet 334:1192–1193.
Rose, G.A. (1962). The diagnosis of ischaemic heart pain and intermittent claudication in field surveys. Bull. World Health Organ. 27:645–658.

Rowell, L.B. (1986). The nature of the exercise stimulus. Acta Physiol. Scand. 556:7–14.

Rowell, L.B., and O'Learly, D.S. (1990). Reflex control of the circulation during exercise: chemoreflexes and mechanoreflexes. J. Appl. Physiol. 69:407–418.

Rubin, S.A., and Brown, H.V. (1984). Ventilation and gas exchange during exercise in severe chronic heart failure. Am. Rev. Respir. Dis. (Suppl.) 129:S63–S64.

Rubin, S.A., Brown, H.V., and Swan, H.J.C. (1982). Arterial oxygenation and arterial oxygen transport in chronic myocardial failure at rest, during exercise and after hydralazine treatment. Circulation 66:143–148.

Schoenmackers, J. (1960). Über Bronchialvenen und ihre Stellung zwischen groeen und kleinen Kreislauf. Arch. Kreisaufforsch. 32:1–86.

Sinoway, L.I., Minotti, J.R., Davis, D., Pennock, J.L., Burg, J.E., Musch, T.I., and Zelis, R. (1988). Delayed reversal of impaired vasodilation in congestive heart failure after heart transplantation. Am. J. Cardiol. 61:1076–1079.

Sullivan, M.J., and Cobb, F.R. (1990). The anaerobic threshold in chronic heart failure. Circulation 81 (Suppl. II):II47–II58.

Sullivan, M.J., Higginbotham, M.R., and Cobb, F.R. (1988). Increased exercise ventilation in patients with chronic heart failure: intact ventilatory control despite haemodynamic and pulmonary abnormalities. Circulation 77:552–559.

Sullivan, M.J., Green, H.J., and Cobb, F.R. (1990). Skeletal muscle biochemistry and histology in ambulatory patients with long-term heart failure. Circulation 81: 518–527.

Sullivan, M.J., Green, H.J., and Cobb, F.R. (1991). Altered skeletal muscle response to exercise in chronic heart failure. Relation to skeletal muscle aerobic enzyme activity. Circulation 84:1597–1607.

Szlachcic, J., Massie, B.M., Kramer, B.L., Topic, N., and Tubau, J. (1985). Correlates and prognostic implication of exercise capacity in chronic congestive heart failure. Am. J. Cardiol. 55:1037–1042.

Taki, J., Yasuda, T., Flamm, S.D., Hutter, A., Gold, H.K., Leinbach, R., and Strauss, H.W., (1992). Comparison of painful and painless left ventricular dysfunction recorded during ambulatory ventricular function monitoring in angina pectoris secondary to coronary artery disease. Am. J. Cardiol. 70:1555–1558.

Tallarida, G., Baldoni, F., Peruzzi, G., Raimondi, G., Di Nardo, P., Massaro, M., Visigalli, G., Franconi, G., and Sangiorgi, M. (1985). Cardiorespiratory reflex from muscles during dynamic and static exercise in the dog. J. Appl. Physiol. 58:844–850.

Tibes, U., Hemmer, B., and Boning, D. (1977). Heart rate and ventilation in relation to venous [K^+], osmolality, pH, Pco_2, Po_2, [orthophosphate], and [lactate] at transition from rest to exercise in athletes and non-athletes. Eur. J. Appl. Physiol. 36:127–140.

Uren, N.G., Davies, S.W., Jordan, S.L., and Lipkin, D.P. (1991). Increased exercise capacity after nebulised diamorphine in chronic heart failure (abstract). Br. Heart J. 66:112.

Uren, N.G., Davies, S.W., Agnew, J.E., Irwin, A.G., Jordan, S.L., Hilson, A.J.W., and Lipkin, D.P. (1993). Reduction of mismatch of global ventilation and perfusion on exercise is related to exercise capacity in chronic heart failure. Eur. Heart J. 70: 241–246.

Volterrani, M., Clark, A.L., Ludman, P.F., Swan, J.W., Adamopoulos, S., Piepoli, M., and Coats, A.J.S. (1994). Determinants of exercise capacity in chronic heart failure. Eur. Heart J. 15:801–809.

Weber, K.T., Kinasewitz, G.T., Janicki, J.S., and Fishman, A.P. (1982). Oxygen utilisation and ventilation during exercise in patients with chronic cardiac failure. Circulation 65:1213–1223.

Weber, K.T., Wilson, J.R., Janicki, J., and Likoff, M.J. (1984). Exercise testing in the evaluation of the patient with chronic cardiac failure. Am. Rev. Respir. Dis. (Suppl.) 129:S60–S62.

Weil, M.H., and Afifi, A.A. (1970). Experimental and clinical studies on lactate and pyruvate as indicators of the severity of acute circulatory failure (shock). Circulation 41:989–1001.

Whipp, B.J. (1983). Ventilatory control during exercise in humans. Annu. Rev. Physiol. 45:393–413.

White, H.C., Butler, J., and Donald, K.W. (1958). Lung compliance in patients with mitral stenosis. Clin. Sci. 17:667–679.

Wilson, J.R., Mancini, D.M., Ferraro, N., and Egler, J. (1988). Effect of dichloroacetate on the exercise performance of patients with heart failure. J. Am. Coll. Cardiol. 12:1464–1469.

Yeh, M.P., Gardner, M.R., Adams, T.D., Yanowitz, F.G., and Crapo, R.O. (1983). "Anaerobic threshold": problems of determination and validation. J. Appl. Physiol. 55: 1178–1186.

12

Perception of Asthma

CHRISTOPHER M. B. HIGGS

Dorothy House Foundation
Bath, England

GABRIEL LASZLO

Bristol Royal Infirmary
and University of Bristol
Bristol, England

I. Relationship Between Subjective and Objective Measurements in Bronchial Asthma

Bronchial asthma is characterized by variability in airway caliber with similarly variable respiratory sensations that include shortness of breath. Some asthmatics are more aware of these symptoms than others, even when lung mechanics are similar. This phenomenon has been studied from time to time since techniques have been available to measure lung function, but its clinical importance has not yet been determined (Bates, 1952; McFadden et al., 1973; Rubinfeld and Pain, 1976).

In clinical practice, a minority of patients take inappropriate amounts of medication for the relief of seemingly mild airflow obstruction; others cause their physicians to despair at their habitually late reporting of disabling exacerbations. Overmedication has been demonstrated among many patients with a tendency to panic during attacks (Dahlem et al., 1977). Jansen-Bjerklie and her colleagues (1992) confirmed that most asthmatics sought help during severe exacerbations in an appropriate manner: these authors regarded "panic" and "fear" as useful information heralding the onset of an attack.

Failure to report for treatment has been implicated as a cause of death in asthma in retrospective surveys (Ormerod and Stableforth, 1980; Johnson et al., 1984; Sears, 1991). It is very difficult to study deaths from asthma prospectively because they are, fortunately, relatively rare. Nevertheless, it is important to determine epidemiologically whether regular treatment, as opposed to symptom control relying on self-assessment, results in an improvement in the morbidity and mortality of asthma. Until this question has been settled, clinicians and researchers need to determine in some way the perceptive threshold and the relationship between symptoms and pulmonary function (Nana and Pain, 1985). Case histories, diary cards, and lung function measurements yield separate items of information about the individual with bronchial asthma. These can be combined and analyzed to produce a picture of that individual's perception of bronchial narrowing.

II. Overview of Past Studies

The relationship between subjective self-assessment of asthma and objective measurement of lung function has been studied in a number of ways.

A. During Acute Severe Asthma and Recovery

In 1973, a study was performed in patients admitted with acute severe asthma, comparing symptoms of dyspnea and wheeze with clinical examination, spirometry, lung volumes, and airways resistance (McFadden et al., 1973). There was poor correlation between symptoms and objective lung function; dyspnea and wheezing did not consistently identify those who had severe impairment of pulmonary function. This was consistent with previous studies showing asthmatics can be asymptomatic despite impairment in respiratory function (Bates, 1952). More recently, a study of acute severe asthma and recovery comparing visual analog scores of breathlessness with peak expiratory flow rate showed that there can be considerable correlation in some but not all patients (Dhand et al., 1988). This study also showed that correlation between breathlessness and peak expiratory flow rate is less during acute asthma than during stable asthma. From our own observations, we also agree that perception of asthma occurring during rapid alterations in physiological state, as in acute severe asthma and exercise-induced asthma, is very different from perception of day-to-day variation in the condition of the airways.

B. Added Resistive Loads to Breathing in Asthma

Studies of the effect of external expiratory resistive loading on breathlessness in normal subjects have contributed little to the subject of perception of asthma. This is partly because of conflicting results and partly because symptoms of asthma cannot be adequately simulated by resistive loads that have little effect on vital capacity. An external expiratory resistive load in excess of the internal load of a severe asthmatic attack can be handled with little breathlessness by breathing slowly and deeply. Furthermore, during external loading there is no increase in lung volume, which is an integral part of the sensation of chest tightness in asthma (Permutt, 1992) and probably in induced bronchoconstriction (Lougheed et al., 1993).

There is a wide variation in the perception of added resistive loads to breathing by patients with asthma (Burki et al., 1978; Burdon et al., 1982), but this is not necessarily different from that found in normal subjects (Burki et al., 1978; Gottfried et al., 1981; Hudgel et al., 1982). Some of the variation and reported differences between normal and asthmatic subjects (Bonnel et al., 1985; del Volgo-Mathiot and Bonnel, 1991) may be a result of psychological factors (Hudgel et al., 1982; Tiller et al., 1987) and the effect of background chronic airflow obstruction (Burki et al., 1978; Gottfried et al., 1978; Mathiot et al., 1986). Kikuchi et al. (1994) studied 11 subjects who had lost consciousness or required mechanical ventilation; these individuals recorded less severe breathlessness when breathing against resistances than asthmatics without near-fatal attacks, who did not differ greatly from normal subjects.

C. Induced Bronchoconstriction

The first major investigation into the perception of bronchoconstriction was by Rubinfeld and Pain (1976). They asked 82 asthmatics to indicate at that point during methacholine challenge they first perceived tightness, and 15% of subjects failed to sense bronchoconstriction at a time when forced expiratory volume in one second (FEV_1) was 20% below starting value.

Other studies have looked at threshold detection of tightness (Rubinfeld and Pain, 1977a, b) and the sensation of breathlessness (Burdon et al., 1982; Orehek et al., 1982; Turcotte et al., 1990) compared with spirometry, lung volumes, or airways conductance. Burdon et al. demonstrated a correlation between Borg scores and respiratory function during histamine challenges and again noted the occasional presence of a very low threshold and widely differing use of the scores at each step in the bronchial challenge procedure. Individuals with greater hyper-reactivity and those with initial airflow obstruction recorded lower scores for the same degree of airflow obstruction. They explained these findings by postulating some form of temporal adaptation or acclimatization. Orehek et al. performed a simpler experiment in which they recorded the presence or absence of dyspnea during the sequential inhalation of inert aerosol, carbachol-induced bronchoconstriction, and subsequent bronchodilatation with salbutamol. All the subjects had asthma: those without initial airflow obstruction responded appropriately.

Those with airflow obstruction at the start were given only placebo and salbutamol; only half of these detected any change in the presence or absence of breathlessness. Lung function was similar in those who sensed bronchodilatation and those who did not. The conclusion was that chronic airflow obstruction impairs the perception of changes in airway tone. Turcotte et al. found no difference in the perception of breathlessness between bronchoconstriction induced by histamine challenge, antigen exposure, or exercise but found a difference between the early and late asthmatic responses, again suggesting a difference in perception of rapidly evolving and slowly developing physiological changes. Killian et al. (1991) studied a large number of asthmatics during exercise and during artificially induced bronchoconstriction. Lougheed et al. questioned this interpretation; they studied 21 patients with mild asthma during bronchoprovocation and found that the best predictor of discomfort was the degree of change in lung inflation. Those who found the pharmacological challenge excessively uncomfortable tended also to experience the greatest degree of dyspnea during exercise.

Although the sensation of tightness experienced during induced bronchoconstriction is closer to the sensation of asthma than external resistive loads, there are some differences and these sensations are probably not strictly comparable. Rather specific terms, such as "chest tightness," correlate better with FEV_1 during bronchial challenge than inquiries about asthma (Marks et al., 1993). In another study of 21 subjects, the descriptions used varied greatly; the most frequent responses were restriction to deep inspiration (95% methacholine, 70% spontaneous asthma); increased work of breathing (90% methacholine, 85% asthma); and difficulty inspiring (90% methacholine, 70% asthma). "Tightness" and "difficulty breathing out" were less commonly mentioned. "Inspiratory difficulty" equated with "asthma breathlessness" in correlating with falls in FEV_1 during the challenge (Lougheed et al., 1993). This problem has led to attempts to study perception during spontaneously occurring asthmatic attacks, which are reviewed critically in Sec. III.

III. Measurement of Perception of Asthma

A. Symptoms Used

Symptoms reported by asthmatics include the sensations of tightness, breathlessness, wheeze, and cough. Some diagnostic confusion arises when the only symptoms are cough and/or exertional dyspnea (McFadden, 1975). In current practice, asthma is diagnosed when one or more symptoms are present in conjunction with variability in lung function over time.

Diary cards for recording patients' symptoms of asthma have been in use for some time in the diagnosis and evaluation of their condition and as an adjunct to pharmaceutical trials (Turner-Warwick, 1977). There are remarkably few reports on the frequency of the various symptoms of asthma and their relationship to the severity of asthma. The first recorded symptoms of "asthma" are in the works of Aretaeus the Cappadocian, circa second century C.E. (Adams, 1860): "The symptoms of its approach are heaviness of the chest, sluggishness to one's accustomed work, difficulty in breathing . . .; they are troubled by cough, flatulence . . . and restlessness. Sometimes a pain comes into the back." The asthma was probably synonymous with breathlessness, and we cannot be sure that Aretaeus was describing asthma as we understand it today. Sir John Floyer, who suffered from typical bronchial asthma, describes "straitness of breathing, . . . convulsive cough, . . . some wheezing, . . . sometimes a little phlegm . . . . the limbs appear quite heavy." (Floyer, 1698). A brief survey of modern textbooks reveals that breathlessness and wheeze are always mentioned. Many mention chest tightness, some mention cough, and a few mention nocturnal waking. Kinsman et al. (1973), using a psychologically oriented questionnaire, the asthma symptom checklist, have shown in 175 patients the wide variety of symptoms that patients report experiencing with asthma if questioned closely.

It is apparent when interviewing patients with asthma that each experiences different combinations of symptoms that vary with the severity of the asthma. A variety of diary cards in use record breathlessness, cough, nocturnal waking, limitation of activity, or wheeze in various combinations. Scores for these symptoms may not consequently relate to severity of asthma. Higgs et al. (1985) interviewed 56 patients with asthma, 31 males and 25 females aged 18–74 years. The patients were asked, "What symptoms do you experience with your asthma?" and "What symptoms do you use to judge the severity of your asthma?" The answers are shown in Table 1. They were then asked specifically which symptoms

Table 1 Symptoms Experienced with Asthma as Reported by 56 Patients (Expressed as %)

Symptom	Percentage reported
Breathlessness	95
Tightness	86
Wheeze	88
Cough	48
Chest pain	46
Limitation of activity	16
Nocturnal waking	13
Panic	11
Sputum	7

Table 2 Symptoms Used to Judge the Severity of Asthma as Reported by 56 Patients (Expressed as %)

Symptom	Percentage used to judge severity
Breathlessness	75
Tightness	70
Wheeze	52
Cough	30
Chest pain	30
Limitation of activity	16
Nocturnal waking	13
Loss of inhaler response	6
Fast pulse rate	4
Sputum	4

they experienced or used to judge the severity of the asthma. The answers are shown in Table 2. Also, 20 patients were asked which symptoms increased or decreased as the asthma worsened. During an attack they reported that breathlessness (100%), tightness (92%), and chest pain (33%) increased. As expected, wheeze worsened in 71% but lessened in 18% during an attack, but change in the severity of cough was unpredictable. We obtained similar results in a much larger study of patients recruited in general practice (unpublished). This implied that if symptoms are to be used in self-assessment of asthma, they must be individually selected and their relationship to severity of asthma assessed.

For this reason, in our studies and some others (Fritz et al., 1990), it was decided to measure the answer to one question—How is your asthma?—rather than score separate symptoms or even the single symptom of breathlessness. It is likely, however, that the results of such studies are comparable to those in which breathlessness was chosen as the marker of airflow obstruction.

B. Scaling Methods

A variety of methods have been used for scaling subjective sensation. They can be classified into ordinal or category scales, interval scales, and ratio scales (Stevens, 1975). The type of scale used depends on the question being asked and the sensitivity required.

Symptoms of asthma are often scored on diary cards using an ordinal scale or a category scale; the number of ordinals or categories determines the sensitivity. The visual analog scale (VAS) is a 10 cm line with marks only at either end. It was first used for scoring mood by Freyd (1923), but it had gained common use when

Aitken (1969) described its use in measuring feelings and then applied it to measure the sensation of breathing with added resistive loads (Aitken et al., 1970).

Accepting that assessment of breathlessness, like self-assessment of asthma, is subjective, with no satisfactory objective substitute, VAS has been employed to assess breathlessness in normal subjects with satisfactory within-subject reproducibility (Stark and Gambles, 1980; Adams et al., 1985) and adequate sensitivity (Stark et al., 1981). The VAS has subsequently been used extensively in the symptomatic assessment of asthma.

The ratio scaling for magnitude estimation commonly used for studies of breathlessness in normal subjects (Killian et al., 1981) is extremely difficult to apply in untrained asthmatics. The modified Borg scale use in the study of breathlessness with acute changes in asthma (Burdon et al., 1982) is a form of category scale with ratio properties that seems to work fairly well in the laboratory (Nana and Pain, 1985). Its ratio bias limits its sensitivity in patients who are generally not experiencing severe asthma.

In a comparison of the VAS and magnitude estimation in assessing breathlessness in normal subjects, Adams et al. (1985) found that both methods yield valid information, but subjects regarded the VAS as a more appropriate means of rating breathlessness. Wilson and Jones (1989) preferred the Borg scale because of its slightly greater stability for measuring dyspnea in normal subjects. Ratio scaling for magnitude estimation is relatively independent of absolute intensities of sensation. The VAS attempts to quantify a sensory level in terms of arbitrary and, it is hoped, constant extremes. It cannot be a truly quantitative scale, but its relative simplicity and apparent reproducibility over time and its ease of application to therapeutic trials have made it the technique of choice. In long-term studies its reproducibility may be limited by the stability of the ends of the scales. For the VAS measuring How is your asthma? the maximum end is anchored to the "most severe asthma" ever experienced by the individual. Assuming that this sensation is not very recent and is not superseded during the course of the study, this extreme can be constant over long periods of time. We therefore chose to use this technique in our studies of the impact of spontaneously occurring asthma in stable clinical situations. Others have scored breathlessness in a similar fashion. Subjects tend to overscore when first introduced to a scale, regardless of which method is used (Wilson and Jones, 1989).

C. Measurement of Airflow Obstruction

No test of airway function is an absolute measure of the asthmatic stimulus. They all yield an approximate estimate, and there is no physiological reason this should be linear. The sensation is judged according to an internal standard—the most severe asthma ever experienced.

Peak expiratory flow (PEF) is generally used to measure spontaneous variations in bronchial caliber in asthma. The equipment is portable and relatively inexpensive. Experience shows that the measurement is sensitive to changes of clinical importance. It can be made repeatedly without inducing bronchoconstriction, which may complicate repeated attempts at measuring FEV_1 or other derivatives of the forced vital capacity. Most, although not all, patients can be taught to measure it reliably (Hetzel et al., 1979).

There is no inexpensive portable device that measures changes in airway resistance during quiet breathing. Fortunately, this measurement correlates fairly well with PEF (Wigal et al., 1986). The original observations of McFadden et al. (1973) were made using a body plethysmograph. FEV_1 is usually employed to measure bronchoconstriction induced in the laboratory by methacholine or histamine, although the measurement of airways resistance offers an attractive and sensitive alternative.

D. Breathlessness in Airflow Obstruction: Relationship to Objective Measurements of Pulmonary Function

The relationship between breathlessness, measured on a Borg scale, and FEV_1 is more or less linear (Burdon et al., 1982).

Experience shows that there is a surprising degree of fairly linear correlation in the number of individuals between subjective assessments of breathlessness and PEF, even in individuals who have not had experience of home measurements. This is useful but hard to understand. Peak flow cannot be considered a linear scale of lung function (Sec. III.C). Furthermore, in some subjects, other indices of airflow obstruction, such as residual volume and total lung capacity, may vary without any change in FEV_1 and probably therefore in PEF (Woolcock and Read, 1966).

The problem of breathing in moderate or severe airflow obstruction is readily explained by mechanical factors.

1. Airway narrowing increases inspiratory resistance and thus work of breathing.
2. Most patients with airflow obstruction show airway closure by functional residual capacity (FRC) and in some instances increases in total lung capacity. The increase in FRC is probably achieved by persistent inspiratory muscle activity throughout expiration and is thought to improve ventilation by increasing airway dimensions. The disadvantage of this adjustment is that the inspiratory muscles are shortened and thus rendered less efficient, the chest wall is close to its resting position, and therefore total compliance of the lungs and chest is increased. These factors combine to make inspiration more uncomfortable and difficult. The addition of continuous positive airway pressure reduces

inspiratory work but does not relieve the sensation of dyspnea, emphasizing the contribution of hyperinflation to the total discomfort of acute asthma (Permutt, 1992).

3. A reduction in midexpiratory flow rates can result in flow limitation during quiet breathing. If the time required for expiration is prolonged or if FRC is never reached, this shortens the time available for inspiration when ventilation increases during exercise.

These factors combine to make the work of the inspiratory muscles approach their maximal capacity when there is airflow obstruction.

In all probability, PEF is a reliable indicator of the varying severity of bronchial asthma because most of the measurements deteriorate and improve together in the majority of subjects. Thus, there is at least crude correlation between changes in PEF, maximal inspiratory flow, functional residual capacity, and residual volume in the majority of subjects under stable conditions. Further studies are required during recovery from acute severe asthma to determine the changing relationship between symptoms and different indices of airflow obstruction.

E. Obscuring the Test

In about one-quarter of asthmatics, self-assessment of asthma may be influenced by a knowledge of PEF (Higgs et al., 1986). In this study, 12 subjects recorded the severity of their asthma using a visual analog scale, with other diary card entries, before making triplicate measurements of PEF on a linear electronic device that allowed the results to be shown to the subject or printed in code. In one-quarter of these patients, there was significant and clinically important improvement in the linear correlation between visual analog scores and PEF. In addition, all the subjects except 1 showed an increase in the numerical value of the correlation coefficient between these variables, indicating that, across the board, there was some influence of knowledge of recent trends in PEF on subjective self-assessment of asthma.

Electronic rotating vane peak flow meters are robust, and they can be rendered acceptably linear by digital computing techniques that allow for the inertia of the device as flow is initiated (and, in volume measurements, for the momentum of the vane after flow has ceased). Devices are now available that are capable of storing 2–4 weeks results in electronic memory for subsequent computer analysis. This avoids the need for coding. They can be programmed to store diary information at the same time and also allow the results of the tests to be concealed or shown to the subject. There is a theoretical risk that a patient may become seriously ill or even die after deteriorating over a period of time, with distressing consequences if the peak flow readings were subsequently decoded and the event shown to have been preventable. For this reason, memorizing meters should incorporate a "low reading" warning, which is shown to the patient even if the readout is supposed to be concealed.

The evidence of whether the measurement of PEF improves the ability of patients to judge changes in airflow obstruction subjectively is contradictory (Sly et al., 1985; Silverman et al., 1990; Clark et al., 1992). In theory, the peak flow meter should be useful as an educational tool as well as a monitoring device, but it may not necessarily be better than training the patients simply to recognize the importance of their symptoms (Charlton et al., 1990).

F. Perception of Bronchoconstriction and Discrimination of Changes in Bronchial Caliber: Methods of Analysis

Two major aspects of perception of asthma have been investigated:

1. The threshold of lung function below which the individual notices abnormal respiratory sensations (threshold of perception).
2. The ability of individual asthmatics to detect changes in the magnitude of the airflow obstruction or, conversely, to predict their lung function (perception of change or discrimination).

In the pioneering study of perceptive threshold (Rubinfeld and Pain, 1976), individuals were asked to score their respiratory sensations using Borg's category scale before the measurement of FEV_1. Bronchoconstriction was induced by the inhalation of methacholine. The threshold of detection was the single point at which a score of higher than 0 was recorded. The observation that 15% of the subjects failed to detect bronchoconstriction at any stage was the stimulus to further work, reviewed in Sec. I.C.

In recent years, a number of investigations have been published employing visual analog techniques to scale the respiratory sensation of asthma during spontaneous variations in peak flow. Interaction between subjective and objective recordings was avoided in various ways. Higgs studied 22 subjects for periods of 2 weeks, asking the question, How is your asthma? by means of a visual analog scale anchored at each end. Results were measured in millimeters (maximum 100) and plotted against PEF measured on a coded meter. Fritz et al. (1990) carried out a similar investigation asking the same question of children in a summer camp. The problem of blinding the peak flow results did not arise, because the measurements were made by trained observers and the children similarly instructed in the use of the visual analog score. We have studied 255 asthmatics recruited in general practice using coded peak flow meters (Kendrick et al., 1993).

Peiffer et al. (1989) posed a similar question relating to breathlessness, which was answered on a visual analog scale and sealed, after which the peak flow measurement was recorded. These results were posted to the investigator. Again, several readings were taken on each day of the study.

The simplest way to consider these results is to measure the correlation coefficient between subjective and objective measurements. This has some validity, provided that it is used carefully. Higgs et al. (1986) showed an improved correlation when PEF was not coded. Fritz et al. (1990) used this to study "perceptual accuracy" among 37 schoolchildren, who provided a mean of 34 observations. Poor correlation is found if the numbers are distributed randomly, but in addition it can be limited by a restriction of the range of either measurement. Clearly, those with a restricted range of PEF may not have important asthma and should be excluded, but those who use only a limited range of VAS demonstrate insensitivity to their physiological status.

The results of this type of experiment are illustrated by some examples of measurements made over a 2-week period by three of our asthmatic subjects who had not recently used an uncoded peak flow meter (Fig. 1). In example A, there is a strong linear correlation between the visual analog scores and coded PEF, expressed here as a percentage of the reference value. In example B the scatter is wider and the correlation is weaker. Subject C had a very poor ability to detect bronchoconstriction, and in this instance the correlation coefficient was close to 0.

Fritz et al. divided their subjects into those with high accuracy ($r = -0.6$ and better, 6 of 31 subjects), medium accuracy (-0.3 to -0.59, 17 of 31 subjects), and low accuracy (below -0.3, 13 of 31 subjects). Peiffer et al. required a correlation coefficient of 0.7 to define good perception, which seems rather stringent. This yielded a figure of over 60% of subjects with poor ability to detect changes in their airflow obstruction. We have allowed for the different number of observations in each subjects by examining significance levels: again, the cutoff point is arbitrary and a value of 5% is probably too stringent. We found a range of correlations similar to those of Fritz et al. in our earlier studies of patients who were attending a hospital clinic. As might be expected, a much lower proportion (40%) of patients recruited in general practice showed significant correlations between their visual analog scores and coded peak flow rates.

As stated earlier, the plots of VAS on PEF are, fortuitously, sufficiently symmetrical to allow linear correlation analysis to be used, and there is no need to employ nonparametric regression. Approximately 10% of individuals in our series appeared to change the way in which they use the visual analog scale during the first 24–48 h of the period of observation. These subjects record high scores at first but gradually settle down to using a more limited range of visual analog scores to mark the severity of the diurnal variation. It is therefore wise to discard the observations made in the first 48 h.

Other derivatives of these plots can be useful under certain circumstances, according to the problem under study.

1. Standard error of VAS on PEF. This is the ability of the individual to predict PEF from symptoms in a way that allows for the fact that those who use a narrower range of VAS necessarily show lower values of r.

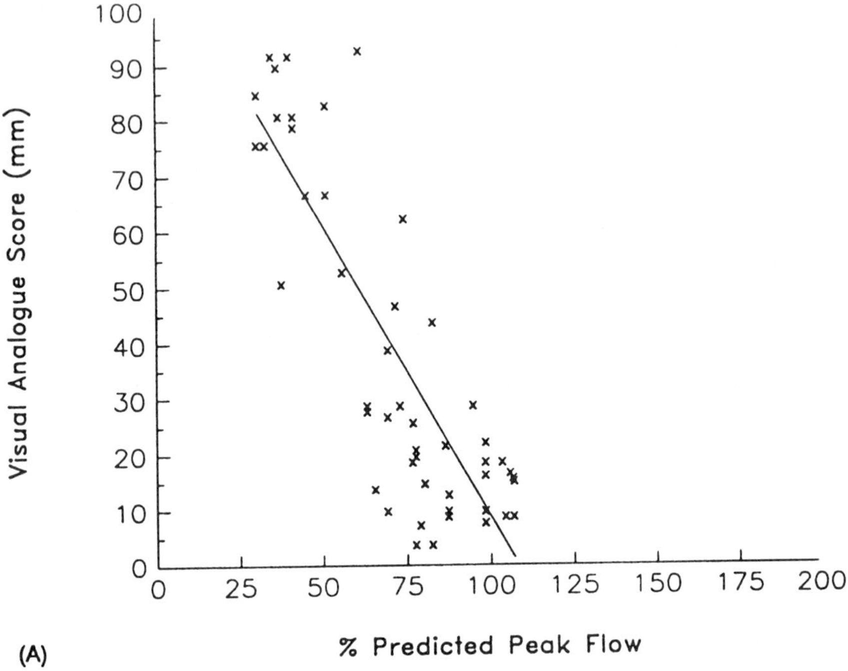
Visual Analogue Score (mm)
100
90
80
70
60
50
40
30
20
10
0
0 25 50 75 100 125 150 175 200
% Predicted Peak Flow

(A)

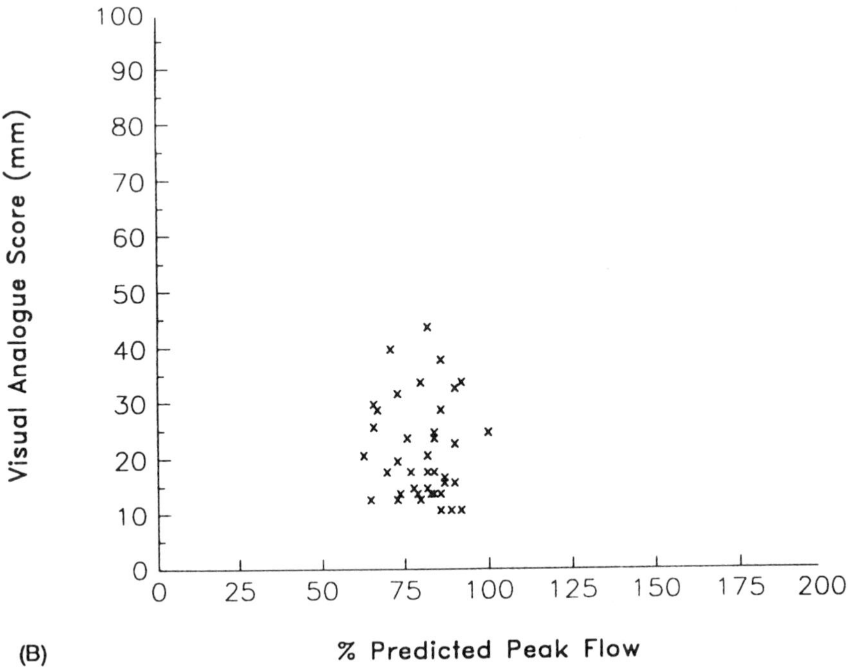
Visual Analogue Score (mm)
100
90
80
70
60
50
40
30
20
10
0
0 25 50 75 100 125 150 175 200
% Predicted Peak Flow

(B)

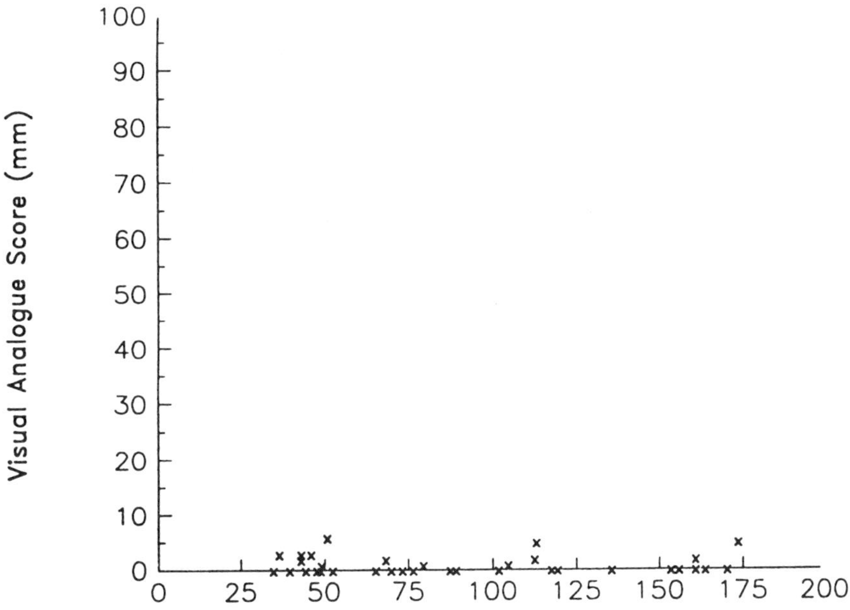

(C)

Figure 1 (A). Good perception of asthma and discrimination of changes in bronchial caliber. Visual analog asthma score plotted against simultaneous measurement of peak expiratory flow recorded by the subject on a meter with a coded readout. In this subject, visual analog asthma scores correlate strongly and in a linear fashion peak expiratory flow. There were 50 measurements, made approximately four times daily over a period of 2 weeks. (B) Poor discrimination of changes in lung function in a subject who was continuously aware of the presence of asthma but in whom there was no significant correlation between peak expiratory flow and visual analog asthma scores. There were 38 observations over 2 weeks. (C) Poor perception of asthma. This subject, who participated in the same study, had large diurnal swings in peak expiratory flow, but most of the visual analog scores were close to the end of the line marked no asthma. There were 34 observations over 2 weeks. The participants were asked to make records four times daily over this period. (Supplied by Dr. A. H. Kendrick.)

2. Slope of VAS on PEF. This can be used to measure the psychological impact of changes in PEF and appears to be sensitive to treatment, as discussed later. It is determined to a major degree by the maximum value of VAS but corrects this for the severity of airflow obstruction.
3. Slope of VAS against the logarithm of PEF (expressed as a percentage of predicted normal). This calculation emphasizes changes in PEF at the lower end of the range: in other words, a fall in PEF from 50 to 25% of predicted normal is allowed the same importance as a fall from

100 to 50%. In our combined series of over 270 sets of measurements, the correlation coefficients were higher when this transformation was applied. This index is most useful for comparisons between individuals.

4. Perceptive threshold. We recently explored the possibility of measuring perceptive threshold from home readings using coded measurements of PEF (Kendrick et al., 1994). The method consists of dividing the range of PEF recorded into five equal compartments and identifying the highest compartment in which at least 50% of the visual analog scores lie above a threshold near zero. Using this approach, we identified 41 subjects of the total of 255 whose visual analog scores did not leave the baseline throughout the experiment. All these subjects had significant asthma. It is possible that some may have failed to understand the idea of visual analog scores, but they comprise 16% of the total, which corresponds closely to the proportion of asthmatic subjects with poor perception of bronchoconstriction induced by pharmacological challenge. The proportion is similar in healthy individuals without asthma (James et al., 1993).

We suggest that a distinction be made between poor perception of bronchoconstriction (acclimatization, lack of awareness, or subconscious denial of any symptom of asthma) and poor discrimination of changes in airway caliber.

IV. Possible Factors Influencing Accuracy of Symptom Perception in Asthma

The differing methods of studying perception of asthma and the lack of consensus about what constitutes excessive, normal, and poor perception of asthma make it difficult to bring together all the data so far available. However, some generalizations are possible.

A. Epidemiology

Since the first demonstration by Rubinfeld and Pain in 1976 that 15% of their group of asthmatics were unable to sense major changes in airflow obstruction, there has been fairly consistent agreement that 15–20% of asthmatics fail to detect bronchoconstriction when it is moderately severe (Nana et al., 1983; Higgs, 1987; Dhand et al., 1988; Irie et al., 1991; Ruffin et al., 1991). A much higher percentage may be aware of their asthma but are not very good at predicting lung function from their symptoms.

There is some evidence that poor perception is more common in asthmatics who suffer nearly fatal asthma attacks (Ruffin et al., 1991) or fatal attacks of asthma (Zach and Karner, 1989). A case-controlled study, mentioned earlier, of 11 subjects who had experienced "near-miss asthma death" showed that these individuals were less dyspneic than other asthmatics and normal subjects when breathing through a circuit with a high inspiratory resistance. Moreover, their ventilatory and inspiratory pressure responses to induced hypoxemia were markedly blunted compared with the control group's. The subjects with the lowest ventilatory responses also had low breathlessness scores during loaded breathing. The authors concluded that their results could not be explained by acclimatization to airflow obstruction, because all three groups experienced the same dyspnea during CO_2-loaded breathing, which generally does not affect airway resistance adversely. The conclusion from this experimental study is that a combination of impaired perception of loaded breathing and a poor ventilatory response to hypoxemia is a risk factor for a severe attack (Kikuchi et al., 1994).

Near-miss sudden death is rare, and case-controlled studies like this are needed to investigate it. Our preliminary results suggest that in the population as a whole, poor discrimination is not associated with near-miss sudden death or a history of severe asthma. Many such individuals appear to have mild asthma: in these instances poor ability to discriminate changes in peak flow may simply represent adaption to a tolerable disorder. In a study from rural France, although a high proportion of asthmatics admitted to regular symptoms, one-quarter believed they required no treatment and 60% failed to seek medical help during attacks (Taytard et al., 1990). Perception of the need for treatment must be distinguished from perception of symptoms.

B. Age and Sex

There is no significant difference between the sexes in perception of asthma. Studies relating asthma symptom score to peak flow have not found any correlation with age (Nana and Pain, 1985; Peiffer et al., 1989; Higgs, 1987), but Connolly et al. (1992) showed impaired perception of bronchoconstriction in elderly asthmatics and elderly normals, suggesting that this is a feature of age. Our own recent studies confirm that up to 60 years age has no influence on perception of bronchoconstriction but that a higher proportion of subjects recruited from an elderly population fall into the category of poor discriminators of changes in peak flow (Kendrick and Laszlo, 1991b, Kendrick et al., 1992). It has been suggested that this reduced perception of asthma in the elderly (over 60) is a factor in their increased mortality (Barnes, 1992).

C. Severity and Duration of Asthma

There seems to be no relationship between perception of asthma and the duration of the presence of asthma (Nana and Pain, 1985; Higgs, 1987; Peiffer et al., 1989; Connolly et al., 1992). Studies relating asthma symptom scores to peak flow have also not identified a relationship with the background severity of asthma. However, other studies indicate a significant influence of background airflow obstruction on the ability of asthma to perceive the severity of their asthma (Burdon et al., 1982; Orehek et al., 1982). It is likely that this is a result of the process of temporal adaptation; that is, background chronic airflow obstruction reduces the magnitude estimation of the severity of asthma (Nana and Pain, 1985; Boulet et al., 1991; Burdon et al., 1982; Connolly et al., 1992). This effect seems to be on the perception of magnitude of bronchoconstriction, not on the discrimination of changes in severity of bronchoconstriction. This may explain why VAS scores and peak flow studies did not identify this relationship. The reduction in sensory magnitude may be an adaptive response (Pain, 1983).

D. Diurnal Variability

The accuracy of perception of symptoms seems to be increased when there is an increased diurnal variation in peak flow (Nana and Pain, 1985; Peiffer et al., 1989; Higgs, 1987), and there is some suggestion that the diminished perception found when there is a background of chronic airflow obstruction is much more marked when there is little reversibility and variability in peak flow. This phenomenon is probably anchored to the minimum peak flow experienced by the patient, as demonstrated by Peiffer et al. (1989), who showed that the highest accuracy in perception within an individual occurs during the period when the peak flow is at its lowest.

E. Bronchial Reactivity

Surprisingly, in view of the relationship between diurnal variability in peak flow and bronchial reactivity, higher bronchial reactivity has been associated with diminished perception of the magnitude of severity of asthma (Burdon et al., 1982), a finding not confirmed by Peiffer et al. (1992) or by our own recent studies (Kendrick and Laszlo, 1991a).

F. Effects of Treatment

There has been very little work directly studying the effects of antiasthma therapy on the perception of asthma. It is possible that bronchodilator drugs and anti-inflammatory agents not only improve bronchoconstriction and airflow obstruction but also have a local effect on afferent sensation (see Sec. V). Also, there are some approaches to asthma therapy, such as acupuncture, hypnosis, and behavioral therapy, that improve asthma symptomatically predominantly by central effects on perception rather than airflow obstruction. It is likely that central sedatives would impair perception of asthma.

The only direct study of effects of drug medication on perception of asthma compared the effects of inhaled cromoglycate, inhaled beclomethasone, and oral theophylline (Higgs, 1987). Cromoglycate seemed to have little effect on perception of asthma; theophylline increased perception of symptoms, in some cases quite markedly, presumably as a result of central stimulatory action, but beclomethasone reduced perception in most patients (Fig. 2). Although the studies were done in the first weeks after treatment, before there was much improvement in lung function, it is possible that part of the effect of beclomethasone was caused by a reduction in minimum peak flow experienced by the patients. There remains the possibility that there was some local or central effect of this drug on perception of asthma.

Although there are several anecdotal report of the effects of hypnosis, yoga, acupuncture, and behavioral therapy on individual cases of asthma, there are few properly controlled trials (Lane and Lane, 1991). The trials that have been done show more improvement in symptoms than in airflow obstruction (Edwards, 1960; Yorkston et al., 1974; Dias et al., 1982). The alteration in perception of asthma that occurs with these treatments may be therapeutic and beneficial, but theoretically there are pitfalls in those patients in whom asthma is brittle and potentially dangerous (Kinsman et al., 1980).

G. Regular Peak Flow Monitoring

It has been shown that making the peak flow result blind to the patient can alter the level of perception of asthma. Conversely, it might be expected that regular monitoring of peak flow by patients would improve their perception of the severity of asthma. Studies of the effect of training patients to recognize their own peak flows on the perception of asthma give interesting results. Patients can be trained to estimate peak flow with a high degree of accuracy (Silverman et al., 1990). They are generally better than their doctors (Shim and Williams, 1980), but their estimated peak flow was found not to be closely correlated with a verbal breathing score. Also, when Reeder et al. (1990) studied patients starting regular peak flow monitoring, they could not find a significant improvement in these patients' perception of the severity of their asthma. It is clear that the relationship between symptom perception and airflow obstruction is complex.

H. Psychological Profiles

It is generally accepted that psychological factors contribute to the symptomatology of asthma. Much work has been done on the relationship between personality and the medical outcome of asthma (Jones et al., 1979). Perception of added resistive loads to breathing in asthma seems more related to psychological characteristics than the presence or absence of asthma (Hudgel et al., 1982). Some of the variability in resistive load perception in asthma may be accounted for by disordered perception, usually involving diminished sensitivity, that is found in anxiety (Tiller et al., 1987). Personality traits assessed from psychological questionnaires have been related to recognition of the asthma state, particularly the "panic fear" state (Kinsman et al., 1982). Others have found high levels of denial are related to minimization of symptoms and to near-miss asthma deaths (Yellow-

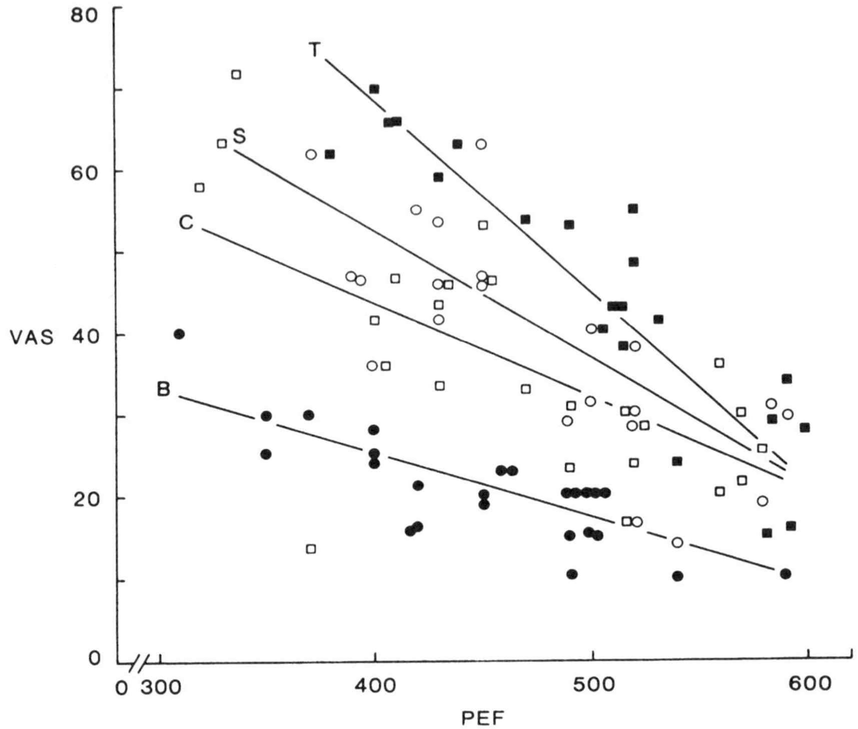

Figure 2 Visual analog asthma score plotted against peak expiratory flow recorded on a meter with a coded readout for 1 of 12 subjects who participated in a study on the effects of standard antiasthma treatment on perception of symptoms. Measurements made four times daily on the last 7 days of each trial period were analyzed. S, regression line for salbutamol alone; T, regular treatment with theophylline; salbutamol as required; C, sodium cromoglycate, with salbutamol as required; B, regular treatment with inhaled beclomethasone dipropionate for 2 weeks, with salbutamol as required. This example illustrates the findings of this study, which showed that sodium cromoglycate did not alter the relationship between asthma scores and peak expiratory flow. Theophylline improved lung function, but 6 of the subjects allocated worse scores to their asthma for the same level of peak expiratory flow, as shown here. Beclomethasone inhalation had little overall effect on the diurnal variation of asthma in the 2 weeks of the study, but 11 of the 12 subjects noted a beneficial effect on symptoms, with a marked reduction in the slope or a downward parallel shift in the regression line. (From Higgs, 1987.)

lees and Ruffin, 1989), and characteristics of repression have been specifically related to poor perception of asthma as measured by the relationship between asthma score and peak flow (Steiner et al., 1987). The presence of asthma is a physical and emotional stress, and perception of asthma seems to be related to perception of emotional arousal (Steiner et al., 1987).

V. Possible Mechanisms of Perception of Asthma

At present, theories on the possible mechanisms of perception of asthma can only be speculative. Asthma is not a single sensation, and its perception must involve central processing of a number of different afferent sensory pathways and neural effects.

Evidence from qualitative studies of the symptoms used in the perception of asthma indicate that breathlessness and tightness constitute a major part but not all of the conscious sensory perception. Part of this must be related to lung mechanics, particularly hyperinflation (Permutt, 1992; Lougheed et al., 1993). The pathways and influence of lung mechanics on breathlessness in nonasthmatics are discussed in other chapters, and presumably the pathways are the same in patients with asthma. There is good evidence that the sensation of asthma has very little to do with the sensation of external added resistive loads (Schwartzstein et al., 1991), and the sensation of asthma is much closer to that sensation of tightness induced by methacholine-induced bronchoconstriction (Rubinfeld and Pain, 1977c).

Apart from the influence of lung mechanics mediated partly by chest wall afferents, there may also be contributions to the sensation of tightness or other sensation of asthma from afferent signals coming from nerve fibers situated within the airways and stimulated by inflammation or bronchoconstriction (Permutt, 1992; Barnes, 1992). These afferents include A and C fibers, some of which function as cough receptors.

Whatever sensory inputs are involved in the perception of asthma, the major component explaining the wide differences found between individuals must be the central processing. Support for this concept comes from the effect of theophylline, a stimulator of higher centers, in increasing perception of asthma (Higgs, 1987) and the association between perception and psychological characteristics, mentioned in Sec. IV. F. The relationship between perception of asthma and perception of other sensations has not yet been properly explored, but the similarity between the perception of physiological changes in asthma and in emotional arousal indicates involvement by similar higher neural centers (Steiner et al., 1987). The possible impairment in perception of bronchoconstriction in elderly people may be explained by impairment in central processing with age (Barnes, 1992). The reduction in perception of asthma with inhaled steroids (Higgs, 1987) could be the result of a local airways effect, but the absence of effect of sodium cromoglycate, which is also supposed to inhibit airway sensory nerves (Barnes, 1992), suggests a more central effect. A steroid effect on central processing is possible (Schraa and Dirks, 1982), but it seems likely that the inhaled steroid produces a rise in the minimum peak flow experienced. Unpublished results from our recent larger study suggests that this is an important factor in the use of visual analog scales for scoring asthma.

In summary, the perception of asthma probably involves a number of higher neural centers in the central processing of sensations related to chest wall mechanics, the effort of breathing, bronchoconstriction, and airway sensitivity. Recent and long-term experience can modify the impact of any level of bronchoconstriction.

VI. Conclusion

The symptoms of bronchial asthma represent one of the most common and distressing examples of a disorder of respiratory sensation. The episodic nature of the condition makes it difficult to investigate but provides us with a naturally occurring model of dyspnea that is amenable to intervention and repays detailed study.

There is increasing interest in this area of investigation because of its potential relevance to morbidity and mortality (Barnes, 1994). All the approaches reviewed are useful. In studies of the perception of spontaneously occurring asthma, the subjects should be unaware of the results of objective tests.

As with other respiratory disorders, patients with bronchial asthma acclimatize readily to mild or moderate departures from normal lung function. Effective treatment is available, but only those who recognize that they are deteriorating can be expected to ask for or to use it. On the basis that the underlying cause of asthma is airway inflammation, current guidelines recommend that asthmatics should take anti-inflammatory medication to keep lung function as near normal as is compatible with acceptable side effects. Clinical experience quickly shows that this approach results in fewer symptoms and less frequent exacerbations. It has been accepted widely in recent years, although little epidemiological evidence exists so far to show that it affects mortality or progression to chronic airflow obstruction.

Many asthmatics are not very good at estimating changes in their lung function, and a significant minority appear to notice airflow obstruction only when it is very severe. There are simple tests that can identify these individuals. The obvious solution is to ask them to measure and record their peak flow at home, although some pose a challenge to their medical advisers because they think they are being offered treatment for a non-disease (*Lancet*, 1983). Those who readily sense changes in peak flow or who have high levels of anxiety during attacks are generally grateful for effective treatment, most reliably with inhaled steroids, which appear to reduce the sensory and psychological impact of the frequent episodes of bronchoconstriction.

Acknowledgments

We thank Dr. Adrian Kendrick for access to unpublished results and Dr. Brian Stonebridge of the Department of Computer Science, University of Bristol for helpful collaboration. We are grateful for generous support from the Special Trustees of the Bristol Royal Infirmary and the National Asthma Campaign of the United Kingdom. We thank Janice Cooper for preparing the manuscript.

References

Adams, F. (1860). The extant works of Aretaeus the Cappadocian. London, Sydenham Society.

Adams, L., Chronos, N., Lane, R., and Guz, A. (1985). Measurement of breathlessness induced in normals: validity of two scaling techniques. Clin. Sci. 69:7–16.

Aitken, R.C.B. (1969). Measurement of feelings using visual analogue scales. Proc. R. Soc. Med. 62:989–993.

Aitken, R.C.B., Zealley, A.K., and Rosenthal, S.W. (1970). Some psychological and physiological considerations of breathlessness. In: Hering-Breuer Centenery Symposium. Breathing. Edited by R. Porter. Churchill, London, pp. 253–267.

Barnes, P.J. (1992). Poorly perceived asthma. Thorax 47:408–409.

Barnes, P.J. (1994). Blunted perception and death from asthma. N. Engl. J. Med. 330:1383–1384.

Bates, D.V. (1952). Respiratory function in asthma. Clin. Sci. 11:203–207.

Bonnel, A.M., Mathiot, M.J., and Grimaud, C. (1985). Inspiratory and expiratory resistive load detection in normal and asthmatic subjects. Respiration 48:12–23.

Boulet, L.-P., Milot, J., and Turcotte, H. (1991). Relationship between changes in diurnal variation of expiratory flows, lung volumes and respiratory symptoms after acute asthma. Respir. Med. 85:487–493.

Burdon, J.G.W., Juniper, E.F., Killian, K.J., Hargreave, F.W., and Campbell, E.J.M. (1982). The perception of breathlessness in asthma. Am. Rev. Respir. Dis. 126: 825–828.

Burki, N.K., Mitchell, K., Chaudhary, B.A., and Zechman, F.W. (1978). The ability of asthmatics to detect added resistive loads. Am. Rev. Respir. Dis. 117:71–75.

Charlton I., Charlton, G., Bloomfield, J., and Mullee, M.A. (1990). Evaluation of peak flow and symptoms only self-management plans for control of asthma in general practice. Br. Med. J. 301:1355–1359.

Clark, N.M., Evans, D., and Williams, R.B. (1992). Patient use of peak flow monitoring. Am. Rev. Respir. Dis. 145:722–725.

Connolly, M.J., Crowley, J.J., Charan, N.B., Nielsen, C.P., and Vestal, R.E. (1992). Reduced subjective awareness of bronchoconstriction provoked by methacholine in elderly asthmatic and normal subjects as measured on a simple awareness scale. Thorax 47:410–413.

Dahlem, N.W., Kinsman, R.A., and Horton, D.J. (1977). Panic-fear in asthma: requests for as needed medications in relation to pulmonary function measurement. J. Allergy Clin. Immunol. 60:295–300.

Del Volgo-Mathiot, M.J., and Bonnel, A.-M. (1991). Suprathreshold resistive load perception in normal and asthmatic subjects. Respiration 58:49–56.

Dhand, R., Kalra, S., and Malik, S.K. (1988). Use of visual analogue scales for assessment of the severity of asthma. Respiration 54:255–262.

Dias, P.L.R., Subramaniam, S., and Lionel, N.D.W. (1982). The effect of acupuncture in bronchial asthma—preliminary assessment. J. R. Soc. Med. 75:245–248.

Edwards, G. (1960). Hypnotic treatment in asthma: real and illusory results. Br. Med. J. 2: 292–297.

Floyer, J.A. (1698). Treatise of the Asthma. Wilkin, London.

Freyd, M. (1923). Measurement of vocational education; an outline of research procedure. J. Ed. Psychol. 14:83–87.

Fritz, G., Klein, R.B., and Overholser, J.C. (1990). Accuracy of symptom perception in childhood asthma. Dev. Behav. Pediatr. 11:69–72.

Gottfried, S.B., Altose, M.D., Kelsen, S.G., Fogarty, C.M., and Cherniack, N.S. (1978). The perception of changes in airflow resistance in normal subjects in patients with chronic airways obstruction. Chest 73(Suppl. 2):286–288.

Gottfried, S.B., Altose, M.D., Kelsen, S.G., and Cherniack, N.S. (1981). Perception of changes in airflow resistance in obstructive pulmonary disorders. Am. Rev. Respir. Dis. 24:566–570.

Hetzel, M., Williams, I.P., and Shakespeare, C.M. (1979). Can patients keep their own peak flow records reliably? Lancet 1:597–599.

Higgs, C.M.B. (1987). Studies on the Perception of Asthma. M.D. Thesis, University of Cambridge.

Higgs, C.M.B., Jones, P., Tanser, A.R., and Laszlo, G. (1985). What are the symptoms of asthma and their importance? (abstract) Thorax 40:688.

Higgs, C.M.B., Richardson, R.B., Lea, D.A., Lewis, G.T.R., and Laszlo, G. (1986). Influence of knowledge of peak flow on self-assessment of asthma: studies with a coded peak flow meter. Thorax 41:671–675.

Hudgel, D.W., Cooperson, D.M., and Kinsman, R.A. (1982). Recognition of added resistive loads in asthma. The importance of behavioural styles. Am. Rev. Respir. Dis. 126: 121–125.

Irie, M., Kubo, C., Sogawa, H., Kihara, H., Kawamura, H., Teshima, H., and Nakagawa, T. (1991). Psychosomatic study of inhalation therapy in patients with bronchial asthma. II. Relationship between subjective self-assessment of dyspnea and peak expiratory flow rates. Jpn. J. Allergy 40:1384–1390.

James, A., Carroll, N., Ryan, G., and Musk, A.W. (1993). Perception of symptoms during high dose methacholine challenge. Am. Rev. Respir. Dis. 147:A831.

Jansen-Bjerklie, S., Ferketich, S., Benner, P., and Becker, G. (1992). Clinical markers of asthma severity and risk: the importance of subjective as well as objective factors. Heart Lung 21:265–272.

Johnson, A.J., Nunn, A.J., Somner, A.R., Stableforth, D.E., and Stewart, C.J. (1984). Circumstances of death from asthma. Br. Med. J. 288:1870–1872.

Jones, N.F., Kinsman, R.A., Dirks, J.F., and Dahlem, N.W. (1979). Psychological contributions to chronicity in asthma patient response style influencing medical treatment and its outcome. Med. Care 17:1103–1117.

Kendrick, A.H., and Laszlo, G. (1991a). Bronchial hyperreactivity and perception of asthma (abstract). Thorax 46:760.

Kendrick, A.H., and Laszlo, G. (1991b). Perception of asthma: effects of age (abstract). Thorax 46:760.

Kendrick, A.H., Dawe, C.N., Pounsford, J.C., and Laszlo, G. (1992). Reduced perception of symptoms in elderly asthmatics (abstract). Eur. Respir. J. 5:30.

Kendrick, A.H., Higgs, C.M.B., Whitfield, M.J., and Laszlo, G. (1993). Accuracy of perception of asthma: patients treated in general practice. Br. Med. J. 307:422–429.

Kikuchi, Y., Okabe, S., Tamura, G., Hida, W., Homma, M., Shirato, K., and Takashima, T. (1994). Chemosensitivity and perception of dyspnea in patients with a history of near-fatal asthma. N. Engl. J. Med. 330:1329–1334.

Killian, K.J., Mahutte, C.K., and Campbell, E.J.M. (1981). Magnitude estimation of externally added loads to breathing. Am. Rev. Respir. Dis. 123:12–15.

Kinsman, R.A., O'Banion, K., Resnikoff, P., Luparello, T.J., and Spector, S.L. (1973). Subjective symptoms of acute asthma within a heterogeneous sample of asthmatics. J. Allergy Clin. Immunol. 52:284–296.

Kinsman, R.A., Dirks, J.F., Jones, N.T., and Dahlem, N.W. (1980). Anxiety reduction in asthma: four catches to general application. Psychosom. Med. 42:397–405.

Kinsman, R.A., Dirks, J.F., and Jones, N. (1982). Psychomaintenance of chronic physical illness: clinical assessment of personal styles affecting medical management. In: Handbook of Clinical Health Psychology. Edited by T. Millon, C. Grew, and R. Meagler. Plenum Press, New York, pp. 435–466.

Lancet. (1983). Perception of breathlessness in asthma (editorial). 1:912–913.

Lane, D.J., and Lane, T.V. (1991). Alternative and complementary medicine for asthma. Thorax 46:787–797.

Lougheed, M.D., Lam, M., Forkert, L., Webb, K.A., and O'Donnell, D.E. (1993). Breathlessness during acute bronchoconstriction in asthma: pathophysiologic mechanisms. Am. Rev. Respir. Dis. 148:1452–1459.

Marks, G., Yates, D., Wordsell, M., and Barnes, P. (1993). Respiratory discomfort during bronchial challenge testing: selecting the appropriate descriptive phrase. Eur. Respir. J. 6(Suppl. 17):469S.

Mathiot, M.J., Bonnel, A.M., and Grimaud, C. (1986). Effects of airflow resistance variations on resistive load detection in normal subjects. Bull. Eur. Physiopathol. Respir. 22:99–105.

McFadden, E.R., Jr. (1975). Exertional dyspnoea and cough as preludes to acute attacks of bronchial asthma. N. Engl. J. Med. 292:555–559.

McFadden, E. R., Jr., Kiser, R., and DeGroot, W.J. (1973). Acute bronchial asthma. Relations between clinical and physiologic manifestations. N. Engl. J. Med. 288: 221–225.

Nana, A., and Pain, M.C.F. (1985). Clinical importance of evaluating the asthmatic patient's sense of breathlessness. Pract. Cardiol. 11:83–87.

Nana, A., Burdon, J.G.W., and Pain, M.C.F. (1983). Assessment of breathlessness in asthma. Aust. N.Z. J. Med. 13:543–544.

Orehek, J., Beaupré, A., Badier, M., Nicoli, M.M., and Delpierre, S. (1982). Perception of airway tone by asthmatic patients. Bull. Eur. Physiopathol. Respir. 18:601–607.

Ormerod, L.P., and Stableforth, D.E. (1980). Asthma mortality in Birmingham 1975–7: 53 deaths. Br. Med. J. 280:687–690.

Pain, M.C.F. (1983). Measurement of the asthmatic state. In: Steroids in Asthma. Edited by T.J.H. Clark. Adis Press, Auckland, p. 35.

Peiffer, C., Marsac, J., and Lockhart, A. (1989). Chronobiological study of the relationship between dyspnoea and airway obstruction in symptomatic asthmatic subjects. Clin. Sci. 77:237–244.

Peiffer, C., Toumi, M., Razzouk, H., Marsac, J., and Lockhart, A. (1992). Relationship between spontaneous dyspnoea and lability of airway obstruction in asthma. Clin. Sci. 82:717–724.

Permutt, S. (1992). Breathlessness in asthma. In: The Campbell Symposium. Breathlessness. Edited by N.L. Jones and K.J. Killian. pp. 60–65. Hamilton, Ontario.

Reeder, K.P., Dolce, J.J., Duke, L., Raczynski, J.M., and Bailey, W.C. (1990). Peak flow meters: are they monitoring tools or training devices? J. Asthma 27:219–227.

Rubinfeld, A.R., and Pain, M.C.F. (1976). Perception of asthma. Lancet 1:882–884.

Rubinfeld, A.R., and Pain, M.C.F. (1977a). How mild is mild asthma? Thorax 32:177–181.

Rubinfeld, A.R., and Pain, M.C.F. (1977b). Relationship between bronchial reactivity, airway caliber, and severity of asthma. Am. Rev. Respir. Dis. 115:381–387.

Rubinfeld, A.R., and Pain, M.C.F. (1977c). Bronchial provocation in the study of sensations associated with disordered breathing. Clin. Sci. Mol. Med. 52:423–428.

Ruffin, R.E., Latimer, K.M., and Schembri, D.A. (1991). Longitudinal study of near fatal asthma. Chest 99:77–83.

Schraa, J., and Dirks, J.F. (1982). The influence of corticosteroids and theophylline on cerebral function. A review. Chest 82:181–185.

Schwartzstein, R., Lilly, J., Israel, E., and Basner, R., Sparrow, D., Weinberger, S., and Weiss, J.W. (1991). Breathlessness of asthma differs from that of external resistive loading. Am. Rev. Respir. Dis. 143:A-596.

Sears, M.R. (1991). Epidemiological trends in bronchial asthma. In: Asthma: Its Pathology and Treatment. Edited by M.A. Kaliner, P.J. Barnes, and C.G.A. Persson. Dekker, New York, pp. 1–49.

Shim, C.S., and Williams, M.H. (1980). Evaluation of the severity of asthma: patients versus physicians. Am. J. Med. 68:11–13.

Silverman, B., James, C., Misra, S., Schneider, A.T., and Chiaramonte, L.T. (1990). Training perception of acute airflow obstruction. Ann. Allergy 64:373–375.

Sly, P.D., Landau, L.I., and Weymouth, R. (1985). Home recording of peak expiratory flow tests and perception of asthma. Am. J. Dis. Child. 139:479–482.

Stark, R.D., and Gambles, S.A. (1980). A new system for assessing the effects of drugs on breathlessness. J. Clin. Respir. Physiol. 16:244–250.

Stark, R.D., Gambles, S.A., and Lewis, J.A. (1981). Methods to assess breathlessness in healthy subjects: a critical evaluation and application to analyse the acute effects of diazepam and promethazine on breathlessness induced by exercise or by exposure to raised levels of carbon dioxide. Clin. Sci. 61:429–439.

Steiner, H., Higgs, C.M.B., Fritz, G.K., Laszlo, G., and Harvey, J.E. (1987). Defense style and the perception of asthma. Psychosom. Med. 49:35–44.

Stevens, S.S. (1975). Partition scales and paradoxes. In: Psychophysics. Edited by G. Stevens. Wiley, New York, pp. 134–171.

Taytard, A., Tessier, J.F., Gervais, M., Gachie, J.P., Douet, C., Kombou, L., Vergeret, J., and Freour, P. (1990). Actual usage of medical facilities by asthmatics in two French rural settings: a preliminary study. Eur. Respir. J. 3:856–860.

Tiller, J., Pain, M., and Biddle, N. (1987). Anxiety disorder and perception of inspiratory resistive loads. Chest 91:547–551.

Turcotte, H., Corbeil, F., and Boulet, L.-P. (1990). Perception of breathlessness during bronchoconstriction induced by antigen, exercise, and histamine challenges. Thorax 45:914–918.

Turner-Warwick, M. (1977). The use of diary cards in asthma. Methods in clinical trials in asthma: Proceedings of a British Thoracic and Tuberculosis Association meeting. Br. J. Dis. Chest 71:228–230.

Wigal, J.K., Kotses, H., Green, T.L., Hann, D.L., and Tinker, T.R. (1986). Total respiratory resistance and peak expiratory flow rate: an intra-subject study. J. Asthma 23: 11–13.

Wilson, R.C., and Jones, P.W. (1989). A comparison of the visual analogue scale and modified Borg scale for the measurement of dyspnoea in normal subjects. Clin. Sci. 76:277–282.

Woolcock, A., and Read, J. (1966). Lung volumes in exacerbations of asthma. Am. J. Med. 41:259–273.

Yellowlees, P.M., and Ruffin, R.E. (1989). Psychological defenses and coping styles in patients following a life-threatening attack of asthma. Chest 95:1298–1303.

Yorkston, N.J., McHugh, R.B., Brady, R., Serber, M., and Sergeant, H.G.S. (1974). Verbal desensitisation in bronchial asthma. J. Psychosom. Res. 18:371–376.

Zach, M.S., and Karner, U. (1989). Sudden death in asthma. Arch. Dis. Child. 64:1446–1451.

13

Cognitive Aspects of Breathlessness

PAUL W. JONES and RACHEL C. WILSON

St. George's Hospital Medical School
London, England

I. Introduction

It is necessary for us to define what we mean by a cognitive approach to breathlessness and explain why such an approach might be useful. The *Oxford English Dictionary* defines cognition as "the action or faculty of knowing and perceiving, conceiving as opposed to emotional and volition; a perception, sensation, notion or intuition." This definition is too broad for specialist use; more usefully, Helson has suggested that the attributes of perception and cognition are quite distinct when used in a psychological or psychophysical context (Helson, 1964). In his view, perception is predominantly concerned with current sensations, usually caused by stimulation by external forces. The sensation being perceived is caused by a single stimulus, and it is not possible to substitute one stimulus for another and still perceive the same sensation. Perception is concerned with current experience: "what is" and the "real." He argues that it is limited to a two-valued logic: a thing either is or is not, with no intermediate values. The detection of a difference between two inspiratory resistances is an example. In contrast, Helson suggests that thinking (cognition) has predominantly central components but may be triggered by external or internal stimuli. It is concerned with the past, present, or future. It may have multiple determinants and be labile. It may also substitute one determinant for another. Thinking deals with contingencies and possibilities, the real and the imagined. It allows for a wide range of values and can operate with probabilities. It seems to us that this is a reasonable description of the process needed to evaluate breathlessness.

Breathlessness occurs only in thinking humans, but in itself this is not evidence for the involvement of cognitive processes. Dyspnea sufficient to stop exercise is an overwhelming experience that does not require any detached intellectual judgments about its character, magnitude, and tolerability. Even during levels of submaximal exercise, patients probably do not engage in self-analysis of their breathlessness to make decisions about changing their work level. These commonsense observations suggest that emotional aspects of breathlessness (judged by the *Oxford English Dictionary* to be the antithesis of cognition) are potentially more important to patients. This view is supported by a recent observation that a majority of patients with chronic obstructive airways disease scored submaximal breathlessness at the point at which they stopped their dyspnea-limited test (Killian et al., 1992a). Tolerability is part of the emotional or affective aspects of breathlessness, not the cognitive domain.

This is not the end of the matter, however. Knowledge of the processes of breathlessness generation comes largely from studies in which patients or experimental subjects are asked to examine critically their respiratory sensations. This requires thought and introspection. Breathlessness results from a number of sensory inputs but is an abstract concept that gains reality through the words used to describe and define it. Abstract concepts and language reside within the sphere of cognition. The process of matching a prevailing sensation to a description provided by an experimenter requires thought. Similarly, the use of a scale with which to convey to an observer the intensity of the sensation being experienced also requires thought. Finally, the process of scaling may require the operation of memory and imagination, both of which are cognitive functions.

Some of the studies reviewed in this chapter were specifically concerned with testing, either directly or indirectly, the involvement of cognitive processes in subjects' assessment of their breathlessness. A greater number were not so designed, but we have attempted to interpret them in the recognition that they all were performed in subjects who were actively thinking about their breathlessness at the time they were studied. The approach that we follow is largely sympathetic with Helson's epistemology of cognition, although we confess to a certain laxity in the use of the term "perception."

II. Development of Conscious Sensation

The process of generating a sensation is conventionally viewed as a sequence with three or four stages: detection, discrimination, recognition, and scaling. A moment's thought reveals that these labels all have strong cognitive associations.

A. Detection of Breathlessness

There are many studies concerning the detection of respiratory sensations. Nearly all these involve the application of loads of different type. Load detection of airway resistances appears to follow Weber's law, because the just noticeable difference (JND) for added resistances increases in proportion to the background resistance (Wiley and Zechman, 1966; Gottfried et al., 1981). The awareness of increased breathing is also amenable to testing using JNDs (Plassman and Lansing, 1990). Even high-level quadriplegics have been shown to detect small changes in tidal volume using a forced-choice method (Banzett et al., 1987). In contrast, the measurement of JNDs in the sensation of breathlessness has attracted little attention. It is known that in most individuals, a threshold level of ventilation must be crossed before breathlessness is registered (Ward and Stubbing, 1985). This threshold may be quite high, but it appears to be repeatable (Simon et al., 1990). The transition from no breathlessness to detectable breathlessness is clearly a boundary state that warrants further investigation.

Stevens suggested that sensations may be classified into two types: class I continua, such as loudness, in which excitation is added to excitation, and class II, in which one excitation is substituted for another (Stevens, 1957). His classification system raises interesting analogies in the context of respiratory sensations. Estimation of the magnitude of inspiratory loads appears to form a class I continuum; however, dyspnea perception is more complex. It may be more akin to Stevens' class II continua, because its character may change with changing intensity. We know of no work to examine this formally, but subjective experience suggests that additional feelings are recruited as magnitude increases. If this were confirmed experimentally, it would then be necessary to test whether the onset of just noticeable breathlessness reflected both a change in the intensity and quality of respiratory sensations.

B. Recognition and Discrimination in Breathlessness

The processes of recognition and discrimination are interrelated, because recognition may require both affirmation—that what is being felt has the attributes of the sensation under inquiry—and refutation—that it lacks the attributes of other sensations. This is a cognitive process. The subject must analyze aspects of a variety of related sensations and then make decisions concerning the unique qualities of the sensation of interest that allow it to be identified reliably. Such decisions are made using criteria established by the subject or provided by the experimenter. A number of different descriptions have been applied to respiratory sensations, and it is worth examining them in some detail.

Dyspnea or Effort?

The most widely held model for the generation of breathlessness was developed from the motor command hypothesis for the perception of effort during voluntary contraction of limb muscles (reviewed in McCloskey, 1978). Terminology from this work was first transferred to respiratory sensation in an experiment to test the effect of respiratory muscle fatigue. In this study, such phrases as "how big is your command or effort?" were introduced (Gandevia et al., 1981). Subsequently there have been numerous studies concerned with perception of applied respiratory loads using such terms as "effort," "load," "resistance," or "force" (Gottfried, et al., 1981, 1985; Altose et al., 1982; Tack et al., 1982; Ward and Stubbing, 1985; Silverman et al., 1988).

It has been suggested that breathlessness and perceived effort are mediated by the same mechanism and are therefore the same (Killian et al., 1984). Implicit in this statement is the assumption that the words *breathlessness* and *effort* are synonymous. It must be appreciated, however, that both are abstract concepts that are given an external reality only through the words used to describe them and through their effects on the individual. The very existence of the terms "breathlessness" and "respiratory effort" implies that these convey different ideas. Results from experimental studies support this view. The term "effort" appears as a feature of the sensation of dyspnea in two of three lists of descriptors provided by patients with cardiopulmonary diseases, but these also contain many other descriptions (Kinsman et al., 1983; Simon et al., 1989; Elliott et al., 1991). Breathlessness in chronic obstructive airways disease was associated with a sense of effort and work but also with gasping for breath, air hunger, out of breath, insufficient air, and a sense of heaviness (Simon et al., 1990). In another list of 45 items, the effort descriptor was at 14 in terms of frequency of occurrence (Elliott et al., 1991).

These studies show that the concept of dyspnea is not adequately defined simply in terms of perceived effort. Direct evidence for this comes from a study of hypercapnia on a background of targeted volitional ventilation. In this experiment, perceived effort and perceived breathlessness (defined as an unpleasant urge to breathe) changed in opposite directions (Demediuk et al., 1992). In a very different study, in patients with chronic obstructive airways disease, the perception of added inspiratory resistance was unrelated to the patients' level of breathlessness-induced disability (Mahler et al., 1987).

In summary, effort sensation results from a volitional muscle contraction. In contrast, breathlessness may arise from a reflex drive to breathe or from a disease process. It is hardly surprising that they are described using different words and phrases. The studies discussed here provide empirical evidence that they are not synonymous and that they may address quite different aspects of the respiratory sensory experience.

Varieties of Breathlessness

Clusters of breathlessness descriptors appear to be loosely linked to particular diseases (Simon et al., 1990; Elliott et al., 1991). Some tests of the validity of these clusters have been performed. Elliott et al. examined the repeatability of their list of descriptor items and found it to be reasonably good, although a number of items were rather unstable (Elliott et al., 1991). Simon et al. examined the concurrent validity of their descriptors by asking normal subjects and patients to apply them to a range of experimental stimuli. Their findings seem to be intuitively appropriate. One particular description, air hunger during constrained ventilation on a background of hypercapnia, agrees with observations made in quadriplegic patients and curarized normal subjects (Banzett et al., 1989, 1990).

These interesting early observations on descriptor clustering require confirmation. Methods that are used to group questionnaire items, such as cluster analysis or factor analysis, all involve a number of decisions by the investigators. In the field of questionnaire design, it has not always proved possible to replicate the original factor structure of a questionnaire when it has been applied to a second population of patients with the same disease. It would be valuable to test the stability and generalizability of the clusters already identified (Simon et al., 1990; Elliott et al., 1991). This could be done in two ways: first by analyzing the existing data using another approach, such as principal component analysis, and second by studying further groups of patients.

Language is the method of entry into the breathlessness experience, but it cannot be assumed that all individuals share a common understanding of the same descriptors. Differences between languages may shed further light in this area, because there appear to be divisions between cultures in the manner in which concepts of symptoms and disease are held. For example, in German there no simple description for a symptom easily described in English as "wheeze" (Burney et al., 1989). There may also be differences in the ways in which psychological states are related to bodily feelings in different languages and cultures. In an international study in asthma, the relationship between impact of the disease on daily life and general health did not vary between countries (Jones et al., 1994). In contrast, the relationship between the general health score and anxiety, measured using the hospital anxiety and depression questionnaire (Zigmond and Snaith, 1983), did vary. This observation may be of particular relevance, because several features of anxiety are expressed in terms of bodily sensations using a range of different descriptors and similes. An attempt has been made to replicate the study of Elliott et al. (1991) in France using the same descriptors after a careful and idiomatic translation into French. However, to date, it has not been possible to replicate the clusters found in England (C. Peiffer, personal communication).

Cognitive Interpretation of Air Hunger Caused by Hypercapnia

Studies on the sensation of air hunger produced by hypercapnia in quadriplegic patients and curarized ventilated normal subjects provide some interesting insights into the perception of respiratory sensations (Banzett et al., 1989, 1990). The patients agreed that the sensation felt as if it were harder to breathe, although they were incapable of breathing. Among the normal subjects there was no consensus over this simile, but they were all in agreement that the sensation was like breath holding. This is an interesting divergence because in these studies both patients and normals were in essentially the same physiological state. These apparent differences may have been conditioned by experience. Breath holding may have been quite familiar to the four normal subjects, and even one of the patients likened the sensation to that of holding one's breath under water. The normal subjects presumably would also have had clear recent memories of how it felt to be breathing harder under physiological circumstances. Because of this, it is likely that they were able to discriminate the experimentally induced sensation from breathlessness caused by more normal stimuli. In contrast, the patients may have lost a clear memory for "normal" breathlessness and assumed that the unpleasant sensation during the experiment was the same as sensations related to breathing that they could recall from the past. It may be significant that one patient believed that normal experiences were too distant for her to make satisfactory comparisons with the experimentally evoked sensation.

These studies may provide one further insight into the generation of dyspnea. There was a clear but not universal tendency for both the normals and the patients to locate the sensation of air hunger in or around the chest. Previous studies on breath holding have related the associated sensations to small involuntary diaphragmatic contractions that develop before the breakpoint (Campbell et al., 1969). There is evidence for the projection of phrenic nerve afferents to the sensory cortex in the cat (Davenport et al., 1985), but in the studies by Banzett et al. it is unlikely that such afferents could have been excited. The most reasonable hypothesis is that the stimulus causing the sensation of air hunger arose in central chemoreceptors. This signal was then projected to the sensory cortex, either directly or through pathways involving the brain stem respiratory motor neurons. Regardless of source, the sensation was interpreted by some subjects as located around or within the chest, despite the absence of any additional afferent information arising from a visceral or somatic structure. Two different mechanisms may be proposed to account for this referred sensation. One is the existence of "hard-wired" pathways involving an area of the associative cortex concerned chiefly with the appreciation of afferents from receptors in the chest. The other invokes a process of learning or conditioning. In physiological circumstances, the stimuli that cause air hunger would not arise in isolation but would be accompanied by other afferent information, including that from the diaphragm. Because the two signals are normally associated, the presence of one may still lead to the interpretation that both were present despite the absence of the other.

In summary, we hypothesize that dyspnea results from the interpretation and association of different sensations, feelings, and cues. Breathlessness caused by the same stimulus may differ between individuals and be described in different ways, depending on an individual's experience. If this is correct, it follows that experience and learning may influence the way in which each individual forms his or her personal idea of breathlessness.

Descriptors for Scaling Breathlessness

The diverse nature of breathlessness has led to a number of different definitions. Some works have simply asked their subjects to measure breathlessness without defining the sensation (El-Manshawi et al., 1986); others have provided various definitions ranging from those relating to difficulty (Mahler et al., 1987) and effort (Silverman et al., 1988; Muza et al., 1990) to shortness of breath (Wolkove et al., 1989) and severity, intensity, and/or discomfort (Belman et al., 1991). It is noteworthy that "intensity of discomfort" was used recently by a group (Killian et al., 1992a, b), who originally equated breathlessness with perceived effort (Killian et al., 1984). Two other groups have used another definition: an uncomfortable need to breathe (Adams et al., 1985a; Wilson and Jones, 1989, 1990; Lane et al., 1990), and a third group used the same phrase, substituting *urge* for *need* (Demediuk et al., 1992). There is evidence that subjects may distinguish between breathlessness (described as an uncomfortable urge to breathe) and respiratory effort (like lifting a weight) (Demediuk et al., 1992), which suggests that the various definitions may not be synonymous. If this is the case, these different studies may have been measuring different aspects of dyspnea. This implies that results using one type of descriptor may not be comparable directly to results obtained with another.

Multidimensional Nature of Breathlessness

As outlined earlier, a number of descriptors may be applied to breathlessness. This does not necessarily imply that it has more than one dimension but simply that there is more than one variety. In many respects, recent studies concerning the semantics of breathlessness follow similar work on the language of pain and the development of such instruments as the McGill pain questionnaire (Melzack and Torgerson, 1971; Melzack, 1975). Pain is multidimensional, and it is well established that it has an affective component that is concerned with feelings and emotions. It has been shown that this aspect of pain is relatively independent of its intensity (Price et al., 1980; Kremer et al., 1982; Jamner and Tursky, 1987).

We have investigated the possibility that distress caused by breathlessness is different from its intensity (Wilson and Jones, 1991a). To measure distress, the word *distress* was added to all the descriptors on the modified Borg scale. The subjects were asked to scale "how much distress your breathing is causing you, or how much it bothers you." The intensity of breathlessness was described to the subjects as a feeling of an uncomfortable need to breathe. Distress and minute ventilation were well correlated in all subjects, and the distress scores were highly repeatable on retesting after an interval of several days. At any given level of ventilation, distress was generally scored lower than intensity, but there was a wide scatter between subjects (Fig. 1). These studies showed that intensity and distress were scaled as if they were different aspects of breathlessness. This supports Comroe's suggestion that an estimation of perceived breathlessness may involve an individual's perception of the sensation and his or her reaction to it (Comroe, 1966). If Comroe's proposition is correct and our findings are confirmed, then it appears that breathlessness has both a level of intensity and an affective component that may be relatively independent of each other.

It is not known which is more important in reducing exercise tolerance: the intensity of breathlessness or the distress it evokes. If it were a high level of distress, our studies indicate that patients would score highly for both distress and intensity at the point of stopping exercise. This may suggest that intensity and distress converged and became synonymous at high levels of work. However, such convergence could be a property of the scale and the way it is used by the patient rather than a characteristic of the sensation. Scales, such as the Borg scale, are closed at both ends; that is, they have maximum and minimum levels. This may predispose them to exhibit ceiling effects because high scores would be constrained by the upper point on the scale (discussed further later). Because intensity generally appears to be scaled higher than distress, it may reach its ceiling at lower levels of ventilation. If exercise continued beyond this point, the level of distress may continue to rise and the two scores would converge. Clearly, it is important to establish the relative importance of intensity and distress in causing exercise limitation, but it will be necessary to study a wide range of work rates, not simply confine observations to the point at which exercise stops.

Definition for Dyspnea

In this chapter, the words *breathlessness* and *dyspnea* have been used apparently interchangeably, as in many writings on the subject. Linguistic studies have shown that there are different ways of describing breathlessness, and there is evidence that subjects can distinguish between different respiratory sensations. There is also emerging evidence that breathlessness or dyspnea is multidimensional and has an associated affective component that is distinct from the intensity of discomfort. There may be varieties of breathlessness, but we suggest that the term "dyspnea" should be reserved for the presence of unpleasant feelings or emotions about prevailing respiratory sensations. To return to an issue raised earlier, we argue that the transition between an awareness that breathing has increased and the development of dyspnea would be signaled by the emergence of a just detectable affective component.

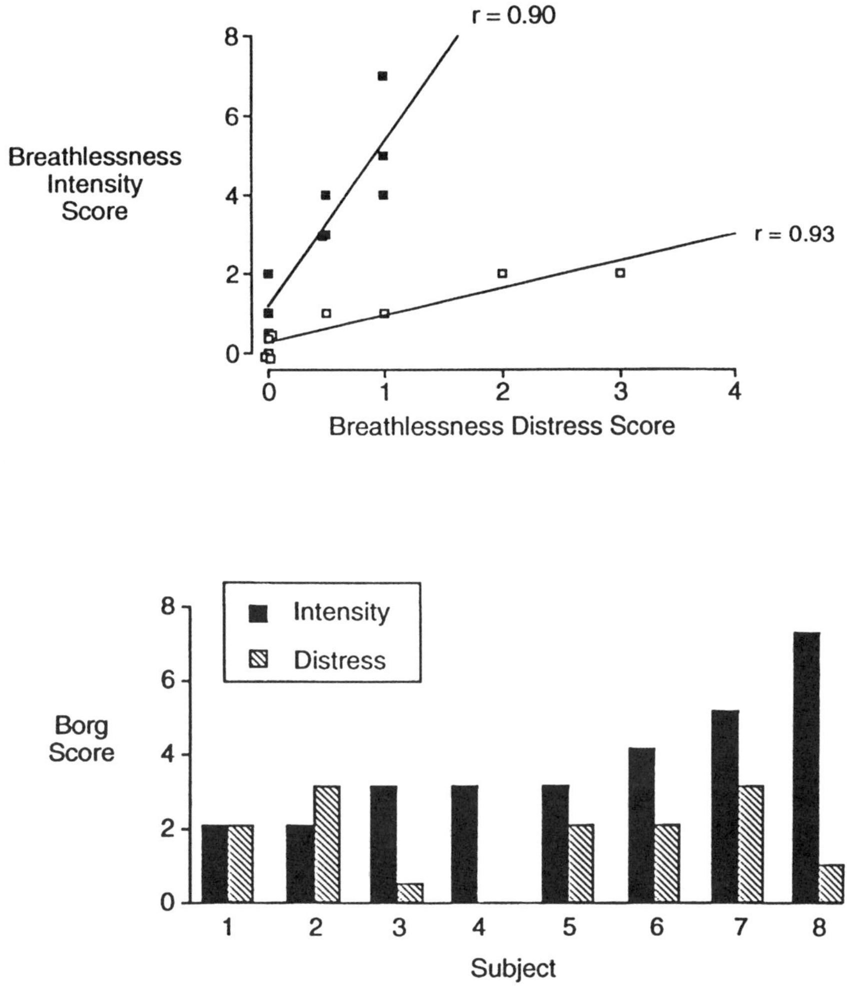

Figure 1 Borg scores for breathlessness intensity and distress caused by breathlessness in normal subjects during incremental exercise. (Top) Distress score plotted against intensity score at the same level of ventilation. Regressions from two subjects are shown, one with a low level of distress relative to intensity and the other with greatest distress. All other subjects lay between these two extremes, except one who registered no distress at all. (Bottom) Maximum Borg scores for distress and intensity obtained at the end of exercise. (From Wilson and Jones, 1991a.)

III. Cognitive Aspects of Breathlessness Scaling

Techniques for scaling respiratory sensations are discussed in detail elsewhere in this book. This section is concerned with factors that may influence scaling. The discussion is restricted to closed scales, such as the visual analog scale (VAS) and Borg scale, in which the scaling range is constrained within limits.

A. Anchoring the Upper and Lower Limits of a Breathlessness Scale

Closed scales have upper and lower limits. The lower limit is usually defined as no breathlessness and the upper as the worst experienced, worst imaginable, or maximal. These limits have sometimes been described as anchor points, and some investigators have tried to establish them before a study by providing an experience of severe breathlessness (Stark et al., 1981). There appears to be little value in doing this, in part because breathlessness scores have proved to be repeatable without such anchoring and in part because most patients and normals do not report maximum breathlessness intensity during a maximal laboratory exercise test (Killian et al., 1992a, b).

B. Stability of Breathlessness Scores

A number of studies have examined the repeatability of breathlessness estimation in normals over periods ranging from 1 day to 1 year (Adams et al., 1985a; Wilson and Jones, 1989, 1991b). Similar studies in patients with obstructive airways disease have been restricted to several days (Silverman et al., 1988; Belman et al., 1991) or a few weeks (Muza et al., 1990). The overall picture is one of good repeatability (Fig. 2). The effects of repeated testing on the magnitude of perceived breathlessness appear to be small, although in one study in patients a progressive fall was observed on daily exercise testing (Belman et al., 1991). Two studies have compared the repeatability and sensitivity of the Borg scale and the VAS. The Borg scale has a number of descriptors attached to its category points that could result in better repeatability compared with the VAS. This theoretical advantage appears to be relatively small in practice, although comparisons between the two scales have not covered study periods longer than 2 weeks (Wilson and Jones, 1989; Muza et al., 1990).

C. Reference Points for High and Low Breathlessness

Stability in breathlessness estimation is a useful property for the experimenter, but it is not known why the measurements are so repeatable. The act of relating a

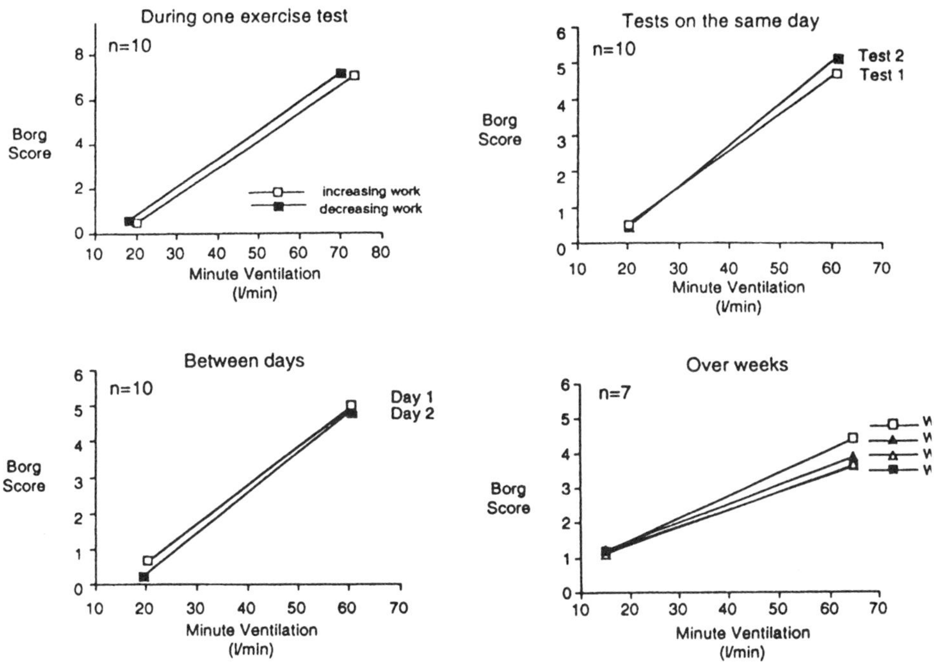

Figure 2 Repeatability of the relationship between breathlessness and ventilation in normal subjects during incremental exercise, obtained at different intervals. In each panel, the slopes are the mean slopes derived from all subjects. There were no significant differences in mean level of breathlessness or the slope of the breathlessness-ventilation relationship, tested using multiple analysis of covariance controlling for between-subject differences (From Wilson and Jones, 1989, 1991b.)

sensory stimulus to a point on a scale requires a number of cognitive processes. The precise nature of these is unclear, but certain stages may reasonably be hypothesized. At the very least, the subject will have to relate the maximum and minimum descriptors on the scale to corresponding levels drawn from their own sensory experiences. Factors influencing these may be different at the upper and lower ends of the scale. At the lower end, each individual must decide at which point the increasing respiratory-related sensations gain an additional quality or quantity that allows them to be judged on a scale labeled breathlessness. There are at least two mechanisms by which this could be achieved. The first is that a sense of dyspnea is triggered on reaching a particular level of respiratory sensation. As discussed earlier, most subjects are aware of their increased breathing before they register breathlessness, so this process would not be simply the detection of a liminal stimulus. A second mechanism could involve the emergence of a specific dyspnea component to the respiratory sensation that characterized the onset of breathlessness. We have suggested that the recruitment of an affective component to the sensation could be one such signal. Both these postulated mechanisms may involve a process of learning. Individuals may recognize a threshold event because they have learned, through experience, that it will progress to unequivocal dyspnea if they proceed to higher work levels.

The problems involved in defining the upper limit on a scale are different from those at the bottom and arise with both the Borg scale and VAS. It has been stated that the Borg scale is basically an interval scale with some ratio scaling properties (Killian, 1985). This explanation does not provide any insight into the way in which subjects may use it. All scales are applied with the assumption that they are internally reliable; that is, their scaling properties do not change with position along the scale. If the maximal reference point of a closed scale is changed, however, the properties of the entire scale are then altered. In virtually all studies of breathlessness, maximal breathlessness is never reached at the beginning of the study. This means that the reliable performance of a scale is dependent on accurate recall or imagination of what it feels like to experience maximal breathlessness. This may not be imaginable until it is experienced. Having read the descriptions of what it feels like to be paralyzed with fixed ventilation and a rising hypercapnia (Banzett et al., 1990), it is very clear to us that we have never experienced a sensation that could be called maximal.

Let us examine a theoretical scenario. Normal subjects, whose previous experience of breathlessness has been limited to recreational sport, agree to take part in an experiment similar to that just mentioned. At maximum levels of hypercapnia they experience levels of breathlessness and distress greater than anything that they have known hitherto. As the sensation worsens, they run out of room on the scale with which to indicate its level. They wish to go supramaximal to indicate how bad they feel, but the closed scale does not allow this. At the beginning of the experiment, they estimate their prevailing level of breathlessness relative to an imagined or remembered maximum. At the end, their maximum reference point has changed, so the relationship between measurements made at the beginning and the ends of the experiment are different. The scale has not performed reliably throughout the study. If the subjects then agree to undergo the same experiment a second time, it is likely that they will be conservative in their use of the lower end of the scale so that they can reserve sufficient room on the scale to express their level of sensation fully when close to maximal. During this experimental run, the scale may perform more reliably. This would not necessarily mean that the subjects were less breathless at lower levels of hypercapnia, merely that they were using the scale differently with a different idea of maximum. It is possible that they would transfer their new reference points to breathlessness experienced in other settings. These effects of experience may occur potentially with any closed scale. Borg recognized this and, in his modified scale, placed maximal above the upper limit to diminish the ceiling effect that tended to happen (Borg, 1982). This is not a satisfactory solution because the use of "maximal" in this way casts doubt upon the reliability of all the submaximal estimates that the subject will have made. Open-magnitude scales do not have this problem but are difficult to apply to dyspnea.

D. Effect of Changing References for Breathlessness Estimation

There are a number of ways in which the relationship between breathlessness and ventilation may change following a revision of maximum and minimum reference points. Four possibilities are illustrated in Fig. 3. In Fig. 3, the breathlessness-ventilation relationship is assumed to be linear, because a number of studies have shown this to be a reasonable approximation for incremental exercise tests

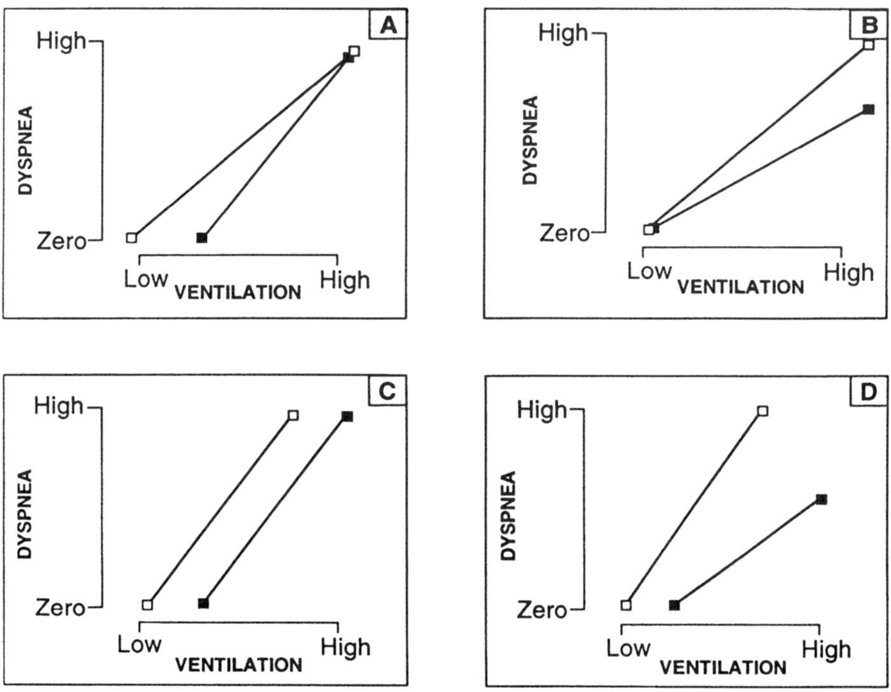

Figure 3 Four theoretical models to illustrate changes that would occur in the breathlessness-ventilation relationship following changes in a subject's threshold for the detection of breathlessness or their set point for maximal breathlessness. See text for full explanation.

(Adams et al., 1986; Wilson and Jones, 1989, 1991a). Change in the reference points could be confined to the threshold for breathlessness, that is, the lower set point, as shown in Fig. 3A, or the upper reference set point (Fig. 3B). Alternatively, both the threshold and the upper reference points could change. There are three possible patterns for this: an equal shift in both threshold and maximal points in the same direction (Fig. 3C), a nonequal shift in the same direction (Fig. 3D), or shifts in opposite directions (not illustrated).

E. Effects of Experience on Breathlessness Estimation in Normals

We have argued that the selection of reference points for scaling will depend on memory and experience, and we have predicted that a period of greater than usual breathlessness may reduce subsequent estimates. This hypothesis was tested in a series of experiments carried out in normal subjects during incremental exercise (Wilson and Jones, 1990). Breathlessness was defined as an uncomfortable need to breathe and measured using the modified Borg scale. We found that subjects could be conditioned to increase or decrease the perceived magnitude of their breathlessness in the second (measurement) section of an exercise test by the presence or absence of a small inspiratory resistance during the first (conditioning) section of the test. Prior experience of breathing with the inspiratory load caused a subsequent underestimation of breathlessness once it was removed compared with estimates made during an identical test that had not been preceded by loaded breathing. In a complementary series of experiments in which the pattern of loading and unloading was reversed, breathlessness estimation changed in the opposite direction. The changes in breathlessness-ventilation relationship with conditioning corresponded to the pattern in Fig. 3C.

The conditioning period in these experiments was only 8 minutes, and the test period took place immediately afterward. The effect of longer periods of conditioning was difficult to test because there are few suitable models that allow a sustained increase in breathlessness for conditioning purposes. We had the opportunity to study a group of mountaineers who were planning to spend 4 weeks walking and climbing above 4000 m. At this altitude, the inspired O_2 is ~90 torr and is sufficiently low to ensure that all activities require higher levels of ventilation compared with the same level of work at sea level. Nearly all individuals who exercise at this altitude are aware that they breathe more during habitual levels of daily exercise. We measured the breathlessness of our mountaineers during incremental ergometer exercise on four occasions over a 5 month period before the expedition and on four occasions over 6 months after their return (Wilson et al., 1993). On return to sea level, there was a significant reduction in the slope of the breathlessness-ventilation relationship that followed the pattern of Fig. 3D. In the first 6 weeks following return to sea level, breathlessness remained significantly below prealtitude levels (Fig. 4), but after 6 months it had returned to prealtitude values.

These two studies suggest that a period of increased respiratory sensation may lead to a reduction in perceived breathlessness during exercise on return to normal conditions. Similar evidence for adaptation can be found in two studies concerned with perception of inspiratory loads. One study was designed specifically to test for adaptation and found that a period of breathing against a very high inspiratory resistance led to a reduction in the perceived magnitude of the load (Revelette and Wiley, 1987). In a similar study, not specifically designed for this purpose, the same pattern can be seen in the results, and the effect appears to have persisted for 1 or 2 days (El-Manshawi et al., 1986).

In all these studies, breathlessness estimation was reduced following a conditioning period in which the subjects experienced an increased level of breathlessness compared with levels to which they were accustomed. This change from "usual" levels of breathlessness may be necessary for adaptation to occur. As mentioned previously, there is little evidence for a reduction in perceived breathlessness on repeated testing (Wilson and Jones, 1989, 1991b), and similarly there was no change in the breathlessness in our mountaineers during their preexpedition training period (Wilson et al., 1993). We also failed to find a hysteresis effect on scaling increasing and decreasing breathlessness during a single exercise test (Wilson and Jones, 1989). A reduction in perceived breathlessness has been observed in patients with chronic obstructive airways disease when tested at daily intervals (Belman et al., 1991). In this case, it may be argued that the high level of dyspnea produced during the exercise tests was a major change from the habitual level of activity in this relatively elderly group of patients. An alternative interpretation of the findings from this study is presented below.

F. Effects of Experience on Breathlessness Perception in Patients

In patients with chronic obstructive airways disease, estimates of breathlessness obtained during cycle ergometer exercise have been reported to be stable within and between days (Silverman et al., 1988). A progressive reduction in score on repeated testing has also been reported (Belman et al., 1991). These differences between the two studies may have been a result of the manner in which breathlessness was recorded. In the study of Silverman et al., the patients scaled sense of effort required to breathe using the Borg ratio of perceived exertion scale, whereas in Belman's study the patients scaled discomfort with breathing. The authors of this paper speculated that the experience of breathlessness may have caused a fall in perceived breathlessness by a process of desensitization (Belman et al., 1991). We support this conclusion in general but offer another possible mechanism. In this study, the patients were asked to anchor the upper limit of the modified Borg

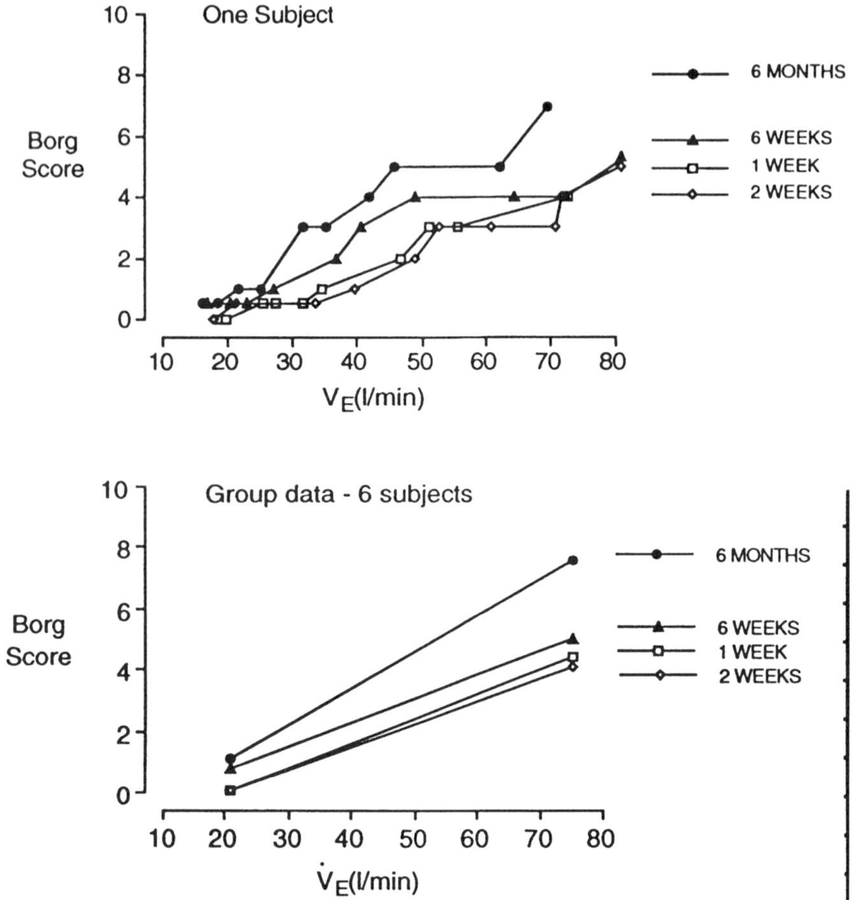

Figure 4 Change in the relationship between breathlessness and ventilation over 6 months following return from a 4 week period spent at an altitude of 4000 m. (Top) Results from one subject. (Bottom) Summary results from all six subjects. There were no significant differences between the first three measurements made over 6 weeks. At 6 months following the return to sea level, the mean level of breathlessness and the slope of the breathlessness-ventilation relationship were significantly higher than the three earlier measurements ($p < 0.0001$, multiple analysis of covariance, controlling for between-subject differences). The mean level of breathlessness and the slope, measured 6 months after the return to sea level, were the same as those recorded immediately before the period at altitude. (From Wilson et al., 1993.)

scale by first imagining a situation or past experience which has caused the worst breathlessness for you—an equivalent sensation should represent a 10 on the scale. During the first exercise test, the patients will have been using a maximum reference level of breathlessness drawn from an experience at some point in the past. Such recollections may be unreliable: there is evidence from studies of labor pain that recalled estimates of pain intensity were lower than estimates obtained at the time (Norvell et al., 1987). During the second and subsequent tests of Belman's study, the patients' memory of a high level of breathlessness will have been only 1 day old, giving them potentially a clearer idea of high levels of dyspnea than they held during their first test.

An incidental observation from a study in asthma also shows evidence of changes in breathlessness estimation. During an investigation of the effects of antigen challenge, dyspnea increased with the immediate airways response to challenge and then recovered as airway caliber improved. In two patients, a late response to antigen also occurred. Despite an increase in airways obstruction similar to that during the immediate response, there was no change in breathlessness (Turcotte et al., 1990). A possible explanation is that the first challenge reduced the sensitivity of the patients' breathlessness perception so that they were unable subsequently to detect an early recurrence of bronchoconstriction.

None of these studies in patients provide conclusive proof of the effects of experience on breathlessness, and intercurrent changes in lung function may make such studies difficult to perform. Nevertheless, it remains a distinct possibility that experience of breathlessness may alter estimates of its magnitude and patients' responses to it.

G. Mechanisms for Changes in Breathlessness Estimation

It has been observed that adaptation appears to be a nearly universal sensory phenomenon (Marks, 1974) and has been reported in modalities as varied as loudness (Stevens, 1956), brightness (Stevens and Stevens, 1963), cutaneous vibration (Gescheider and Wright, 1968), taste (McBurney, 1966), and even cutaneous pain (Burns and Dallenbach, 1933). For a lucid and very comprehensive review of sensory adaptation, the reader is referred to Helson (1964). Breathlessness is not due to a unique sensory input, however, and we briefly review some possible mechanisms that could result in changes in its perceived magnitude.

Change in the Drive to Breathe

The motor command theory of breathlessness would predict that a change in respiratory effort caused by changes in lung mechanics, chemoreceptor drive, or respiratory muscle fatigue would alter the magnitude of dyspnea. Such a process could not account for the changes in breathlessness seen in our loading studies, because we ensured that breathlessness measurements were made under the same conditions of load (Wilson and Jones, 1990). In these experiments, muscle fatigue was not a possible explanation, either, because if this were present, breathlessness should have increased rather than decreased after a conditioning period of breathing against a resistance. Changes in respiratory drive cannot account for the results from our study on the effects of altitude. We observed that the ventilatory equivalent for oxygen on return to sea level was somewhat increased compared with prealtitude levels (Wilson et al., 1993), yet breathlessness for a given level of ventilation or oxygen consumption was lower. Again, the changes in breathlessness were in the opposite direction from those predicted on the basis of any change in respiratory drive. It does not appear that changes in motor command could account for the changes in breathlessness observed in our studies, but under other circumstances it may be difficult to exclude this mechanism completely.

Peripheral Adaptation

In physiology, the term "adaptation" is retained to describe the decline in rate of firing of receptors under constant stimulation. Such adaptation has been well documented for vagally mediated lung stretch receptors. In addition, muscle and tendon organs of respiratory muscles probably possess adaptation characteristics similar to those of receptors in other striated muscles. However, these adaptation characteristics apply to sustained stimuli. Receptors in the ventilatory apparatus are under continual phasic stimulation. It is not known whether there are sustained changes in response characteristics of the receptors following maintained changes in ventilation or loading of the respiratory muscles. It seems unlikely that peripheral adaptation could account for the reduction in breathlessness that we observed for 6 weeks after our subjects returned from altitude to sea level.

Change in the Overall Motor Sensory Experience

Breathlessness arises on a background of other respiratory sensations, and it is possible that it may change as part of a general reduction in sensation. This in itself would imply an adaptive change in the perception of other respiratory sensations. Against this proposal is the observation that, under certain experimental conditions, breathlessness may increase yet the perception of respiratory effort may fall (Demediuk et al., 1992).

Change in the Type of Sensation Being Scaled

Linguistic studies suggest that there may be varieties of breathlessness. It is possible that experiences of different types of breathlessness may cause subjects to change their internal criteria for the qualitative nature of the respiratory sensation being scaled. This could result in them scaling a different part of their respiratory experience, for example a shift from the intensity of discomfort to an affective component.

Change in the Scaling of Breathlessness

This hypothesis proposes that the sensory experience and the quality of the sensation being scaled remain the same, but the subjects change the reference points that they use for scaling. Direct evidence for this mechanism comes from a study involving magnitude estimation of inspiratory loads. Following a period of breathing against high resistive loads, there was a reduction in perceived magnitude of the resistive loads on retesting (Revelette and Wiley, 1987). In this study, unlike studies of dyspnea, the inspiratory load provided a specific sensation resulting from a specific stimulus. The perceived magnitude of the load was measured by requiring the subjects to squeeze a hand grip dynamometer to achieve a sense of effort that corresponded to the effort required to overcome the inspiratory load. They were given no visual feedback of the grip achieved. Thus, the process of sensing the respiratory load and the method of expressing its perceived magnitude were very similar. This methodology should have increased the probability that the subjects were responding to exactly the same respiratory sensation before and after the period of conditioning. In the absence of any other mechanism, we believe that a change in scaling caused by a change in reference points could account for the changes in breathlessness measured in our studies (Wilson and Jones, 1990; Wilson et al., 1993).

IV. Nonrespiratory Influences on Breathlessness Perception

Breathlessness has been shown to be higher during hypercapnia than at an equivalent level of ventilation during exercise (Stark et al., 1981). These and similar observations led to the argument that dyspnea may seem to be more "appropriate" during exercise than while inhaling carbon dioxide at rest. This could lead to it being rated lower in intensity. This is a valid argument, but in hypercapnic and exercise-induced dyspnea, it hinges on the assumption that different respiratory drives produce the same degree of breathlessness for a given level of ventilation. This issue remains unresolved (Swinburn et al., 1984; Ward and Whipp, 1989; Lane et al., 1990). Furthermore, there appear to be different varieties of ventilatory experience depending on the type of stimulus to breathing (Simon et al., 1989, 1990). It remains possible that breathlessness is environmentally conditioned, but it is not yet clear whether other mechanisms could be responsible for apparent differences in breathlessness during different types of reflexively driven breathing.

Respiratory sensations may be influenced by other nonrespiratory factors.

For example, breath holding time was extended by having the subjects perform cognitive and psychomotor tasks at the same time (Matthews, 1982). The same workers subsequently showed that breathlessness could be prolonged by a negative incentive (threat of an electric shock) but not by a positive incentive in the form of a monetary reward or a neutral distraction, such as performing a mantra (Alpher and Blanton, 1991). Mood state may also be a factor in the perception of inspiratory loads, with the surprising observation that anxiety was negatively correlated with the exponent for inspiratory load perception (Tiller et al., 1987). This is contrary to what might be expected with breathlessness. A number of studies have shown that anxiety scores are raised in patients with chronic obstructive airways disease and correlate well with disability (Jones et al., 1989). We have also found a low but significant positive correlation between anxiety and Borg score for dyspnea on exercise (C. M. Baveystock and P. W. Jones, unpublished observations).

Stimuli not directly related to the act of breathing have been shown to influence direct measurements of breathlessness. Blowing cold air onto the cheek has reduced the intensity of breathlessness in subjects breathing against an inspiratory resistance during hypercapnia (Schwartzstein et al., 1987). Interestingly, the same effect was not found with air blown against the leg. Nasal airflow also appears to be a factor. In patients with chronic obstructive airways disease receiving air or oxygen through nasal cannulae, topical anesthesia to the nose increased perceived dyspnea (Liss and Grant, 1988). This finding suggests that the sensation of airflow through the nasal space may reduce breathlessness. Finally, we have observed that breathlessness estimates were higher when subjects were exercised while fasting compared with when they were exercised after a liquid meal, whether mainly fat or mainly carbohydrate (Wilson et al., 1990). This difference was not caused by substrate effects on the ventilatory response to exercise.

In asthma, a large proportion of patients may fail to detect deteriorating airways obstruction, and this has led to the concept of poor perceivers. It has been reported that patients' VAS scores for asthma severity correlated more closely with peak expiratory flow rate when the patients were given access to their peak flow measurement than when it was hidden from them by coding (Higgs et al., 1986). This observation indicates that patients may be inclined to adjust their perception of asthma severity to match other cues, suggesting that they integrate information from sources other than respiratory sensations in forming their estimate of symptom severity.

In conclusion, breathlessness estimation does not occur in isolation and there is evidence that it is subject to a number of influences, some quite unrelated to the act of breathing or respiratory effort. These include experience of breathlessness and recall of those experiences, incentives, mood, influences from other somatic and possibly visceral sources, and other cues. In an experiment, is important to control for these factors, but in daily life they are largely uncontrolled yet may have a significant impact on a patient's perception of their dyspnea and their response to it.

V. Studies of Volitional Hyperventilation and Breathlessness

There have been a number of studies in which breathlessness has been measured during volitional hyperventilation. These are very interesting for the light that they throw on the generation of dyspnea, but they are also conceptually some of the most difficult experiments to interpret in this field.

In studies from Guz's group, it was observed that breathlessness during volitional hyperventilation was very much lower than during hypercapnia and exercise: indeed, it was almost negligible (Adams et al., 1985b; Freedman et al., 1987). This general pattern was not found in studies from another group, who recorded substantial breathlessness during volitional hyperventilation, albeit less than that induced by hypercapnia (Chonan et al., 1990). These workers found no difference between exercise and volitional hyperventilation. During hypercapnia, breathlessness was greater while the subjects were asked to constrain their breathing voluntarily than during free breathing (Chonan et al., 1987). These studies were later extended to show that all volitional departures from the spontaneous level of breathing during hypercapnia were accompanied by a proportional increase in breathlessness (Chonan et al., 1990).

One reason for the apparent discrepancy between these results may have been the description of the sensation given to the subjects. Guz's group defined breathlessness as an uncomfortable need to breathe; Chonan et al. asked their subjects to scale the intensity of the sensation of difficulty in breathing. These two definitions appear to be quite different. *Need* implies a necessity or compulsion. Any action resulting from a need could be largely independent of a subject's desire to do it. On the other hand, *difficulty* implies that an obstacle, activity, or task can be achieved only by effort or an effort of will. If the experimental subjects of these research groups shared the same associations that we have drawn with these two words, it would suggest that they were scaling different aspects of breathlessness. It is not possible to be firm in this conclusion, because the subjects were not presented with both descriptions with instructions to follow one and reject the other. In another study of similar design, however, the same group of subjects were asked to scale two different aspects of their respiratory sensations, one using the word *urge* and the other implying effort. This had a very significant effect on the results (Demediuk et al., 1992).

There may be a broader problem than language with regard to the perception of volitional changes in breathing. The motor command theory for the generation of breathlessness (Gandevia et al., 1981) postulates the existence of pathways carrying afferent information about the level of respiratory motor drive from these motoneurons to the cortex. The ventilatory responses to exercise and chemoreceptor stimulation are reflex activities mediated through the motoneurons in the brain stem respiratory center. In contrast to reflexively driven breathing, volitional respiratory activity must originate in the cerebral cortex. Premotor potentials, recorded from an area of the cerebral cortex associated with respiratory motor activity, were not found during spontaneous breathing (Macefield and Gandevia, 1991). Volitional respiratory activity may be transmitted through separate motor pathways from those involved in reflex breathing (Plum, 1970); the activity of the brain stem respiratory motoneurons during voluntary breathing is not known. It cannot be assumed that afferent neuronal traffic to the associative cerebral cortex is derived from the same source in both reflex and volitional ventilation, and neither can it be assumed that such traffic will be processed or interpreted in the same manner if it comes from different sources.

A cognitive approach to this issue would recognize that the human is a reasoning being and that thinking about breathlessness is an interpretative act. Volitional hyperventilation is premeditated, whereas reflexively driven breathing is not. Is it possible for a thinking being to ignore that it is wilfully overriding reflex respiratory control processes and still conclude that the resulting respiratory sensation is breathlessness? The answer to this may depend on the definition of breathlessness. The word *effort* implies volitional activity. A sense of effort is an appropriate description of the process required to overcome an inspiratory resistance applied to a single breath. Similarly, effort may be an appropriate description for the sensation produced in the process of maintaining a predetermined pattern and depth of breathing. If breathlessness were synonymous with volitional effort, then the issues would be clearer. The act of breathing produced during reflexively driven breathing is not volitional, however, and cannot be suppressed at will. During breathlessness, subjects experience respiratory sensations that they cannot control because they cannot choose to reduce their level of breathing immediately. Lack of control over breathing is associated with a high level of distress (Quirk and Jones, 1990). In certain respects, breathlessness may be analogous to the sensation of tickle. It is perfectly possibly for an individual to replicate the stimulation of their own skin exactly, but this does not induce the feeling of tickle that results when the same stimulus is applied by someone else.

We conclude that the volitional control of breathing is an interesting experimental tool with which to examine respiratory sensations. Results from studies using this tool are not entirely consistent. This may reflect differences in the instructions to the subjects but may point to more fundamental differences in the way individuals interpret the sensations experienced during reflex and voluntary changes in breathing.

VI. Nonlinear Model of Breathlessness

At the beginning of this chapter we presented a standard model for the formation of conscious sensation. In it, the process of breathlessness estimation was viewed as a sequence of steps in which inputs from a number of sources are detected, discriminated, recognized, and then scaled. Some of the studies discussed in this chapter lead us to conclude that this concept is too simple and that it should include feedback pathways. For example, there is direct evidence that prior experience of breathlessness may influence subsequent estimates, both in the short term (Revelette and Wiley, 1987; Wilson and Jones, 1990) and over several weeks (Wilson et al., 1993). We have also discussed observations that suggest that an individual's qualitative description of breathlessness may be altered by experience (Banzett et al., 1989, 1990), pointing to an influence on the discrimination and recognition step. In addition, a chance finding from a further study (Turcotte et al., 1990) implicates a possible effect of breathlessness on the detection step. These various observations suggest the existence of one or more pathways by which breathlessness may modulate the processes responsible for its generation (Fig. 5).

We suggest that the process by which breathlessness is perceived may be described best as a nonlinear model in which the output (breathlessness) can feed back to modify the processes by which it was generated (i.e., detection, discrimination, recognition, and scaling). This has important implications for an understanding of the mechanisms by which breathlessness is perceived. In a linear model, the size of the output may be predicted from the size of the input if the operating characteristics of the system are known. This is not possible with a nonlinear system, because its operating characteristics are not constant. For example, the effect of feedback from the output of the system (i.e., breathlessness) to an earlier stage (e.g., magnitude scaling) would be to alter the performance characteristics of the scaling step, thereby changing the perceived level of breathlessness, which in turn modifies the scaling step, with consequent effect on the perceived level of breathlessness, and so on. When nonlinear systems are modeled mathematically, the usual method of estimating the response to a given input is to allow the model to iterate (i.e., cycle) until a stable value for the output is achieved. Nonlinear models may be studied using computer programs relatively easily, but nonlinear systems are difficult to investigate experimentally. One approach is to assume that small changes in input and output will produce similarly small feedback effects, so that the overall performance characteristics of the pathway will be close to those of a linear system. Indeed, this assumption underlies a very great deal of work on physiological control systems.

We hypothesize that the processes by which the magnitude of breathlessness is estimated together form a nonlinear system. If correct, this means that breathlessness is perceived by a mechanism whose operating characteristics may be

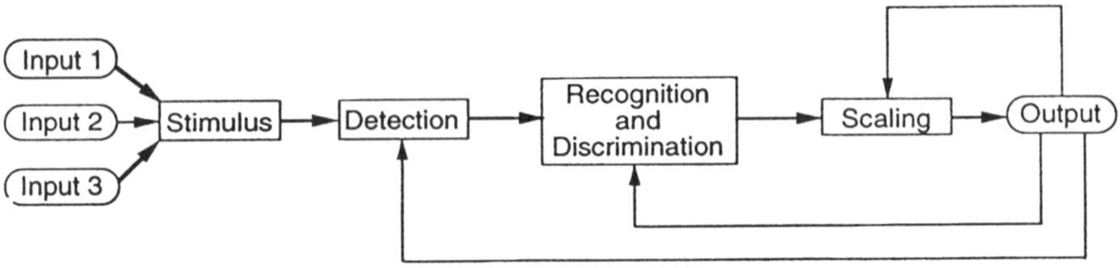

Figure 5 Model for the formation of breathlessness in which feedback from the output influences the gain of earlier steps in the pathway. It is apparent that such feedback influences the gain of the whole system and thereby alters the size of the output; that is, the size of the output may in turn determine its own magnitude. These are properties of a nonlinear system. The nature of the feedback pathways, as positive or negative, is not specified, but experimental findings suggest that feedback to the scaling stage is may be largely negative, that is, causing a reduction in sensitivity.

continually changing. These changes could become large over the period of time that characterizes the development of chronic lung disease. The effect of feedback to alter the gain of a particular step in the pathway of breathlessness estimation is only one way in which the performance of system may change. Even the gain of a linear system may appear to change if a large change in stimulus intensity moves it from the slope to the plateau of a response curve. In addition, inputs external to the system may also influence its operating characteristics. For example, a signal derived from a disease process, although not contributing directly to the sensation, may alter the gain of a particular step and change the magnitude of perceived breathlessness. In this context, we have observed that breathlessness estimation in normal subjects was influenced by whether the subject was studied fasting or following a small liquid meal (Wilson et al., 1990).

In conclusion, it is quite possible that responses to small experimental stimuli in normal subjects may be different from those measured in patients with established disease. This could imply differences in mechanism between perception of breathlessness in health and dyspnea in disease. However, an alternative hypothesis is that the basic structural pathways responsible for breathlessness and dyspnea do not change as disease develops or progresses, merely that the operating characteristics of the system by which they are perceived are changed. Experience of breathlessness may be one factor contributing to such changes.

VII. Concluding Observations

In this chapter we have approached breathlessness from a cognitive viewpoint. We have critically examined a number of experiments concerned with respiratory sensations. Each of these studies was performed on subjects who had been asked to think about and analyze their prevailing sensory experience. Most of these experiments were not designed to test a cognitive theory of breathlessness, but most are open to reasoned speculation concerning the processes that underlie the way in which the subjects reported their experience. Cognitive factors appear to influence every step in the generation of breathlessness. This has important implications for the design of experimental studies and may lead to better therapeutic approaches toward modifying the symptom that forms the critical link between cardiopulmonary diseases and disability.

References

Adams, L., Chronos, N., Lane, R., and Guz, A. (1985a). The measurement of breathlessness induced in normal subjects: validity of two scaling techniques. Clin Sci. 69:7–16.

Adams, L., Lane, R., Shea, S.A., Cockcroft, A., and Guz, A. (1985b). Breathlessness during different forms of ventilatory stimulation: a study of mechanisms in normal subjects and respiratory patients. Clin. Sci. 69:663–672.

Adams, L., Chronos, N. Lane, R., and Guz, A. (1986). The measurement of breathlessness in normal subjects: individual differences. Clin. Sci. 70:131–140.

Alpher, V.S., and Blanton, R.L. (1991). Motivational processes and behavioral inhibition in breath holding. J. Psychol. 125:71–81.

Altose, M.D., Dimarco, A.F., Gottfreid, S.B., and Strohl, K.P. (1982). The sensation of respiratory muscle force. Am. Rev. Respir. Dis. 126:807–811.

Banzett, R.B., Lansing, R.W., and Brown, R. (1987). High-level quadraplegics perceive lung volume change. J. Appl. Physiol. 62:567–573.

Banzett, R.B., Lansing, R.W., Reid, M.B., Adams, L., and Brown, R. (1989). "Air hunger" arising from increased P_{CO_2} in mechanically ventilated quadriplegics. Respir. Physiol. 76:53–67.

Banzett, R.B., Lansing, R.W., Brown, R., Topulos, G.P., Yager, D., Steele, S.M., Londono, B., Loring, S.H., Reid, M.B., Adams, L., et al. (1990). "Air hunger" from increased P_{CO_2} persists after complete neuromuscular block in humans. Respir. Physiol. 81: 1–17.

Belman, M.J., Brooks, L.R., Ross, D.J., and Mohsenifar, Z. (1991). Variability of breathlessness measurement in patients with chronic obstructive pulmonary disease. Chest 99:566–571.

Borg, G.A.V. (1982). A category scale with ratio properties for intermodal and interindividual comparisons. In: Psychophysical Judgement and the Process of Perception. VEB Deutscher Verlag der Wissenschaften, Berlin, pp. 25–34.

Burney, P.G.J., Laitinen, L.A., Perdrizet, S., Huckauf, H., Tattersfield, A.E., Chinn, S., Poisson, N., Heeren, A., Britton, J.R., and Jones T. (1989). Validity and repeatability of the IUATLD (1984) Bronchial Symptoms Questionnaire: an international comparison. Eur. Respir. J. 2:940–945.

Burns, M., and Dallenbach, K.M. (1933). The adaptation of cutaneous pain. Am. J. Psychol. 45:111–117.

Campbell, E.J.M., Godfrey, S., Clark, T.J.H., Freedman, S., and Norman, J. (1969). The effect of muscular paralysis induced by tubocurarine on the duration and sensation of breath-holding during hypercapnia. Clin. Sci. 36:323–328.
Chonan, T., Mulholland, M.B., Cherniack, N.S., and Altose, M.D. (1987). Effects of voluntary constraining of thoracic displacement during hypercapnia. J. Appl. Physiol. 63:1822–1828.
Chonan, T., Mulholland, M.B., Altose, M.D., and Cherniack, N.S. (1990a). Effects of changes in level and pattern of breathing on the sensation of dyspnea. J. Appl. Physiol. 69:1290–1295.
Chonan, T., Mulholland, M.B., Leitner, J., Altose, M.D., and Cherniack, N.S. (1990b). Sensation of dyspnea during hypercapnia, exercise, and voluntary hyperventilation. J. Appl. Physiol. 68:2100–2106.
Comroe, J.H. (1966). Some Theories of the Mechanism of Dyspnea. Blackwell Scientific, Oxford.
Davenport, P.W., Thompson, F.J., Reep, R.L., and Freed, A.N. (1985). Projection of phrenic nerve afferents to the cat sensory motor cortex. Brain Res. 328:150–153.
Demediuk, B.H., Manning, H., Lilly, J., Fencl, V., Weinberger, S.E., Weis, J.W., and Schwartzstein, R.M. (1992). Dissociation between dyspnea and respiratory effort. Am. Rev. Respir. Dis. 146:1222–1225.
Elliott, M.W., Adams, L., Cockcroft, A., MacRae, K.D., Murphy, K., and Guz, A. (1991). The language of breathlessness. Use of verbal descriptors by patients with cardiopulmonary disease. Am. Rev. Respir. Dis. 144:826–832.
El-Manshawi, A., Killian, K.J., Summers, E., and Jones, N.L. (1986). Breathlessness during exercise with and without resistive loading. J. Appl. Physiol. 61:896–905.
Freedman, S., Lane, R., and Guz, A. (1987). Breathlessness and respiratory mechanics during reflex or voluntary hyperventilation in patients with chronic airflow limitation. Clin. Sci. 73:311–318.
Gandevia, S.C., Killian, K.J., and Campbell, E.J.M. (1981). The effect respiratory muscle fatigue on respiratory sensations. Clin. Sci. 60:463–466.
Gescheider, G.A., and Wright, J.W. (1968). Effects of sensory adaptation on the form of the psychophysical magnitude function for cutaneous vibration. J. Exp. Psychol. 77:308–313.
Gottfried, D.S.B., Altose, M.D., Kelsen, S.G., and Cherniak, N.S. (1981). Perception of changes in airflow resistance in obstructive pulmonary disorders. Am. Rev. Respir. Dis. 124:566–570.
Gottfried, S.B., Redline, S., and Altose, M.D. (1985). Respiratory sensation in chronic obstructive pulmonary disease. Am. Rev. Respir. Dis. 132:954–959.
Helson, H. (1964). Adaptation-Level Theory: An Experimental and Systematic Approach to Behavior. Harper and Row, New York.
Higgs, C.M.B., Richardson, R.B., Lea, D.A., Lewis, C.T.G., and Laszlo, G. (1986). Influence of knowledge of peak flow on self assessment of asthma: studies with a coded peak flow meter. Thorax 41:671–675.
Jamner, L.D., and Tursky, B. (1987). Discrimination between intensity and affective pain descriptors: a psychophysiological evaluation. Pain 30:271–283.
Jones, P.W., Baveystock, C.M., and Littlejohns, P. (1989). Relationships between general

health measured with the sickness impact profile and respiratory symptoms, physiological measures and mood in patients with chronic airflow limitation. Am. Rev. Respir. Dis. 140:1538–1543.

Jones, P.W. and the Nedocromil Sodium Quality of Life Study Group (1994). Quality of Life, symptoms and pulmonary function in asthma: long-term treatment with nedocromil sodium examined in a controlled multicentre trial. Eur Respir J 7:55–62.

Killian, K.J. (1985). The objective measurement of breathlessness. Chest 88:84–90.

Killian, K.J., Gandevia, S.C., Summers, E., and Campbell, E.J.M. (1984). Effect of lung volume on perception of breathlessness, effort and tension. J. Appl. Physiol. 57: 686–691.

Killian, K.J., Leblanc, P., Martin, D.H., Summers, E., Jones, N.L., and Campbell, E.J.M. (1992a). Exercise capacity and ventilatory, circulatory and symptom limitation in patients with chronic airflow limitation. Am. Rev. Respir. Dis. 146:935–940.

Killian, K.J., Summers, E., Jones, N.L., and Campbell, E.J. (1992b). Dyspnea and leg effort during incremental cycle ergometry. Am. Rev. Respir. Dis. 145:1339–1345.

Kinsman, R.A., Yaroush, R.A., Fernandez, E., Dirks, J.F., Schocket, M., and Fukuhara, J. (1983). Symptoms and experiences in chronic bronchitis and emphysema. Chest 83:755–761.

Kremer, E.F., Atkinson, J.H., and Ignelzi, R.J. (1982). Pain measurement: the affective dimensional measure of the McGill pain questionnaire with a cancer pain population. Pain 12:153–163.

Lane, R., Adams, L., and Guz, A. (1990). The effects of hypoxia and hypercapnia on perceived breathlessness during exercise in humans. J. Physiol. (Lond.) 428:579–593.

Liss, H.P., and Grant, B.J.B. (1988). The effect of nasal flow on breathlessness in patients with chronic obstructive pulmonary disease. Am. Rev. Respir. Dis. 137:1285–1288.

Macefield, G., and Gandevia, S.C. (1991). The cortical drive to human respiratory muscles in the awake state assessed by premotor cerebral potentials. J. Physiol. (Lond.) 439:545–558.

Mahler, D.A., Rosiello, R.A., Harver, A., Lentine, T., McGovern, J.F., and Daubenspeck, J.A. (1987). Comparison of clinical dyspnea ratings and psychophysical measurements of respiratory sensation in obstructive airways disease. Am. Rev. Respir. Dis. 135:1229–1233.

Marks, L.E. (1974). Sensory Processes: The New Psychophysics. Academic Press, London.

Matthews, P.B.C. (1982). Where does Sherrington's "muscular sense" originate? Muscles, joints, corollary discharges? Annu. Rev. Neurosci. 5:189–218.

McBurney, D.H. (1966). Magnitude estimation of the taste of sodium chloride after adaptation to sodium chloride J. Exp. Psychol. 72:869–873.

McCloskey, D.I. (1978). Kinesthetic sensibility. Physiol. Rev. 58:763–820.

Melzack, R. (1975). The McGill pain questionnaire: major properties and scoring methods. Pain 1:275–299.

Melzack, R., and Torgerson, W.S. (1971). On the language of pain. Anaesthesiology 34: 50–59.

Muza, S.R., Silverman, M.T., Gilmore, G.C., and Hellerstein, H.K. (1990). Comparison of scales used to quantitate the sense of effort to breathe in patients with chronic obstructive pulmonary disease. Am. Rev. Respir. Dis. 141:909–913.

Norvell, K.T., Gaston-Johansson, F., and Fridh, G. (1987). Remembrance of labor pain: how valid are retrospective pain measurements? Pain 31:77–86.

Plassman, B.L., and Lansing, R.W. (1990). Peptual cues used to reproduce an inspired lung volume. J. Appl. Physiol. 69:11233–11130.

Plum, F. (1970). Neurological integration of behavioural and metabolic control of breathing. Breathing: Hering-Bruer Centenary Symposium. Churchill, London, pp. 159–181.

Price, D.D., Barrell, J.J., and Gracely, R.H. (1980). A psychophysical analysis of experiential factors that selectively influence the affective dimension of pain. Pain 8:137–149.

Quirk, F.H., and Jones, P.W. (1990). Patients' perception of distress due to symptoms and effects of asthma on daily living and an investigation of possible influential factors. Clin. Sci. 79:17–21.

Revelette, W.R., and Wiley, R.L. (1987). Plasticity of the mechanism subserving inspiratory load perception. J. Appl. Physiol. 62:1901–1906.

Schwartzstein, R.M., Lahive, K., Pope, A., Weinberger, S.E., and Weiss, J.W. (1987). Cold facial stimulation reduces breathlessness induced in normal subjects. Am. Rev. Respir. Dis. 136:58–61.

Silverman, M., Barry, J., Hellerstein, H., Jonos, J., and S.K. (1988). Variability of the perceived sense of effort in breathing during exercise in patients with chronic obstructive airways disease. Am. Rev. Respir. Dis. 137:206–209.

Simon, P.M., Schwartzstein, R.M., Weiss, J.W., Lahive, K., Fencl, V., Teghtsoonian, M., and Weinberger, S.E. (1989). Distinguishable sensations of breathlessness induced in normal volunteers. Am. Rev. Respir. Dis. 140:1021–1027.

Simon, P.M., Schwartzstein, R.M., Weiss, J.W., Fencl, V., Teghtsoonian, M., and Weinberger, S.E. (1990). Distinguishable types of dyspnea in patients with shortness of breath. Am. Rev. Respir. Dis. 142:1009–1014.

Stark, R.D., Gambles, S.A., and Lewis, J.A. (1981). Methods to assess breathlessness in healthy subjects: a critical evaluation and application to analyse the acute effects of diazepam and promathezine on breathlessness induced by exercise or by exposure to raised levels of carbon dioxide. Clin. Sci. 61:429–439.

Stevens, J.C., and Stevens, S.S. (1963). Brightness function: effects of adaptation. J. Opt. Soc. Am. 53:375–385.

Stevens, S.S. (1956). The direct estimation of sensory magnitude—loudness. Am. J. Psychol. 69:1–25.

Stevens, S.S. (1957). On the psychophysical law. Psychol Rev. 64:153–181.

Swinburn, C.R., Wakefield, J.M., and Jones, P.W. (1984). Relationship between ventilation and breathlessness during exercise in chronic obstructive airways disease is not altered by prevention of hypoxaemia. Clin. Sci. 67:515–519.

Tack, M., Altose, M.D., and Cherniak, N.S. (1982). Effect of aging on the perception of resistive loads. Am. Rev. Respir. Dis. 126:463–467.

Tiller, J., Pain, M., and Biddle, N. (1987). Anxiety disorder and perception of inspiratory resistive loads. Chest 91:547–551.

Turcotte, H., Corbeil, F., and Boulet, L.P. (1990). Perception of breathlessness during bronchoconstriction induced by antigen, exercise, and histamine challenges. Thorax 45:914–918.

Ward, M.E., and Stubbing, D.G. (1985). Effect of chronic lung disease on the perception of added inspiratory loads. Am. Rev. Respir. Dis. 132:652–626.

Ward, S.A., and Whipp, B.J. (1989). Effects of peripheral and central chemoreflex activation on the isopnoeic rating of breathing in exercising humans. J. Physiol. (Lond.) 411:27–43.

Wiley, R.L., and Zechman, F.W. (1966). Perception of added airflow resistance in humans. Respir. Physiol. 2:73–87.

Wilson, R.C., and Jones, P.W. (1989). A comparison of the visual analogue scale and modified Borg scale for the measurement of dyspnoea during exercise. Clin. Sci. 76:277–282.

Wilson, R.C., and Jones, P.W. (1990). Influence of prior ventilatory experience on the estimation of breathlessness during exercise. Clin. Sci. 78:149–153.

Wilson, R.C., and Jones, P.W. (1991a). Differentiation between the intensity of breathlessness and the distress it evokes in normal subjects during exercise. Clin. Sci. 80: 65–70.

Wilson, R.C., and Jones, P.W. (1991b). Long-term reproducibility of Borg scale estimates of breathlessness during exercise. Clin. Sci. 80:309–312.

Wilson, R.C., Al-Saady, N.M., Blackmore, C.M., Jones, P.W., and Bennett, P.W. (1990). Effect of fasting on breathlessness during exercise. Eur. Respir. J. 3:155s.

Wilson, R.C., Oldfield, W.L.G., and Jones, P.W. (1993). Effect of residence at altitude on the perception of breathlessness on return to sea level in normal subjects. Clin. Sci. 84:159–167.

Wolkove, N., Dajczman, E., Colacone, A., and Kreisman, H. (1989). The relationship between pulmonary function and dyspnea in obstructive lung disease. Chest 96: 1247–1251.

Zigmond, A.S., and Snaith, R.P. (1983). The hospital anxiety and depression scale. Acta Psychiatr. Scand. 67:361–370.

14

Dyspnea
A Possible Target for Pharmacological Intervention

RONALD D. STARK and NORMAN J. W. RUSSELL

Zeneca Pharmaceuticals
Macclesfield, Cheshire, England

ALISON CLOVA STARK

General Infirmary at Leeds
Leeds, England

I. Introduction

Dyspnea is the most common symptom in patients with cardiorespiratory disease. In addition, up to half of the patients in terminal care for cancer have dyspnea as the main symptom, particularly in the period before death (Higginson and McCarthy, 1989; Fainsinger et al., 1991). Clearly, dyspnea remains an immense clinical problem and a challenge for therapeutics.

An agent that could reduce the sensation of dyspnea without undesirable effects would be expected to improve dramatically the patient's quality of life. Not only would there be a reduction in the distress and anxiety that accompany dyspnea, but the restrictions of many aspects of daily life imposed by breathlessness would be reduced or their onset delayed. Such an agent would never be a substitute for specific therapy directed at the underlying disease process but could be of value when, as frequently is the case, the pathology is irreversible.

Discovery of drugs to reduce dyspnea is hindered because the pathophysiological mechanisms are difficult to investigate in humans and are still in dispute. Animal studies must rely on surrogate end points taken to reflect the relevant sensations. Consequently, research on pharmacological approaches to breathlessness is in its infancy, and at this stage there are no more than hints of possible therapeutic opportunities. Few pharmaceutical companies have shown more than passing interest in dyspnea as a therapeutic target.

The focus of our experimental studies was to use as tools pharmacological agents that might interact with mechanisms possibly implicated in dyspnea (Stark and Guz, 1984; Stark, 1988). Such agents were not designed specifically for dyspnea, and any effect was unlikely to be more than modest. This required precision in the assessment of dyspnea. Expectations were realistic; it was more likely that we would contribute to eliminating candidate mechanisms rather than making a startling breakthrough.

II. Assessing Dyspnea to Detect Drug Effects

Progress in detecting drug effects was dependent on advances in the last 15 years that offered greater precision in the assessment of breathlessness. Any method must be reproducible, sensitive, and, of course, specific for the sensation under study. In view of the inevitable subjectivity in studying breathlessness, rigorous validation of the method and sound experimental design are crucial.

In 1980, visual analog scales (VAS) were applied serially to assess breathlessness during submaximal exercise (Stark and Gambles, 1980). In this way, it was possible to study dyspnea without taking the subjects to the limits of their exercise tolerance. The responses were summarized in terms of the relationship of breathlessness to minute ventilation or to oxygen uptake.

Various procedures were adopted in an attempt to enhance the reliability of the test (Stark et al., 1981; Morton et al., 1983; Stark, 1988). Rather than relying on a single VAS, multiple VAS were used during the period of study to monitor changes in the sensations during and immediately after exercise. In our laboratory, it has been policy to fix or "anchor" the upper end of the VAS by a short period of strenuous exercise. Identical exercise could be undertaken on other days of the study to provide a constant reference point. Thus, the VAS was "calibrated" with respect to both the quantity and the quality of the sensation of breathlessness. Some other laboratories have not followed this practice and may have compromised on the high level of reproducibility it probably achieves.

It is important to avoid bias in the design of the experiments, especially when drugs are studied, and to reduce variation in the experimental results to increase precision. The environment was maintained constant from day to day of the study, and subjects were "naive" before becoming familiar with the test and the VAS during preliminary sessions. The order of treatments was randomized, and comparisons were made on a within-subject basis under double-blind conditions.

Validation of the methods concentrated on reproducibility and sensitivity.

Demonstration that the VAS was reliable in one group of subjects, however, carried no guarantee that other groups of subjects would also use the VAS with reliability. For this reason, validation was performed in each study. Occasional subjects did not show consistency, and the protocol allowed them to be excluded during the preliminary phase of the studies.

Reproducibility was assessed by comparing the responses of subjects to identical periods of exercise performed 1 or 2 weeks apart. In general, individual subjects showed high levels of reproducibility (Stark et al., 1981, 1983; Stark and Gambles, 1981; O'Neill et al., 1984, 1985a, b). Between-subject variations were considerable, however, and this has implications for using VAS to compare responses in parallel groups of subjects. Long-term reproducibility has less relevance to drug studies, most of which are conducted over short periods of time.

The sensitivity of the test concerns the ability of the VAS to detect real changes in breathlessness. In normal subjects this was tested by comparing exercise tests in the presence and absence of a low-value inspiratory resistance under double-blind conditions, with randomization of the order and after "anchoring" of the VAS (see preceding references). It has been a consistent finding that the resistance is not detected at rest but during exercise, the VAS shows greater breathlessness at the highest levels of ventilation.

It is concluded from these studies in healthy subjects that the relationship between breathlessness and ventilation is reproducible and also sensitive to change and therefore should be capable of detecting effects from active pharmacological agents. A final question concerns the specificity of the test; in other words, is the VAS truly recording breathlessness? The approach used in this laboratory has been to induce breathlessness by exercise to calibrate the VAS. Other investigators have used verbal descriptions of the sensation, and it is therefore possible that there are differences between the sensations studied in different laboratories. Rating of perceived exertion (Borg and Linderholm, 1970) is now in wide use. Wilson and Jones (1989) found greater reproducibility with the Borg scale but suggested that the VAS might have greater precision and sensitivity. The specificity of the Borg scale for dyspnea depends critically on the instructions given to the subject.

During studies in patients (Stark et al., 1982; Stark and Chatterjee, 1983), the exercise loads were less and the reference point for the VAS was a recurring activity in the patient's daily life known to induce marked breathlessness. Patients generally required more careful explanation of the VAS, and measurement of ventilation was more difficult, especially in those with moderately severe respiratory impairment. Reproducibility was studied in patients with chronic obstructive pulmonary disease or diffuse parenchymal disease (Stark et al., 1982; O'Neill et al., 1986). In general, patients demonstrated a highly reproducible response to the same graded exercise, but a proportion of patients was unable to use the VAS in a meaningful way. The sensitivity of the test was estimated in asthmatic patients during bronchodilatation induced by salbutamol (Stark et al., 1982). Most of the patients indicated lower VAS scores for dyspnea at given levels of ventilation after salbutamol, but others used the VAS inconsistently. The conclusion must be that a proportion of patients, even after careful explanation of the VAS and familiarization with the test, cannot use the VAS reliably. Protocols for clinical studies on mechanisms or treatment of dyspnea should allow for prospective exclusion of such subjects.

On this critical background it has been possible to explore the effects of a range of pharmacological agents and to detect effects that hitherto would have been missed. Two possible patterns of drug effect on dyspnea have been described (Stark and O'Neill, 1983; Stark, 1988), and these are illustrated in Fig. 1. In the first type of response, there are reductions both in ventilation and in breathlessness. Thus, in comparison with placebo, the drug effect shows a retreat down the line of relationship between breathlessness and ventilation. The second type of response consists of a change in this relationship such that breathlessness is reduced but ventilation is unchanged; this represents a more attractive clinical profile. Thus, the line of relationship moves toward the ventilation axis.

As a rough guide, an agent that reduced breathlessness by 20% at a standard level of ventilation during exercise is likely to be of clinical interest. Effects of this size were seen with salbutamol in patients with asthma (Stark et al., 1982) and in healthy subjects with chlorpromazine (O'Neill et al., 1985a).

It has become clear that there are different sensory components in different

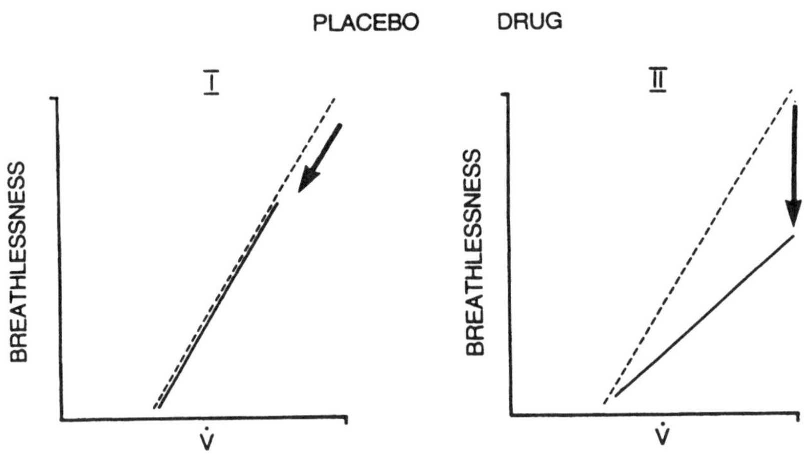

Figure 1 Potential patterns of drug effects on breathlessness. In type I, breathlessness and ventilation both decrease and the line of relationship does not change. In type II, ventilation is unchanged and breathlessness alone decreases. (Reprinted from Stark, 1988.)

patients reporting breathlessness (see Chap. 6). Thus, for example, *difficulty* in breathing in can be distinguished from an *unpleasant urge* to breathe that can be *relieved* by breathing in. It is possible that different pharmacological approaches could be adopted for varying components of what is called breathlessness.

III. Attempts to Modify Dyspnea: Approaches Relating to Respiratory Drives

A. Interest in the Role of the Vagus

The classic studies undertaken in the 1960s and early 1970s on breath holding and hypercapnia examined how various interventions or disease processes affected these particular respiratory sensations. The results are summarized in Tables 1 and 2.

The studies show that normal sensations from breath holding depend on the presence of the vagus nerves and the phrenic nerves. The mechanism may involve activity in vagal sensory nerves reflexly leading to an increase in phrenic nerve activity; the sensation does not appear to arise from vagal activity itself because it is blocked by curare. During exposure to raised levels of carbon dioxide, there

Table 1 Breath Holding: Effects of Neurological Lesions or Interventions

Intervention/ lesion	Breath holding		Conclusions on involvement in breath holding	References
	Duration	Sensation		
Chest wall block	No change	No change	Intercostal muscles: no; sympathetic afferents: no	Noble et al., 1970
C7 transection	No change	No change	Intercostal muscles: no	Noble et al., 1970
Phrenic block	Increased	Decreased	Diaphragm: yes	Noble et al., 1970 Noble et al., 1971
C3 transection	Increased	Decreased	Accessory muscles: no	Noble et al., 1970
Curare	Increased	Decreased	Diaphragmatic contraction: yes	Campbell et al., 1969 Campbell et al., 1967
Vagal block	Increased	Decreased	Vagal afferents: yes	Guz, 1966; Noble et al., 1970

Source: Adapted from Stark and Guz (1984).

Table 2 Hypercapnia: Effects of Interventions or Disease States

Intervention/disease	Respiratory sensation	Ventilatory response	References
Bilateral vagal block	Not detected	Reduced especially frequency	Noble et al., 1970 Guz et al., 1970a
Chest wall block	Detected	Unaffected	Eisele et al., 1968
Phrenic block	Detected	$\dot{V}/CO_2$ relationship moved to left?	Noble et al., 1970
Fixed ventilation after poliomyelitis	Detected? Which sensation?	Not available	Patterson et al., 1962
Fixed ventilation after poliomyelitis and right vagotomy	Not detected	Not available	Noble et al., 1970
Paralysis with D-tubocurarine followed by breath holding to P_{CO_2} of 70 mm Hg	Not detected	Not available	Campbell et al., 1969
C3 transections tracheostomy 1. Breathing spontaneously with accessory muscles	Detected	Not available	Noble et al., 1970
2. Artificially ventilated	Not detected	Not available	Noble et al., 1970

Source: Adapted from Stark and Guz (1984).

appears to be a role for the vagus nerves because blockade of the vagus reduces the sensation and the ventilatory response is reduced as a consequence of a smaller increase in respiratory frequency. Curare is not expected to modify vagal activity but reduced the sensation, suggesting that activity of the respiratory muscles contributes to breathlessness during hypercapnia. This is supported by the reduced sensation in patients who were artificially ventilated. However, the conclusion is challenged by a more recent study that showed that the respiratory sensations during hypercapnia were unaffected by neuromuscular blockade with vecuronium (Banzett et al., 1990).

Overall, such studies on sensations related to dyspnea point to interactions between the vagus and the respiratory muscles in generating the subjective response. It is not surprising, therefore, that there has been some interest over the years on disentangling any role of the vagus in dyspnea.

B. Vagal Block

In patients with severe dyspnea, there may be accompanying rapid shallow breathing and a reduction in breath-holding time. There was keen interest, therefore, to determine the effects of interrupting vagal afferent traffic. The results of blocking the vagus nerves in patients with various diseases, either by local anesthesia or by surgical section, are summarized in Table 3. Generally, the frequency of breathing was reduced and breath holding was prolonged with a reduction in the unpleasant sensation. The more precise methods of assessing dyspnea had not been developed when these studies were performed, but in many cases there was reduction in the sensation of breathlessness; this could be the result of a reduction in vagal drive to breathing.

These findings stimulated a search for other less drastic methods of interfering with afferent nerve activity from the lungs and also led to efforts to distinguish between the various types of pulmonary afferent nerves.

C. Local Anesthetic Aerosols

Local anesthetic agents administered by aerosol, with a particle diameter predominantly in the range 5–20 μm, to patients with various pulmonary disorders, including chronic obstructive airways disease, suppressed cough but did not modify dyspnea (Howard et al., 1977). Similarly, in patients with interstitial lung disease whose oxygen saturations were maintained with supplementary oxygen, inhalation of 5% bupivacaine with a mass median diameter of 4.77 μm did not affect either the pattern of breathing or the perception of breathlessness (Winning et al., 1988). These studies suggest that sensory receptors in the large airways are not major contributors to the generation of dyspnea. The relatively large particles in these aerosols would be expected to have little effect on the unmyelinated vagal afferents that arise in the vicinity of the alveolus and pulmonary capillary. These

Table 3 Effect of Vagal Block or Section (B or S) on Patients with Breathlessness

Diagnosis	Vagal procedure	Breathing frequency	Breath holding		Dyspnea	Reference
			Duration	Sensation		
Pulmonary vascular obstruction	B, S	Decreased	Increased	—	Decreased	Guz et al., 1970b
Left ventricular failure	B	Decreased	—	—	—	Guz et al., 1970b
Rigid chest wall	B	No change	—	—	No change	Guz et al., 1970b
Lymphangitis carcinomatosa	B	Decreased	Increased	Decreased	Decreased	Guz et al., 1970b
Carcinoma bronchus	B, S	Decreased	—	—	—	Guz et al., 1970b
Diffuse pulmonary fibrosis	B, S	No change	Increased	—	No change	Guz et al., 1970b
Sarcoid infiltration	B	No change	No change	Decreased	—	Guz et al., 1970b
Diffuse pulmonary fibrosis	B	Decreased	Increased	—	Decreased	Guz et al., 1970b
Panacinar emphysema	B, S	Decreased	—	—	No change	Guz et al., 1970b
Chronic bronchitis and emphysema	B	No change	Increased	Decreased	No change	Guz et al., 1970b
Chronic bronchitis and emphysema	B	No change	—	—	No change	Guz et al., 1970b
Asthma	B	Decreased	—	—	—	Guz et al., 1970b
Emphysema	S	—	—	—	Decreased	Bradley et al., 1982
Emphysema	S	—	—	—	Decreased	Bradley et al., 1982
Emphysema	S	—	—	—	No change	Bradley et al., 1982
Emphysema	S	—	—	—	Decreased	Bradley et al., 1982
Emphysema	S	—	—	—	Decreased	Bradley et al., 1982

Source: Adapted from Stark and Guz (1984).

are the J receptors described first by Paintal (1969). It is possible that activity of these receptors could explain the beneficial effects of vagal block on dyspnea. This would be consistent with the speculation that J receptors mediate dyspnea in diseases associated with the alveoli or pulmonary circulation (Paintal, 1977).

Testing the J receptor hypothesis involves interrupting the activity of the unmyelinated vagal fibers at their source close to the alveoli of the lung. There is experimental evidence from dogs suggesting that disodium cromoglycate given intravenously reduced the activity of J receptors in response to capsaicin (Dixon et al., 1980). When given by Spinhaler, disodium cromoglycate had no effect on breathlessness in healthy subjects, although this aerosol may not have achieved deposition in the relevant areas (Stark and Gambles, 1981).

Another approach to testing the role of J receptors involves administering local anesthetic by a specially designed aerosol, producing particles small enough for alveolar deposition. Using a modified jet nebulizer, 2% lignocaine solution produced an aerosol with a mass median diameter (MMD) of 1.7 μm (geometric standard deviation, GSD, = 1.2 μm) (Stark et al., 1985). Given to rats made tachypneic by pulmonary microemboli, this aerosol reversed the tachypnea, but a similar quantity of lignocaine given by Wright's nebulizer (MMD 11.2 μm) did not have this effect. Because the tachypnea was probably mediated by pulmonary "C" fibers, these results provided support for the conclusion that the aerosol was achieving deposition at alveolar level in animals. A similar aerosol generator administered 5% lignocaine (MMD 2.5 μm; GSD 1.7 μm) to dyspneic patients with diffuse alveolar disease or chronic airflow obstruction. No dramatic benefit on dyspnea or walking distance was apparent, although the interpretation was hindered by a small reduction in forced expiratory volume in one second (FEV_1) after lignocaine. In addition, given the low mass output of these aerosol generators in relation to the large alveolar surface area and the poor accessibility to areas of the lung with most advanced pathology, there are some concerns on whether sufficient amounts of drug were deposited in the alveoli to achieve a pharmacological effect.

Thus, there are experimental obstacles to assessing the role of J receptors using local anesthetic aerosols in clinical dyspnea. It must be concluded, however, that there is no evidence in support of a major role for them.

D. Benzonatate

This interesting compound provided an alternative, blood-borne approach in efforts to modulate sensory traffic from the lungs.

Benzonatate is a local anesthetic molecule containing a long-chain glycol that possibly assists uptake into nervous tissue. It is an orally active antitussive agent with a duration of action of about 6 h but only moderate performance (Salem and Aviado, 1965; Eddy et al., 1969). Its animal pharmacology is relatively unusual within the local anesthetic class because it is most effective on lung sensory receptors (Bein and Bucher, 1957). This forms the basis for its alleged peripheral mode of action as a cough suppressant.

In one of the clinical studies, Wilson et al. (1958) measured exercise tolerance after a single intramuscular dose and after multiple oral doses of benzonatate (150–200 mg/day) in 30 patients with pulmonary fibrosis or emphysema. In addition to the antitussive effect, exercise tolerance increased and patients reported that they were less dyspneic; the pattern of breathing during exercise suggested higher tidal volumes and lower frequencies. Michelson and Schiller (1957) also reported symptomatic benefit. However, in a randomized, double-blind comparison of benzonatate (100 mg three times per day) and placebo each given for 1 week, Darke et al. (1959) found that 23 patients with chronic pulmonary disease showed no consistent improvement in dyspnea; 6 patients with interstitial pulmonary fibrosis were assessed during exercise, but tolerance was unaffected when receiving benzonatate.

When our attention was drawn to this work (G. M. Lees, personal communication), it seemed appropriate to reinvestigate benzonatate using modern techniques and the more sensitive and precise methods now available for studying breathlessness in humans. We were mindful that there might be opportunities for chemical manipulation of the benzonatate molecule to enhance any therapeutic effect. The findings relating to benzonatate per se have not been published previously.

Animal studies were based principally on models in conscious rats that have been described previously (Stark et al., 1985). Intratracheal instillation of carrageenan produces a pneumonitis characterized by rapid, shallow breathing that is dependent on the integrity of nonmyelinated receptor afferents in the vagus (Trenchard and Guz, 1972). Benzonatate given orally or intravenously was active in this model and caused a reversible, dose-related inhibition of the tachypnea. Intravenous injection of Sephadex G25 microemboli in conscious rats causes an acute tachypnea; previous similar studies in rabbits attributed such tachypnea to activation of pulmonary J receptors (Guz and Trenchard, 1971). Orally administered benzonatate reversed the tachypnea, and when given before embolism, it minimized the subsequent effects. A range of studies including single-fiber neurophysiological recordings supported the hypothesis that benzonatate was acting peripherally and was not causing a general central respiratory depression.

These findings in animals and the earlier clinical reports together provided a strong stimulus for the reassessment of benzonatate in humans.

A group of six healthy volunteers participated in a double-blind, randomized, within-subject comparison of benzonatate and placebo, with each treatment given on two separate occasions. The maximum clinical dose of 200 mg was given by mouth 1 h (three subjects) or 2 h (three subjects) before a standard exercise test.

The severity of the breathlessness was assessed by visual analog scales and was related to the minute ventilation. When the two placebo tests were compared, a high level of reproducibility of the methodology was demonstrated, and this was published previously (Stark et al., 1981; Figs. 1, 2, and 3). Benzonatate, however, did not reduce breathlessness in relation to ventilation during exercise in these subjects.

An alternative model of breathlessness involves exposure to carbon dioxide during rebreathing. A total of six subjects entered a double-blind, randomized, within-subject comparison of single doses of benzonatate (200 mg) and placebo given on two different occasions. The relationship of breathlessness to ventilation was reproducible during the two placebo tests, but no significant effect was detected 1 h after benzonatate. Benzonatate did not alter the ventilatory response to carbon dioxide or breath-holding time.

Finally, the effects of benzonatate were investigated in dyspneic patients. The details on the patients, methods, and validation were published previously (Stark et al., 1982). A group of five patients with chronic bronchitis and FEV_1 values between 0.8 and 2.4 L gave informed consent to participate in a double-blind, randomized, within-subject comparison of benzonatate and placebo. Benzonatate was given at a dose of 100 mg three times daily for 5 days, and placebo was given in a matching way. Exercise was performed 1 h after the first dose of each treatment and 1 h after the final dose. The relationship of dyspnea score to ventilation was reproducible in these patients but was unaltered by benzonatate either as a single dose or after 5 days of treatment. Diary cards completed daily during the study confirmed the lack of effect on dyspnea.

In conclusion, the excitement provoked by the animal studies on this agent was not supported by studies in healthy subjects or in patients. The validity of the methods used was such that any effect of clinical significance should have been detectable. The difficulty of establishing predictive animal models of dyspnea is also emphasized. However, it must be stated that studies have not yet been done on the human analogs of animal models described earlier, for example patients dyspneic with pneumonia, pulmonary embolism, or lung collapse in whom abnormal vagal afferent traffic is likely to be present.

E. Drugs Affecting Prostanoids

The presence of prostanoids in the inflammatory process raises the possibility that they might have effects at a peripheral site of origin for the sensation of dyspnea. In preliminary work on normal subjects, indomethacin, a widely used inhibitor of cyclooxygenase, was given at an oral dose of 50 mg and its effects on exercise were compared with placebo on a double-blind, within-subject basis (O'Neill et al., 1985b). Minute ventilation and the pattern of breathing were not significantly affected by indomethacin, but breathlessness in relation to ventilation was significantly reduced (Fig. 2). The size of the change was not large but seemed to indicate a possible role for prostanoids in normal subjects.

The critical study was in patients likely to have active inflammation present in the lung. It was expected that the role of prostanoids would be exaggerated in this situation. In a double-blind randomized study, the effects of acute and chronic administration of indomethacin were compared with placebo in breathless patients with diffuse parenchymal disease of the lung (O'Neill et al., 1986). Indomethacin had no effect on the relationship of breathlessness to ventilation or on the distance walked in 6 minutes.

This discrepancy between the findings in normal subjects and in patients is of interest. The occurrence of hypoxia during exercise in patients was considered but did not explain the findings. The VAS is probably a less sensitive test in patients than in young, healthy subjects, but the absence of effect on the walking distance provides further evidence that indomethacin lacked an effect in patients.

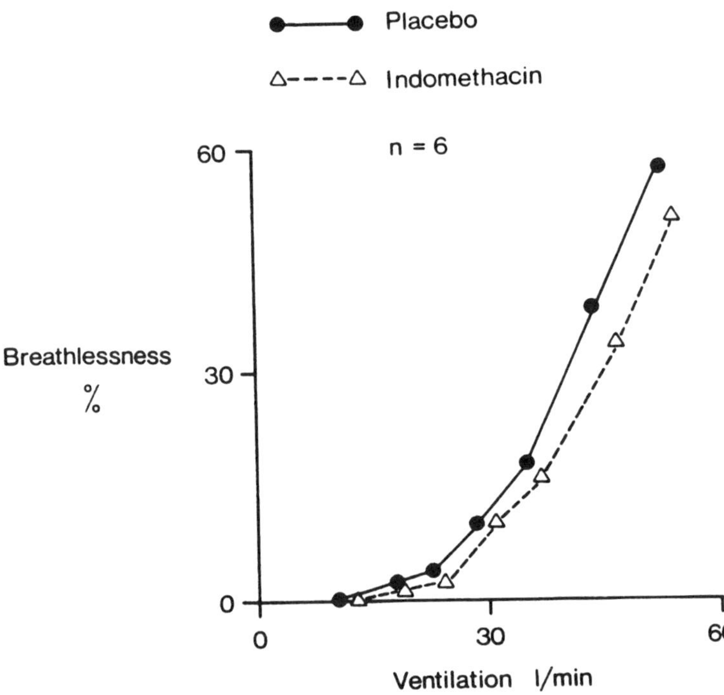

Figure 2 Mean relationship of breathlessness to ventilation during exercise after placebo and after indomethacin in healthy subjects. (Adapted from O'Neill et al., 1985b.)

More recently, normal subjects have been exposed to prostaglandin E_2 inhaled from a Bird nebulizer (Taguchi et al., 1992). Airways resistance and lung volume were unchanged, but during exercise, breathlessness in relation to ventilation increased. This finding with exogenous prostaglandin E_2 increasing breathlessness is compatible with the earlier reported effect of indomethacin decreasing breathlessness in normal subjects (O'Neill et al., 1985b).

F. Pulmonary Denervation

Heart-lung transplant results in complete pulmonary denervation and yields another opportunity to assess neurogenic mechanisms. In the study of Kimoff et al. (1990), four transplant recipients were compared with healthy age-matched controls. Some differences in the ventilatory response to exercise were detected. However, the transplant recipients became breathless during exercise and the relationship of breathlessness to ventilation did not appear to be disturbed. Such findings do not indicate a significant role for pulmonary afferents in the perception of dyspnea during exercise in these patients. We hope that future investigators will report whether pulmonary denervation affects the dyspnea associated with pulmonary pathologies, such as pneumonia or pulmonary embolism, in which abnormal vagal afferent activity is likely to occur.

G. Hypoxia and the Carotid Bodies

Hypoxia has been shown to induce breathlessness in normal subjects (Guz et al., 1981; Adams et al., 1982). During exercise, exposure to an hypoxic gas mixture induced an increase in breathlessness even before there was a change in ventilation (Chronos et al., 1988). Such findings led to the suggestion that hypoxia is a "dyspnogen." Because the ventilatory response to hypoxia is mediated by the carotid bodies, the response to resection of this apparatus is of some interest. There is an extensive literature on the subject, but two more recent papers are of particular interest.

Vermeire et al. (1988) followed 27 patients who had undergone bilateral carotid body resection for dyspnea associated with advanced chronic obstructive pulmonary disease (COPD). In the following 5 years, 12 of the patients died, 10 from respiratory failure; this is in accord with the expected mortality. Of the patients who were still alive, 11 were assessed. Arterial oxygen and carbon dioxide pressures (P_aO_2 and P_aCO_2 were not significantly different from the preoperative values, and patients reported continuing relief of their dyspnea.

Another picture was presented by Stulbarg and Winn (1989), who monitored three patients with COPD after bilateral carotid body resection. FEV_1 was unchanged after surgery, but the arterial blood gas tensions showed deterioration. Ventilation was reduced and was accompanied by relief of dyspnea that persisted until death, which occurred 3–36 months after resection.

Although these studies suggest that dyspnea may benefit from bilateral carotid body resection, the place of this controversial intervention remains uncertain.

The effects of oxygen have received particular attention. In a study of patients with COPD at rest, supplemental oxygen by nasal cannulae increased P_aO_2 and reduced dyspnea, although the effect was not different from that found with air used as a control (Liss and Grant, 1988). During exercise, the provision of oxygen enrichment reduced breathlessness and increased effort tolerance in "pink puffers" (Woodcock et al., 1981a). Others have shown that oxygen produced more rapid recovery from exercise in a majority of patients with COPD (Evans et al., 1986). On this basis, there seems to be a place for bursts of oxygen to assist exercise in certain patients with COPD; suitable candidates can be identified by exercise testing (Strom et al., 1991). In a recent study, Bruera et al. (1993) reported a beneficial effect of oxygen in hypoxemic patients with terminal cancer.

IV. Attempts to Modify Dyspnea: Approaches Relating to Central Mechanisms

A. Opioids

Much of the interest in opioids in dyspnea stemmed from the well-known benefits of such agents as morphine in left ventricular failure. There are several possible modes of action in this situation, none of which has been definitively established.

Knowledge has advanced rapidly in the last 10 years. Some investigators have studied the milder opioids; others have taken the brave step of examining strong opioids in severe dyspnea.

Codeine at a single oral dose of 60 mg was assessed in healthy subjects. Only small effects occurred, but both breathlessness and ventilation during exercise decreased significantly (Stark et al., 1983). Such changes were consistent with the type I profile (Fig. 1). Codeine did not prevent detection of an inspiratory resistance but permitted higher levels of carbon dioxide to be tolerated during breath holding.

Woodcock et al. (1981c) studied dihydrocodeine in patients with the pink puffer syndrome, and although they did not present the results in the form of breathlessness-ventilation plots, it appears that proportionally breathlessness was more affected than ventilation. Such findings suggest a type II effect (Fig. 1), in contrast to the effects of codeine.

To clarify this issue, future studies of opioids should include presentation of the data in terms of the relationship of breathlessness to ventilation. However, the difficulties in measuring ventilation in patients with respiratory impairment are recognized.

Dextromethorphan is an antitussive agent without analgesic properties that has structural similarities to codeine. In a single-blind, nonrandomized study, a 60 mg oral dose of dextromethorphan was compared with placebo in patients with chronic obstructive pulmonary disease (Giron et al., 1991). The maximal exercise, the breathing pattern, and the breathlessness at a given level of ventilation were all unchanged by dextromethorphan.

Several uncontrolled studies showed that morphine given by intravenous infusion (Cohen et al., 1991) or subcutaneously (Bruera et al., 1990) can provide relief of dyspnea in patients with terminal cancer. After intravenous infusion of morphine, P_aCO_2 increased steadily and most of the patients died during treatment; after subcutaneous morphine, respiratory function was maintained. In patients given naloxone, dyspnea and anxiety returned rapidly (Cohen et al., 1991).

Convincing evidence on the antidyspneic effect of morphine comes from a randomized, single-blind study in patients with stable, eucapnic COPD who were assessed during exercise (Light et al., 1989). Morphine was given as an oral solution at the relatively high dose of 0.8 mg/kg, which induced changes in mental function. The workload and oxygen consumption increased by about 20% after morphine, although two of the patients became hypotensive after exercise. At comparable levels of oxygen uptake, ventilation and dyspnea were both significantly lower on morphine compared with placebo. Unfortunately, the data are not presented as a plot of breathlessness against ventilation or oxygen uptake, which would have permitted characterization of the response.

Eiser et al. (1991) assessed diamorphine (diacetylmorphine) on exercise tolerance and dyspnea in pink puffers, with considerable attention to study design and the assessments. Diamorphine had no significant effect on exercise tolerance or on dyspnea, but this probably related to the low dose of diamorphine (2.5–7.5 mg) and the low or absent plasma levels in many of the patients.

Nebulized morphine, providing a mean inhaled dose of about 0.6 mg, was compared with placebo in a double-blind, randomized, crossover study in patients with severe chronic lung disease (Young et al., 1989). Side effects did not occur, and exercise tolerance increased significantly. Dyspnea was not formally assessed in the study, but the authors speculate that, because ventilation was unchanged, a type II response was occurring. Support for this finding in a patient with cancer has been supplied by Tooms et al. (1993), although Beauford et al. (1993) failed to confirm an effect in COPD. Such an interesting profile is obviously worthy of further investigation; the relationship of dyspnea to ventilation should receive particular attention. Sedation is unlikely to be a complicating factor when opioids are given at low doses by inhalation.

Finally, a hint of the possible role of endogenous opioids comes from comparing the effects of naloxone and placebo on methacholine-induced bronchoconstriction (Bellofiore et al., 1990). After naloxone, the breathing frequency and the sensation of dyspnea were significantly greater. These findings suggest a modulating effect from endogenous opioids on respiratory sensations and provide further encouragement that the opioid approach to dyspnea could be fruitful.

B. Phenothiazines

A small and statistically significant reduction in dyspnea occurred after promethazine in pink puffers (Woodcock et al., 1981b), but no significant effects could be demonstrated in healthy subjects (O'Neill et al., 1985a).

Efforts were made to look more closely at the components of the pharmacological activity of promethazine by comparing mebhydroline, a specific H_1 receptor antagonist with minimal sedative properties, and chlorpromazine, the arche-

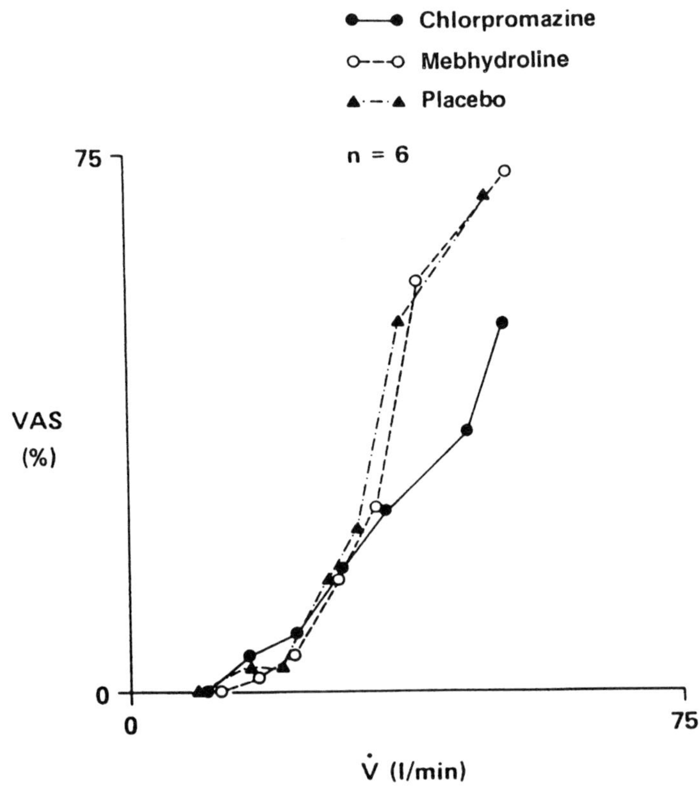

Figure 3 Mean relationships between breathlessness (VAS) and ventilation (V̇) for 6 healthy subjects after placebo, mebhydroline, or chlorpromazine. (Reprinted from O'Neill et al., 1985a.)

typal phenothiazine (O'Neill et al., 1985a). The level of sedation after either agent was not significantly different from that after administration of placebo.

Mebhydroline was without effect, but chlorpromazine depressed the relationship between breathlessness and ventilation (type II; Fig. 3). The mean reduction in breathlessness at the standardized ventilation was almost 20%, and this was achieved without measurable sedation.

Chlorpromazine at a dose of 25 mg together with 10 mg morphine was administered to patients with advanced cancer who had severe dyspnea unaccompanied by pain (Ventafridda et al., 1990). The uncontrolled observations suggested beneficial effects on the dyspnea. The authors question whether a controlled study of each agent and the combination should be undertaken. Clearly, understanding of the contributions made by each of these agents would provide an invaluable basis for any future therapy.

C. Diazepam

Although there were claims that chronic administration of diazepam at doses of about 25 mg/day reduced dyspnea in pink puffers (Mitchell-Heggs et al., 1980), the findings were not confirmed in a later study (Woodcock et al., 1981b). In both studies, drowsiness occurred at the doses used. In normal subjects diazepam did not change breathlessness during exercise or hypercapnia and breath holding was unaffected (Stark et al., 1981).

Clinical experience suggests that breathlessness at rest may improve when patients are drowsy. The ideal treatment should minimize breathlessness without inducing drowsiness. Studies targeted at the treatment of dyspnea should therefore include formal assessment of sedation and related sensations (Stark et al., 1981; O'Neill et al., 1985a).

V. Attempts to Modify Dyspnea: Approaches Relating to Respiratory Muscles

There are many indications that the respiratory muscles play a key role in generating dyspnea and also the sensations associated with breath holding and hypercapnia referred to earlier in this review. There have been few pharmacological studies directed at the respiratory muscles, but this may change in the coming years.

One area of activity concerns the possible effects of theophylline on respiratory muscle strength. Jaeschke et al. (1991) studied patients with chronic airways obstruction given inhaled salbutamol, oral theophylline, or placebo alone or in combination. Correlations between changes in FEV_1, maximum inspiratory pressure (as a measure of respiratory muscle strength), and dyspnea were examined. The authors infer that aminophylline has greater effect on dyspnea than can be accounted for by bronchodilatation and suggest that this might be caused by a beneficial effect on respiratory muscle strength. Murciano et al. (1989) found that chronic administration of theophylline in patients with severe COPD improved pulmonary function, improved respiratory muscle performance by 29%, and reduced dyspnea. They too suggested that the effects on muscle strength may have contributed to the reduction in dyspnea. Opportunities exist for further exploration of this interesting area.

Myotonic dystrophy may affect the inspiratory muscles and cause dyspnea. In a patient with dyspnea and tachypnea but without respiratory failure, procainamide, a recognized treatment for myotonia, reduced diaphragmatic relaxation time and abolished the tachypnea and dyspnea (Fitting and Leuenberger, 1989).

Finally, it is worth recording that progressive muscular relaxation can reduce dyspnea and anxiety in patients with COPD (Renfroe, 1988).

VI. Conclusions

The new phase of research on dyspnea probably started at the Symposium of the European Society for Clinical Respiratory Physiology on breathlessness held in Sheffield in 1980. Since then, momentum has gathered and interest has become more international with the result that dyspnea is now one of the very active areas of pulmonary research. Here, personal views are presented on what has been achieved in the last 15 years.

In the early stages, considerable effort was expended in justifying dyspnea as a therapeutic target. Was it clinically acceptable to treat a symptom? Those working with the terminally ill have brought into focus the dire distress of the dyspnea death. For the multitude of patients with dyspnea related to cardiorespiratory disease, there is the chronic impairment of quality of life. To a large extent, the days of doubt have now passed.

Dyspnea research in the 1960s and 1970s contributed knowledge of potential mechanisms. One tool remained crude during these years, and this was the instrument for assessing the sensation. By the early 1980s, greater precision was on offer and the lesson was quickly learned that subjective methodology had to be handled with care. It is notable how much of the literature has concentrated on the validity of the measurements. Similarly, uncontrolled observations are being replaced with meticulous experimental design involving randomized, double-blind comparisons of treatments. There has been a steady move from study of normal subjects to those who have dyspnea as a result of disease and in whom the relevant mechanisms operate.

For the purposes of this review, the pharmacological approaches have been grouped into three areas. The relative interest in each of these and the therapeutic promise may be showing evolution.

The early studies stimulated interest in the role of the vagus and other respiratory drives. The relative accessibility of the pulmonary afferents was attractive to those considering possible pharmaceutical interventions. The vagus has been tackled from several angles: aerosols of local anesthetic, blood-borne local anesthetic, and pulmonary denervation. Notwithstanding the difficulties in performing definitive studies in humans, especially patients, an adequate mechanistic basis for therapy has not been established. The vagal approach to treating dyspnea is probably untenable.

Early reluctance to evaluate opioids in dyspnea has now been overcome, and there is evidence that systemic administration of morphine may have symptomatic benefit. What is less clear is how this benefit relates to changes in ventilation and the pattern of breathing. If preliminary findings with small doses of morphine by inhalation are confirmed, the door could open to a variety of options, possibly including agents effective on particular receptor subtypes. It is expected that the next decade will see whether effective therapeutic regimens can be developed. The role of phenothiazines in the treatment of dyspnea has been enigmatic for almost 15 years and surely requires urgent resolution.

The ultimate solution to dyspnea, however, may lie with the respiratory muscles and their central connections. Here, pharmacological intervention is in its infancy and real opportunities may occur only when there is fuller understanding of the basic physiology.

We conclude that much has been achieved. It is hard to believe that the worldwide commitment to understanding dyspnea will not bring the therapeutic advances that are keenly awaited.

Acknowledgment

We gratefully acknowledge the help of Ms. Kathryn Beard in preparing the manuscript.

References

Adams, L., Chronos, N., and Guz, A. (1982). Breathlessness during different ventilatory drives in normal subjects. J Physiol. (Lond.) 324:33P.

Banzett, R.B., Lansing, R.W., Brown, R., Topulos, G.P., Yager, D., Steele, S.M., Londono, B., Loring, S.H., Reid, M.B., Adams, L., and Nations, C.S. (1990). "Air hunger" from increased P_{CO_2} persists after complete neuromuscular block in humans. Respir. Physiol. 81:1–18.

Beauford, W., Saylor, T.T., Stansbury, D.W., Avalos, K., and Light, R.W. (1993). Effects of nebulised morphine sulfate on the exercise tolerance of the ventilatory limited COPD patient. Chest 104:175–178.

Bein, H.J., and Bucher, K. (1957). Anasthetische Wirkung an Lungendehnungsrezeptoren und anderen nervosen Substraten. Helv. Physiol. Acta 15:55–62.

Bellofiore, S., Di Maria, G.U., Privitera, S., Sapienza, S., Milic-Emili, J., and Mistretta, A. (1990). Endogenous opioids modulate the increase in ventilatory output and dyspnea during severe acute bronchoconstriction. Am. Rev. Respir. Dis. 142:812–186.

Borg, G., and Linderholm, H. (1970). Exercise performance and perceived exertion in patients with coronary insufficiency, arterial hypertension and vasoregulatory aesthenia. Acta Med. Scand. 187:17–26.

Bradley, G.W., Hale, T., Pimble, J., Rowlandson, R., and Noble, M.I.M. (1982). Effect of vagotomy on the breathing pattern and exercise ability in emphysematous patients. Clin. Sci. 62:311–319.

Bruera, E., MacMillan, K., Pither, J, and MacDonald, R.N. (1990). Effects of morphine on the dyspnea of terminal cancer patients. J. Pain Symptom Manage. 5:341–344.

Bruera, E. de Stoutz, N., Velasco-Leiva, A., Schoeller, T., and Hanson, J. (1993). Effects of oxygen on dyspnea in hypoxaemic terminal-cancer patients. Lancet 342:13–14.

Campbell, E.J.M., Freedman, S., Clark, T.J.H., Robson, J.G., and Norman, J. (1967). The effect of muscular paralysis induced by tubocurarine on the duration and sensation of breath-holding. Clin. Sci. 32:425–432.

Campbell, E.J.M., Godfrey, S., Clark, T.J.H., Freedman, S., and Norman, J. (1969). The effect of muscular paralysis induced by tubocurarine on the duration and sensation of breath-holding during hypercapnia. Clin. Sci. 36:323–328.

Chronos, N. Adams, L., and Guz, A. (1988). Effect of hyperoxia and hypoxia on exercise-induced breathlessness in normal subjects. Clin. Sci. 74:531–537.

Cohen, M.H., Anderson, A.J., Krasnow, S.H., Spagnolo, S.V., Citron, M.L., Payne, M., and Fossieck, B.E. (1991). Continuous intravenous infusion of morphine for severe dyspnea. South. Med. J. 84:229–234.

Darke, C.S., Snowden, B.A., Verel, D., Daly, J.J., and Layland, W.R. (1959). Action of "Tessalon" on the dyspnoea of patients with chronic lung disease. BMJ 1:622–624.

Dixon, M., Jackson, D.M., and Richards, I.M. (1980). The action of sodium cromoglycate on "C" fibre endings in the dog lung. Br. J. Pharmacol. 70:11–13.

Eddy, N.B., Friebel, H., Hahn, K.J., and Halbach, H. (1969). Codeine and its alternates for pain and cough relief. Bull. World Health Organ. 40:639–719.

Eisele, J., Trenchard, D., Burki, N., and Guz, A. (1968). The effect of chest wall block on respiratory sensation and control in man. Clin. Sci. 35:23–33.

Eiser, N., Denman, W.T., West, C., and Luce, P. (1991). Oral diamorphine: lack of effect on dyspnoea and exercise tolerance in the "pink puffer" syndrome. Eur. Respir. J. 4:926–931.

Evans, T.W., Waterhouse, J.C., Carter, A., Nicholl, J.F., and Howard, P. (1986). Short burst oxygen treatment for breathlessness in chronic obstructive airways disease. Thorax 41:611–615.

Fainsinger, R., MacEachem, T., Hanson, J., Miller, M.J., and Bruera, E. (1991). Symptom control during the last week of life on a palliative care unit. J. Palliative Care 7:5–11.

Fitting, J.W., and Leuenberger, P. (1989). Procainamide for dyspnea in myotonic dystrophy. Am. Rev. Respir. Dis. 140:1442–1445.

Giron, A.E., Stansbury, D.W., Fischer, C.E., and Light, R.W. (1991). Lack of effect of dextromethorphan on breathlessness and exercise performance in patients with chronic obstructive pulmonary disease (COPD). Eur. Respir. J. 4:532–535.

Guz, A. (1966). Effects of blocking the vagus nerves in man. In: Breathlessness. Edited by J.B.L. Howell and E.J.M. Campbell. Blackwell, Oxford, pp. 65–71.

Guz, A., and Trenchard, D. (1971). The role of the non-myelinated vagal afferent fibres from the lungs in the genesis of tachypnoea in the rabbit. J. Physiol. (Lond.) 213:345–371.

Guz, A., Noble, M.I.M., Eisele, J.H., and Trenchard, D. (1970a). The role of vagal inflation reflexes in man and other animals. In: Breathing, Hering-Breuer Centenary Symposium. Edited by R. Porter. Churchill, London, pp. 17–40.

Guz, A., Noble, M.I.M., Eisele, J.H., and Trenchard, D. (1970b). Experimental results of vagal block in cardiopulmonary disease. In: Breathing, Hering-Breuer Centenary Symposium. Edited by R. Porter. Churchill, London, pp. 315–329.

Guz, A., Adams, L., Minty, K., and Murphy, K. (1981). Breathlessness and the ventilatory drives of exercise, hypercapnoea and hypoxia. Clin. Sci. 60:17–18P.

Higginson, I., and McCarthy, M. (1989). Measuring symptoms in terminal cancer: are pain and dyspnoea controlled? J. R. Soc. Med. 82:264–267.

Howard, P., Cayton, R.M., Brennan, S.R., and Anderson, P.B. (1977). Lignocaine aerosol and persistent cough. Br. J. Dis. Chest 71:19–24.

Jaeschke, R., Guyatt, G.H., Singer, J., Keller, J., and Newhouse, M.T. (1991). Mechanism of bronchodilator effect in chronic airflow limitation. Can. Med. Assoc. J. 144:35–39.

Kimoff, R.J., Cheong, T.H., Cosio, M.G., Guerraty, A., and Levy, R.D. (1990). Pulmonary denervation in humans. Am. Rev. Respir. Dis. 142:1034–1040.

Light, R.W., Muro, J.R., Sato, R.I., Stansbury, D.W., Fischer, C.E., and Brown, S.E. (1989). Effects of oral morphine on breathlessness and exercise tolerance in patients with chronic obstructive pulmonary disease. Am. Rev. Respir. Dis. 139:126–133.

Liss, H.P., and Grant, B.J.B. (1988). The effect of nasal flow on breathlessness in patients with chronic obstructive pulmonary disease. Am. Rev. Respir. Dis. 137:1285–1288.

Michelson, A.L., and Schiller, I.W. (1957). The effect of methoxypoly(ethyleneoxy)ethyl *p*-butylaminobenzoate (Tessalon) on ventilation and lung volumes. J. Allergy 28:514–518.

Mitchell-Heggs, P., Murphy, K., Minty, K., Guz, A., Patterson, S.C., Minty, P.S.B., and Rosser, R.M. (1980). Diazepam in the treatment of dyspnoea in the "pink puffer" syndrome. Q. J. Med. New Series 49:9–20.

Morton, P.B., O'Neill, P.A., Stark, R.D., and Stretton, T.B. (1983). A demonstration of methods for studying breathlessness. J. Physiol. (Lond.) 342:8–9P.

Murciano, D., Auclair, M.H., Pariente, R., and Aubier, M. (1989). A randomized, controlled trial of theophylline in patients with severe chronic obstructive pulmonary disease. N. Engl. J. Med. 320:1521–1525.

Noble, M.I.M., Eisele, J.H., Trenchard, D., Guz, A. (1970). Effect of selective peripheral nerve blocks on respiratory sensations. In: Breathing, Hering-Breuer Centenary Symposium. Edited by R. Porter. Churchill, London, pp. 233–246.

Noble, M.I.M., Eisele, J.H., Frankel, H.L., Else, W., and Guz, A. (1971). The role of the diaphragm in the sensation of holding the breath. Clin. Sci. 41:275–283.

O'Neill, P.A., Morton, P.B., Sharman, P., Marlow, H.F., and Stark, R.D. (1984). The effects of ICI 118,587 and atenolol on the responses to exercise and on breathlessness in healthy subjects. Br. J. Clin. Pharmacol. 17:37–41.

O'Neill, P.A., Morton, P.B., and Stark, R.D. (1985a). Chlorpromazine—a specific effect on breathlessness? Br. J. Clin. Pharmacol. 19:793–797.

O'Neill, P.A., Stark, R.D., and Morton, P.B. (1985b). Do prostaglandins have a role in breathlessness? Am. Rev. Respir. Dis. 132:22–24.

O'Neill, P.A., Stretton, T.B., Stark, R.D., and Ellis, S.H. (1986). The effect of indomethacin on breathlessness in patients with diffuse parenchymal disease of the lung. Br. J. Dis. Chest 80:72–79.

Paintal, A.C. (1969). Mechanisms of stimulation of type J pulmonary receptors. J. Physiol. (Lond.) 203:511–532.

Paintal, A.C. (1977). Thoracic receptors connected with sensation. Br. Med. Bull. 33: 169–174.

Patterson, J.L., Mullinax, P.F., Bain, T., Kreuger, J.J., and Richardson, D.W. (1962). Carbon dioxide-induced dyspnea in a patient with respiratory muscle paralysis. Am. J. Med. 32:811–816.

Renfroe, K.L. (1988). Effect of progressive relaxation on dyspnea and state of anxiety in patients with chronic obstructive pulmonary disease. Heart Lung 17:408–413.

Salem, H., and Aviado, D.M. (1965). Antitussive agents, local anesthetics. Int. Encyclop. Pharmacol. Ther. 3:635–645.

Stark, R.D. (1988). Dyspnoea: assessment and pharmacological manipulation. Eur. Respir. J. 1:280–287.

Stark, R.D., and Chatterjee, S.S. (1983). A new exercise test for clinical dyspnea. Pract. Cardiol. 9:86–95.

Stark, R.D., and Gambles, S.A. (1980). A new system for assessing the effects of drugs on breathlessness. J. Clin. Respir. Physiol. 16:244P.

Stark, R.D., and Gambles, S.A. (1981). Effects of salbutamol, ipratropium bromide and disodium cromoglycate on breathlessness induced by exercise in normal subjects. Br. J. Clin. Pharmacol. 12:497–501.

Stark, R.D., and Guz, A. (1984). Dyspnoea—symptoms—a continuing monograph series. Edited by J. Conway. Pharmaceuticals Division of ICI, Cheshire, UK.

Stark, R.D., and O'Neill, P.A. (1983). Dihydrocodeine for breathlessness in "pink puffers." Br. Med. J. 286:1280–1281.

Stark, R.D., Gambles, S.A., and Lewis, J.A. (1981). Methods to assess breathlessness in healthy subjects: a critical evaluation and application to analyse the acute effects of diazepam and promethazine on breathlessness induced by exercise or by exposure to raised levels of carbon dioxide. Clin. Sci. 61:429–439.

Stark, R.D., Gambles, S.A., and Chatterjee, S.S. (1982). An exercise test to assess clinical dyspnoea; estimation of reproducibility and sensitivity. Br. J. Dis. Chest 76:269–278.

Stark, R.D., Morton, P.B., Sharman, P., Percival, P.G., and Lewis, J.A. (1983). Effects of codeine on the respiratory responses to exercise in healthy subjects. Br. J. Clin. Pharmacol. 15:355–359.

Stark, R.D., O'Neill, P.A., Russell, N.J.W., Heapy, C.G., and Stretton, T.B. (1985). Effects of small-particle aerosols of local anaesthetic on dyspnoea in patients with respiratory disease. Clin. Sci. 69:29–36.

Strom, K., Boe, J., Boman, G., and Skoogh, B.E. (1991). Expectations of benefit from long-term oxygen therapy. Eur. Respir. Rev. 1:541–549.

Stulbarg, M.S., and Winn, W.R. (1989). Bilateral carotid body resection for the relief of dyspnea in severe chronic obstructive pulmonary disease. Chest 95:1123–1128.

Taguchi, O., Kikuchi, Y., Hida, W., Iwase, N., Okabe, S., Chonan, T., and Takishima, T. (1992). Prostaglandin E_2 inhalation increases the sensation of dyspnea during exercise. Am. Rev. Respir. Dis. 145:1346–1349.

Tooms, A., McKenzie, A., and Grey, H. (1993). Nebulized morphine (letter). Lancet 342:1123–1124.

Trenchard, D., and Guz, A. (1972). The role of pulmonary vagal afferent nerve fibres in the development of rapid shallow breathing in lung inflammation. Clin. Sci. 42: 231–263.

Ventafridda, V., Spoldi, E., and Conno, F.D. (1990). Control of dyspnea in advanced cancer patients. Chest 98:1544–1545.

Vermeire, P., De Backer, W., Van Maele, R., Bal, J., and Van Kerckhoven, W. (1988). Bilateral carotid body resection for severe chronic airway obstruction: a 6 year follow-up. Am. Rev. Respir. Dis. (Suppl.) 137:443.

Wilson, R.C., and Jones, P.W. (1989). A comparison of the visual analogue scale and modified Borg scale for the measurement of dyspnoea during exercise. Clin. Sci. 76:277–282.

Wilson, R.H.L., Farber, S.M., and Mandel, W. (1958). A new agent of therapeutic value in pulmonary insufficiency and irritative cough. Antibiot. Med. 5:567–572.

Winning, A.J., Hamilton, R.D., and Guz, A. (1988). Ventilation and breathlessness on maximal exercise in patients with interstitial lung disease after local anaesthetic aerosol inhalation. Clin. Sci. 74:275–281.

Woodcock, A.A., Gross, E.R., and Geddes, D.M. (1981a). Oxygen relieves breathlessness in "pink puffers." Lancet 1:907–909.

Woodcock, A.A., Gross, E.R., and Geddes, D.M. (1981b). Drug treatment of breathlessness: contrasting effects of diazepam and promethazine in "pink puffers." BMJ 283:343–346.

Woodcock, A.A., Gross, E.R., Gellert, A., Shah, S., Johnson, M., and Geddes, D.M. (1981c). Effects of dihydrocodeine, alcohol, and caffeine on breathlessness and exercise tolerance in patients with chronic obstructive lung disease and normal blood gases. N. Engl. J. Med. 305:1611–1616.

Young, I.H., Daviskas, E., and Keena, V.A. (1989). Effect of low dose nebulised morphine on exercise endurance in patients with chronic lung disease. Thorax 44:387–390.

15

Management of the Breathless Patient

ANNE COCKCROFT

Royal Free Hampstead NHS Trust
and Royal Free Hospital School of Medicine
London, England

ANGELA HESLOP

Charing Cross Hospital
London, England

I. Introduction

Severe breathlessness is frightening for both patients and carers, including health care professionals. Persistent breathlessness can dominate all other aspects of life. This chapter is concerned with the clinical management of the breathless patient in the broadest sense; it is particularly concerned with the management of those patients in whom the underlying condition responsible for breathlessness is not fully treatable, so that management of the symptom itself and life around the symptom becomes a priority. It differs from other chapters in this volume in that it makes relatively little reference to published work on physiological mechanisms; it is based on the combined experience of the two authors in working with breathless patients in the hospital and home setting and helping them to manage their lives despite breathlessness.

Improved understanding of the pathophysiology of breathlessness may eventually lead to specific, effective treatments of these distressing symptoms. This is some way off, but proper application of the knowledge we already have can help to reduce the distress of acute breathlessness and improve the quality of life for patients with chronic breathlessness. Good management requires cooperation between different health care professionals, other caregivers, and the patients themselves. Many aspects must be considered: home and hospital care, acute exacerbations and everyday limitations, physical and psychological aspects, planning for improvement, and preparing for dying. Not all these areas are relevant to all breathless patients: the needs of a young asthmatic are different from those of any elderly person with severe irreversible airways obstruction or intractable heart failure, but for all breathless patients it is important to make an assessment and to plan management of the symptom, not merely the underlying condition, and to go beyond the immediate situation to plan for the future with the patient. Above all, it is important to respond to the differing needs of patients as individuals, so that there can be no set formula to be applied in all cases.

II. Assessment of the Patient

Proper management is based on a full assessment of the patient's condition, both acute and long term. Our experience in looking after breathless patients suggests that this assessment must include psychological and social aspects, as well as the more familiar physical assessment. This is now thought to be true for many conditions but is especially relevant for patients suffering breathlessness, which is a profoundly disturbing symptom with implications for all areas of a patient's life.

A. Physical Assessment

Differential Diagnosis of Underlying Condition

Breathlessness is a prominent symptom in a variety of physical conditions. The differential diagnosis of acute and chronic breathlessness is quite broad (Cockcroft, 1993) and is not reiterated here. It is important to reach a diagnosis because the nature of the underlying condition and, in particular, its likely prognosis in response to treatment will make a great difference to the management appropriate for the symptom of breathlessness. If the condition is likely to be short-lived and non-recurring, such as an episode of bacterial pneumonia in a healthy young adult, then all that is needed is an explanation, some action to reduce the symptom acutely (usually providing oxygen via mask or nasal cannulae), and reassurance that it will rapidly diminish as the pneumonia resolves. In other conditions, breathlessness, although usually responding to immediate treatment, is likely to recur, for example in asthma or in ischemic heart disease with episodes of left ventricular failure. Some advance planning of how to deal with the recurrent symptom is necessary in these conditions. The conditions that pose the greatest challenge for managing breathlessness are those that are chronic and respond poorly to treatment, with a progressive deterioration likely. These include chronic obstructive airways disease, cryptogenic fibrosing alveolitis, various types of industrial pneumonoconiosis, end-stage heart failure, and primary or secondary malignant lung tumors. Thus the planning of management of breathlessness in a particular patient must begin with a thorough understanding of the nature and prognosis of the underlying condition.

Assessment of Severity of Breathlessness

Having established, as far as possible, the details of the underlying condition, the next task is to assess the severity of the symptom of breathlessness in the patient. The quantification of breathlessness can be undertaken at a number of levels (Cockcroft et al., 1989). In managing individual patients, the need is usually to assess breathlessness in the clinical interview and examination. It is surprising how many medical students and doctors still describe breathlessness as part of the examination of the patient, rather than the history, as if it were a clinical sign rather than a symptom. The only way to measure a patient's breathlessness is to ask him or her about it in some way. There are a number of questions that can be included in a clinical interview to solicit useful information about a patient's breathlessness. Some of these are listed in Table 1. Comparisons between patients for level of breathlessness are very difficult to make and not particularly helpful to management of each individual. Comparisons of the symptom over time or in response to treatment in an individual are very important, however, and can be achieved provided the same questions are asked of the individual on different occasions.

The response that patients give to questions about breathlessness may be complicated by their use of language to describe their sensations. Normal subjects may use different descriptors for breathlessness induced by different means (Simon et al., 1989). Among patients with chronic breathlessness, there is evidence of variation in the terms chosen to describe the sensation, with some grouping by underlying diagnosis; the descriptors chosen by individual patients are quite repeatable (Elliott et al., 1991).

Many methods described for quantifying breathlessness, either by standardized questionnaire or by exercise testing, are essentially measures of exercise tolerance, which assume a more or less similar level of the symptom of breathlessness limiting the exercise. The level of breathlessness that limits exercise may actually vary both between and within patients, but level of exercise tolerance is nevertheless an important aspect to assess in breathless patients because it is likely to determine much of the handicap they experience in everyday life. Standardized questionnaires, such as the Medical Research Council respiratory symptoms questionnaire (Medical Research Council, 1986), have the disadvantage that the grades of breathlessness are too broad to reflect small but useful changes in exercise tolerance. Direct measurement of exercise tolerance by means of exercise testing is more troublesome for both patients and health professionals, and progressive exercise tests, in particular, may not reflect limitation of activity imposed by breathlessness in everyday life. Self-paced walking tests (McGavin et al., 1976) may offer a more realistic reflection of disability caused by breathlessness

Table 1 Questions That May Be Useful for Assessing Breathlessness in the Clinical Interview

Question	Advantages	Limitations
What is it that limits your activities?	Establishes the role of breathlessness and usual descriptor	No estimate of severity or variability
How much can you do At your best? At your worst?	Estimate of maximum ability relevant to patient; indication of variability	Needs detail of activity and timing
How does it feel when you have to stop?	Description of the sensation	Language and culture
What are you unable to do now because of your breathing?	Limitation on lifestyle; pointer for rehabilitation	May generate too much information
How much does your breathing vary During the day? From day to day?	More detail of the symptom variability	Does not give overall severity
Is your breathing now the same, better, or worse than a year ago?	Assessment of symptom progression over time	Shorter time scale may be needed for some patients
Does anything make your breathing Better? Worse?	Assessment of effects of therapy, role of cold air, emotion, e.g.	Often produces negative or nonspecific answers

Source: Reprinted from Cockcroft et al. (1989).

in real life; this kind of exercise test can be modified to allow recording of the severity of breathlessness by the subject during the test (Beaumont et al., 1985).

Exercise tests, with or without measurement of accompanying breathlessness, are mainly of research interest. Practical management of a breathless patient requires a simple but reliable means of recording the level of breathlessness experienced by that individual in daily living, so that this can be followed over time. The criteria for defining and recording severity of breathlessness will probably vary between patients, but this does not really matter.

Assessment of Medication

The patient's current medication and its effectiveness are important factors in planning management. Before embarking on, say, an exercise program, it is important to establish the patient on the optimal medication to reduce the level of breathlessness. An important component of the therapeutic regimen is oxygen therapy. It is important to establish what the patient is actually taking, rather than simply what is prescribed, because there may be large discrepancies. There are a number of reasons for this (see later); sometimes there is lack of understanding of the regimen, and sometimes the patient has found that the prescribed regimen has side effects or is not very effective. There is evidence that many patients prescribed long-term oxygen do not use it for the intended period each day (Evans et al., 1983). When prescribing home oxygen for a patient, the physician and the patient must be clear whether this is mainly to relieve episodes of breathlessness or whether its long-term use for many hours each day is intended to improve prognosis (Nocturnal Oxygen Therapy Trial Group, 1980; Medical Research Council Working Party, 1981). Unless this distinction is clearly explained, it is unlikely that the patient will use the oxygen as intended.

Attention to detail is important. This includes, for example, assessing technique of using pressurized inhalers or nebulizers. Patients are often right about problems with their medication. An example is a woman who complained that she got no benefit from her inhaler with spacer (although she had demonstrable reversibility of her airways obstruction); careful examination of the spacer revealed that it was faulty and remained closed so that no drug was delivered to the patient.

Assessment of Related Factors

The level of disability related to a given respiratory impairment varies according to such factors as age and habitual level of fitness. Clinical experience suggests that individuals who are older and/or less used to taking exercise tend to suffer more breathlessness and limitation of activity than those who are younger and fitter. More importantly, they require a less vigorous rehabilitation regimen. Many people who suffer persistent breathlessness are elderly and often have other conditions that can limit their mobility, lead to pain and discomfort, or reduce their ability to take in new information. These conditions include arthritis, ischemic heart disease, peripheral vascular disease, and hearing and sight impairment. Full assessment of a breathless patient must include all these other factors so that a personalized regime can be planned that is appropriate and achievable.

B. Psychological Assessment

Knowledge and Understanding of Condition and Medicines

Whether in a hospital ward or a family practitioner's office or making a home visit, a doctor or a nurse is in a good position to make an assessment of a patient's information needs. A patient who is breathless is not always able to express himself clearly; this can be related to his physical condition or his diminished sense of importance. Taking time and sitting down with him will assist the process of learning about what he needs to know and enable him to assimilate advice given. Inviting the patient to tell his story of recent events, enquiring about what made him call a doctor, and asking him how he feels provide much insight into the knowledge, skill, and interest that he has in his health.

Assessment is the basis on which a doctor makes clinical decisions. A patient who is encouraged to participate in this process is an active learner, and this may enhance the consultation, increase her confidence in future self-care, and develop her individual sense of commitment to decisions in which she has taken part. Lack of privacy, interruptions, impaired vision, and diminished hearing are some of the many features that hinder the patient's interaction with the doctor. Adult learning, of which assessment is the first stage, is based on four assumptions (Knowles, 1973):

1. Adults are self-directing human beings.
2. Adults have accumulated experience and are resources for learning.
3. Adults have a readiness to learn related social roles or tasks to perform.
4. Adults engage in learning activities that are problem centered and that contribute to solutions of current life situations.

If these concepts are borne in mind, the individual and family can be put more at ease in discussing their problems and may have increased potential for rehabilitation and self-care.

Assessing a patient's knowledge and understanding of the condition and medicines may be achieved by asking such questions as the following: What is it you understand is the matter with you, and which medicines seem to help? Can you show me your medicines and inhalers? It may emerge that there are difficulties with dexterity, recalling instructions or converting these to action, dislikes of certain medicines, or use of self-prescribed medicines. As the dialogue develops, the patient's recognition of the connection between treatment and illness may become apparent and, if not, most patients or their caregivers value receiving relevant information. However, many patients report that they have not been expected to learn about their condition or medications (Cockcroft et al., 1987).

Emotional State

The assessment of a patient's emotional state will include his adjustment to illness or disability, his perception of breathlessness, the presence of obvious anxiety or depression, and relationships with those around him.

Breathlessness limits activity, and makes people feel less in control of their everyday lives. However, individuals differ in their subjective experience of breathlessness and their interpretation of its meaning for them. It has been reported that good premorbid coping ability and the presence of psychosocial assets are prognostic of good adjustment to chronic obstructive airways disease (Agle et al., 1973). Stress occurring during illness or recovery period is likely to interfere with recovery (Mayou et al., 1978). Feelings of helplessness, uncertainty, and depression have been found to be associated with poor physical recovery (Viney and Westbrook, 1982).

Coping strategies are required by patients attempting to manage demands consequent upon any chronic illness. Some of these demands, listed by Strauss (1984), are uncertainty associated with prognosis; the requirement for great effort in palliation of the condition; social isolation and the intrusive impact on lives resulting in lifestyle changes; and the need to manage and prevent crises.

Basic assessment of a patient's emotional state is necessary for planning management, whether acute or long term. This assessment includes noting her posture and facial expression, how she tells the story, the presence of obvious anxiety, and the degree of order in her environment. Explorative and open questions enable patients to feel a sense of trust; this is important whether practical strategies or aspects of medical care are being discussed. Some people find the experience of persistent breathlessness overwhelming and are unable to adjust. This may lead to depression and/or panic attacks, presenting the patient with an added burden. Time spent understanding the patient's perspective may assist toward improving the adaptive capacities of individuals living with breathlessness and other forms of disability.

C. Social Assessment

The handicap experienced by a person with chronic illness can be defined as "the disadvantage that limits or prevents fulfillment of a normal role" (Williams and Bury, 1989). The level of disability from a given respiratory impairment is variable; the resulting handicap is even more variable. The patient's capacity to manage the demands of his illness will depend upon his personal resources, such as family, interests, money, and ability to confront psychological or family problems. Assets include adequate housing, money, and education. However, it is suggested that a supportive relative in the home is the single most important factor in adjustment to chronic illness (Barstow, 1974). Assessing a patient at home allows a health care professional to observe how the patient accomplishes a small task, such as removing an item of clothing or the planning required to visit his local shop. It depends on his capacity to calculate the availability of his "mobility resources": time, energy, and money. Fagerhaugh (1975) describes this process as deciding on "routing strategies." For example, a patient may be able to leave his home only later in the day after using treatments, taking time finishing routines, perhaps getting down stairs, and then gauging how long he can stay away within his energy limits. Asking questions about nutrition, finances, and available social outlets and observing how a patient moves about his home are illuminating and may determine whether further aids for living or social support could enhance his rehabilitation or sense of well-being and quality of life.

III. Management of the Patient

Good management of a breathless patient follows on naturally from a full assessment and includes psychosocial aspects as well as simply physical management. We have divided this section into the management of acute exacerbations of breathlessness in hospital and long-term management; in reality the two aspects should be closely allied.

A. Management of Acute Exacerbations in the Hospital

Good management of acute exacerbations of breathlessness treated in the hospital includes not only the treatment given while in the hospital but also preparation for hospital discharge. The stay in the hospital is part of the continuum of the patient's life, or sometimes the last episode of his or her life; treatment in the hospital, even if it successfully deals with the immediate problem precipitating admission, is usually not capable of "curing" the underlying condition responsible for chronic breathlessness. This consideration should lead to moderation of desires to apply the more extreme and heroic therapeutic interventions, which are often extremely uncomfortable for the patient and make no difference to the long-term prognosis.

Management of Symptoms as Well as Pathophysiology

When patients are admitted to the hospital acutely ill, it is all too easy to focus upon the treatment of the underlying condition and pay less attention to treating their symptoms, troublesome as these may be for them. Sometimes this may delay the relief of the problem for which the patient sought help. For example, in treating an episode of acute bacterial pneumonia, antibiotics are clearly vital but they will not improve breathlessness until the pneumonia resolves after some days; supplemental oxygen usually helps to relieve breathlessness by reducing ventilation but is often not indicated as necessary on the basis of arterial blood gas analysis.

Sometimes a focus upon physiology rather than symptoms can lead to treatment that worsens a patient's symptoms. The use of respiratory stimulants in patients with respiratory failure frequently worsens breathlessness because of the increased ventilatory drive. Of course, their use may be justified in circumstances in which a patient is in respiratory failure yet could be returned to a reasonable quality of life if he survives the acute episode. This requires judgments about what is a reasonable quality of life, about the likelihood of recovery with and without the use of stimulants, and about the symptomatic effects that will be produced. The patient and/or family are an important source of information and also have a right to participate in the deliberations. Sometimes the continued presence of a spouse or other near relative can keep a patient with respiratory failure alert and be as effective as a respiratory stimulant, without some of the more unpleasant side effects.

Simple considerations in practical management can greatly increase the comfort of a breathless patient in hospital. A patient in bed in the initial stages of an acute exacerbation is limited in movement from breathlessness, weakness, and debilitation from pyrexia and dehydration. Improving such a patient's position in bed can make her breathing more comfortable and even more efficient. Effective positioning of pillows to support the patient's body shape can enhance ventilation and support the spine, especially the lumbar region, thus avoiding musculoskeletal pain. Assessing her pressure risk score (Waterlow, 1985) may indicate the need to introduce a suitable pressure relief bed. Regular repositioning promotes positional comfort and encourages expectoration and leg muscle activity. Oxygen delivery devices can lead to nasal and oral dryness, and this should be checked; adequate tube length should be provided to avoid awkward postures. Supervision of the use of bedside nebulizers or inhalers should aim to optimize drug delivery and pay attention to cleanliness to reduce the risk of oral thrush or secondary infection. Patients must have a plentiful supply of nutritious liquids within easy reach to improve hydration (dehydration is very uncomfortable as well as sometimes life threatening). The means for summoning help need to be explained and left easily accessible to the patient.

There are particular problems in treating the breathlessness of terminal illness, for example in a patient with lung secondaries from a tumor elsewhere or in a patient with end-stage heart failure. There is evidence that breathlessness is generally more difficult to control than pain in terminally ill patients (Hinton, 1963). Especially if lung disease is present, doctors may be reluctant to use opiates to obtund the sensation of breathlessness, for fear of respiratory depression hastening death. In fact, if opiates are used appropriately to control symptoms, there is little evidence of their producing dangerous respiratory depression. Supplemental oxygen and anxiolytics are useful adjuncts in breathlessness that is hard to control in dying patients. Fear may greatly increase the distress of a breathless, dying patient, and the opportunity to talk about his fears of dying and related events may help to relieve his distress.

Discharging a Patient Home

Discharge from the hospital has been recognized for many years to present problems (Skeet, 1971; Armitage, 1985; Jones, 1984). There is evidence that patient discharge is often unplanned; there is a lack of communication networks and inadequate interpersonal cooperation. All this results in the patient and family having their needs unmet. There seem to be a number of reasons for discharge difficulties: communication between the hospital and primary services is hampered by lack of insight into each other's roles and work activities; medical education is predominantly hospital based; research done into chronic obstructive airways disease is mainly concerned with medical issues or the psychological concomitants of the disease, paying little attention to the social aspects of a patient and family living with chronic illness and disability (Williams, 1989); and, of course, there is pressure on beds.

Successful discharge of any patient requires a plan that is evolved before the patient is moved from one environment to another. This important event is all too often not planned at all. The aims of a discharge plan are to prepare the patient to the highest achievable level of independence physically and emotionally, to facilitate a safe and organized transfer, and to promote continuity of care between hospital and home.

Successful discharge is based on knowing and observing what a patient is able to do within her activities of living and assessing the reasons for any limitations. Deficits in self-care capacities may result from a number of problems, including lack of knowledge, lack of relevant skills, lack of motivation, and the presence of a limited range of behavior (Pritchard and David, 1988).

The potential for reestablishing independence and self-care in the future can be explored through discussion, planning, and testing strategies in the ward. It is necessary to establish realistic and relevant goals that link with the patient's home environment. For example, in considering the goal of the patient being able to get to the lavatory independently at home after discharge, the following questions need to be answered: What distance does he need to walk between bed and lavatory at home? How long will this take? What aids (including supplemental oxygen) will be needed? Will it be possible to accomplish this in safety? Realistic discharge goals need constant review as the patient's condition improves or deteriorates. Patient's need to be given opportunities to practice relevant activities on the ward, under supervision. This improves the assessment that can be made of their capabilities and increases their mobility, which is the first stage of a home exercise program (see later).

An important aim of preparation for discharge is to assist the patient to be independent and to remain fit within his or her capacities. Small adjustments to furniture, wall, or stair rails can help patients to raise themselves from seated positions and help them to walk further by providing opportunities to pause, feel safe, and regain their breath. A walking stick or frame for some patients promotes confidence and improved fitness. Preparing a patient for discharge is part of promoting recovery and restoring confidence as he or she grows more competent in self-care activities. Most daily routines involve a patient in movement and therefore help to improve mobility. Planning goals toward recovery and independence is an educational process that can be continued after discharge. Before discharge there are opportunities to talk with the patient about his or her knowledge of illness and disability and how to recognize deterioration and keep well are important to discuss before going home. Emphasis should be on positive aspects of keeping well, exercise, interests, nutrition, recognizing signs of chest infection, basic structure of lungs, airways, changes in symptoms, and how to respond to them.

B. Long-term Management Plan: Living with Breathlessness

Patient-Centered Approach to Management

The basis of this approach is that management must be tailored to the requirements of individual patients. It will vary according to the nature and severity of the patient's underlying condition causing breathlessness, according to her age and general physical capacities, according to her emotional state and resources, and according to her social circumstances and available support. This is why a careful assessment of the patient, as described earlier, is essential before embarking upon a management plan. It follows that no two patients will have the same plan; the emphasis on different elements varies enormously depending upon their individual requirements and circumstances. A common theme is the idea of progress, however slow, in areas agreed between the patient and health care professional as important. This theme is supported by the setting of goals in key areas, both short and long term. This facilitates follow-up discussions about progress and obstacles to progress.

This patient-centered approach was applied in a controlled trial of a respiratory nurse visiting patients with chronic breathlessness in their homes and found to be effective in educating patients about their condition and medications and in reducing mortality over the short period of the study (Cockcroft et al., 1987). A later controlled study found that patients visited by a respiratory health worker were little different from controls in terms of disability measures but had a reduced mortality over 1 year (Littlejohn et al., 1991). It seems that this sort of personalized care for frail patients can keep them alive longer, despite their disabilities.

The goals that are set in the patient-centered approach relate to specific areas, such as education and use of medication, emotional and social needs, and improvement in mobility. Management in these different areas is described here, followed by some examples of the sorts of goals that might be set with patients.

Many professionals can potentially be involved in the management of a breathless patient, including hospital-based doctors and nurses, general practitioners (GPs) and community nurses, physiotherapists, occupational therapists, psychiatrists and psychiatric nurses, and social workers. Each brings a particular expertise to bear, but it is important that there is good communication between all those concerned with the care of a patient, to avoid duplication, gaps in care, and contradictions. It is helpful to have one person who is the prime point of contact for each patient and coordinates the involvement of all others. Who this should be depends on local circumstances and varies between patients; what matters is to identify this person clearly.

Exercise Training Programs

Controlled studies have demonstrated that a significant improvement in exercise tolerance can be achieved in patients with chronic obstructive airways disease by means of programs of exercise training (McGavin et al., 1977; Sergysels et al., 1979; Cockcroft et al., 1981). Complicated and hospital-based regimens are not necessary to achieve useful results; simple programs of home-based exercises have been shown to be effective (McGavin et al., 1977). Exercise regimens are usually not at a level that would be expected to produce cardiovascular training effects, such as improvement in anaerobic threshold. Despite this, there is evidence of an improvement in exercise efficiency following simple exercise training programs in patients with chronic obstructive airways disease, with reduced ventilation for a given external workload and increased stride length (Cockcroft et al., 1985). This may be caused by effects on skeletal muscle structure and function or improved efficiency of the motion of walking. There is little evidence that exercise training changes the perception of breathlessness for a given level of ventilation, although some evidence that prior experience of breathlessness modifies current experience (Wilson and Jones, 1990). What matters to the patient is to be able to do more before being limited by breathlessness and to be fit enough to perform up to the limits imposed by the disease.

It is suggested by some that the effects of exercise training programs in breathless patients may be the result of psychological improvement (Donner and Howard, 1992). However, a controlled trial that examined this found that psychological improvements occurred in both the exercise and control patients and that the improvement in exercise tolerance in the exercise group was not related to psychological changes (Cockcroft et al., 1982). This study also did not find any psychological factors to be predictive of which patients would benefit most from exercise training.

Health care professionals who might be considering an exercise program for their breathless patients could be discouraged by suggestions that detailed prior physiological assessment of the patient, including exercise testing in the hospital, is required before exercise can be "prescribed" (Donner and Howard, 1992). The reality can be much simpler (Cockcroft, 1985). Both patients and their doctors often have fears about increasing exercise. Patients fear the breathlessness that will accompany exercise, and may believe that severe breathlessness can lead to rapid death. They can be reassured that breathlessness itself is not dangerous and be advised that a sensible exercise program is one that incorporates several spells of exercise each day, sufficient to provoke moderate, not severe, breathlessness, and gradually increasing in length and intensity at a rate that they can manage. Doctors fear that patients with respiratory disease may also have cardiovascular disease and that exercise may precipitate a cardiovascular collapse. They can be reassured that such patients cannot usually exercise at a level that stresses the cardiovascular system, and patients should be instructed to report any symptoms, such as chest pain, when they increase their activity, so that these can be investigated if necessary.

Using the patient-centered approach mentioned earlier, the health care professional can decide with the patient what sort of exercise is most appropriate and set goals for the results to be achieved. For example, if the patient wants to be able to go to and from the post office, a quarter of a mile from his house, then the aim of his training will be to allow him to cover the half-mile there and back in a reasonable time. A more disabled, elderly patient may simply want to be able to get as far as his garden gate, and a younger, fitter patient (say, with asthma) may want to achieve a high level of training so that he can take part in a marathon. Just as quality of life tends to decrease unevenly in a series of step changes with reducing exercise tolerance, so a large increase in quality of life can be achieved with a relatively small increase in exercise tolerance from a rehabilitation exercise program. This is illustrated in Fig. 1. The key to success is to identify, with the patient, the "threshold" he wants to cross with his improved exercise capacity. As with all goals, progress must be monitored and the goals may have to be modified up or down depending on progress.

Any exercise program for patients with chronic breathlessness must be "for life" and must incorporate the idea that setbacks may occur, for example because of intercurrent chest infections. Simple, practical advice about how to make exercise part of a normal daily routine, rather than something quite separate, can help patients to maintain fitness within the limitation imposed by their breathlessness. This can include advice about use of bronchodilators in relation to exercise, use of a walking stick or frame, wearing appropriate clothing for exercise, and eating in relation to exercise. There are no patients for whom some sort of attention to increased mobility is not appropriate, however limited their capacities. In some cases, provision of a wheelchair may be necessary to allow the patient to achieve useful mobility; this should not been seen as "failure" of an exercise program, but rather as another option for improving mobility and quality of life.

Educating Patients About Their Condition and Medication

Many patients with chronic breathlessness are elderly and have only a basic level of general education; they have not been involved in any form of education for many years. Additionally, any form of stress or crisis is expected to reduce the

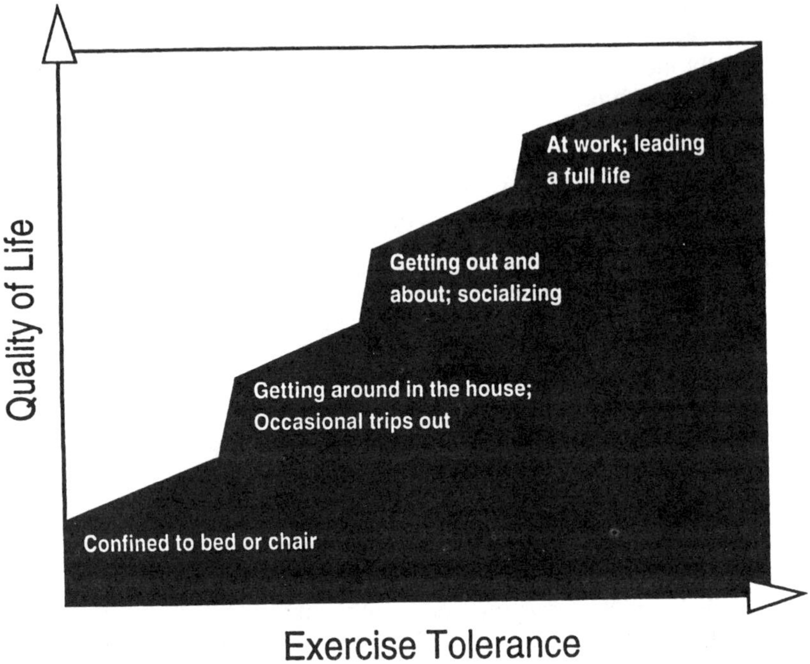

Figure 1 Step changes in quality of life associated with the reduction in exercise tolerance accompanying progression of chronic obstructive pulmonary disease. This process can be reversed in a rehabilitation exercise program, with large improvements in quality of life associated with modest increases in exercise tolerance. (Reprinted from Cockcroft, 1985.)

capacity to assimilate new information (Cohen et al., 1986). Despite these difficulties, individually tailored programs of education for breathless patients (Bagnall and Sigsworth, 1988) can lead to improvements in their knowledge of their condition and medications (Cockcroft et al., 1987; Bagnall and Heslop, 1987). A full initial assessment is essential (see earlier), followed by a program that allows the patient to learn at his or her own pace, provides reinforcement of messages, and concentrates on aspects of interest and practical value to the individual patient.

Visual aids can be very helpful. For example, an illustration might show bronchoconstriction, with the effects of bronchodilators, and include a note of that patient's regimen for using medication and space for the patient to record its use. Examples of charts prepared for individual patients about their medications, to be kept for future reference, are shown in Tables 2 and 3. The process is not so much

Table 2 Example of Teaching Chart Prepared for Individual Patient

Medication	Action	Advice
Bronchodilator inhaler	Opens airways, relaxes airway muscles, allows increased airflow	Take after food; practice good inhaler technique
Steroid inhaler	Opens airways by decreasing swelling of walls; works as a preventive measure	Advice regarding dosage tapering; rinse mouth after steroid inhaler
Amoxicillin tablets	Helps the body to fight infection by killing the bacteria (germs)	Take when signs of infection; take the full 7 day course.

one of giving the patient standard information and instructions to remember but more a dialogue around issues the patient finds confusing or difficult or wishes to learn more about. This might include discussion about difficulties with opening medicine bottles and with devices requiring manual strength or dexterity; difficulty reading the labels on medicines; the need to translate instructions into action relevant to that individual; the patient's usual patterns of medicine taking at home in relation to the instructions from the clinic; and difficulties with getting someone to renew the prescription or collect medicines from the pharmacist for patients

Table 3 Medicine Chart

Starting date: Name: Ted Brown	Key nurse: M. Smith Weight: 128 lbs		Telephone: Peak flow: 250	
Name of medicine and action	Breakfast	Lunchtime	Afternoon snack	Bedtime
Prednisolone helps breathing by reducing swelling in airways	15 mg (3 × 5 mg) 3 tablets	After food		
Bricanyl: breathing	×2 Use before exercise	2	2	2
Atrovent: breathing lasts longer	2	2	2	2
Aminophylline, 225 mg	1 after food			1
Ranitidine, 150 mg	Protects stomach			1

who cannot manage this themselves. The idea is to give information that the patient wants and needs to manage her or his own condition; education is part of the process of empowerment of the patient.

Self-Management of Exacerbations

Part of the education of patients with conditions causing chronic breathlessness is in how to recognize deterioration early and what action to take when this happens. It is important that patients be well-informed about what signs to look out for and what action to take. They also need to have suitable materials immediately available, for example, a course of antibiotics and a supply of oral steroids kept at home to use when necessary. The details of what to do for exacerbations must be tailored to the individual patient. For an elderly, frail patient this may mean supply of a telephone with a number to call in emergencies; for a younger, more able patient a supply of emergency medication and instructions on who to contact if this fails within a set time are appropriate.

Most patients can learn to recognize relatively small changes in their respiratory symptoms and act on them early. There are some people, however, who appear to have low sensitivity to increases in airways obstruction and can become severely ill before they become aware of increased breathlessness (Jones, 1992). These people may need to be provided with such equipment as a peak flow meter and be instructed to take action on the basis of a reduction in peak expiratory flow rate even if they are not aware of worsening symptoms.

Patients can get most support in managing acute exacerbations of their condition from doctors they know well. The doctor gets to know what symptoms are a significant early sign of deterioration in a particular patient, and the doctor and patient come to trust each other. The doctor trusts the patient to recognize and act on signs of deterioration and provides suitable means to do this, and the patient trusts the doctor's judgment and advice. This sort of relationship is best achieved by having one doctor who sees the patient on each occasion he or she attends the surgery or the hospital clinic; unfortunately, this is not always easy to arrange in practice.

Management of Emotional and Social Difficulties

Emotional Difficulties

The stresses with which many patients with chronic breathlessness must cope include life changes, stopping work, decreasing energy levels, routine disruption, stress within relationships, loss of social life, and losses of status or power. The strategies they develop to cope with these stresses often include a tendency to control emotional distress by limiting stressful contacts with their environment. Fear of embarrassment, breathlessness, or other symptoms may lead to the development of repressive psychological defenses (Dudley et al., 1969). Physical help, for example with symptom control, can reduce fear and improve emotional state in many cases. Sometimes more specialized psychological or psychiatric help is needed. A study of patients with chronic obstructive airways disease confirmed that psychological difficulties are common and found that sessions with a respiratory nurse were effective in helping with breathlessness but tended to increase depression, but sessions of supportive therapy with a psychotherapist had more effect on emotional problems (Rosser et al., 1983). A combined approach can address both physical and emotional difficulties.

The emotional needs of those caring for patients with chronic breathlessness, both professionals and nonprofessionals, should not be forgotten. Carers are encouraged to form close professional relationships with their patients and to help them deal with difficult and painful issues concerning loss, guilt, and anger. This can generate powerful emotional responses in the caregivers, and they need to be provided with adequate support to enable them to undertake their work safely and efficiently. In the study of respiratory nurses visiting patients at home reported by Cockcroft et al. (1987), regular meetings were held between the two nurses and a psychotherapist who was familiar with the sort of work they were doing to allow them to discuss difficulties they had encountered with particular patients and also to discuss their own feelings about the work they were doing. Both nurses found these meetings helpful. The same psychotherapist runs meetings for the hospital staff on the respiratory ward, where they discuss difficult patients and their own feelings about these patients (Sigsworth, 1988).

Social Support

According to Barstow (1974), the presence of a supportive friend or family at home is probably the single most important factor in adjustment to a chronic illness. Equally, an ill family member can place enormous demands on the family. The family needs an opportunity to discuss their concerns and be assisted in how to support and care for the sick relative. Chronic sickness will involve changes in the whole family's social life.

Issues of social support in illness have been reviewed by Sarason et al. (1988). Although most researchers consider social support to be a multidimensional concept, most definitions include the idea of emotional closeness or intimacy (Wood, 1984). There is growing evidence that how people appraise the support available to them may be even more important than their actual interpersonal contacts (Heller and Swindle, 1983). This is understandable given individual differences in the need for contacts and the meanings attached to them.

Home respiratory care is not well established in the United Kingdom. The doctor or nurse can begin to review financial need and suggest an application for attendance allowance because many chronically ill patients may well qualify for this allowance. Practical interventions, such as reviewing the comfort and safety of the environment and providing aids for living, may help to minimize breathlessness and improve quality of life. A wheelchair assessment may enable the patient to have greater social opportunities. Social services may assist in housing or sheltered accommodation that may be needed or offer respite periods for relatives engaged in the long-term care of a family member. Some areas have a caregiver association that may provide social support to the carer. A telephone is essential, especially if the patient spends long periods alone, and some patients and relatives benefit from a community alarm system, thus freeing a caregiver to leave the home for periods.

An association for people with long-term lung problems, called the Breathe Easy Club, has been established in recent years. It provides breathless patients with a newspaper about new developments in lung disease and about treatments and services available and gives them an opportunity to share experiences and information with people in a similar situation.

Examples of Goals Set with Patients in Management Plans

Table 4 shows examples of the sorts of goals, both short and long term, that might be set with patients. Patient A is an elderly lady with severe breathlessness caused by emphysema. Patient B is a teenager with asthma.

C. Examples of Good and Bad Management

The following examples are drawn from a number of case histories. They are intended to illustrate that integrated management, tailored to the patient's wishes and needs, is the key to success. Problems occur when care is fragmented and when insufficient attention is paid to the patient's symptoms and physical and psychological needs.

Example of Bad Management

Mr. P. first came into hospital when he was aged 62 years. He had been a heavy smoker all his life and had experienced gradually increasing breathlessness over the last 5 or 10 years, having to retire early from his work as a plumber because of this. He had never been given a diagnosis for his condition but had seen several different general practitioners (GPs) in the practice, each of whom had prescribed drugs for his chest, including tablets and inhalers. The tablets made him feel shaky, so he did not take them, and he had never been shown how to use the inhalers, of which he had been prescribed several varieties. He had no idea of what his medicines were or what they were supposed to do. He admitted that he had a cabinet full of medicines he had not used at home.

Mr. P's wife was also a heavy smoker and died 4 years previously from lung cancer. Mr. P. was secretly very fearful that he, too, had lung cancer, but he had

Table 4 Examples of Goals Set with Patients

Patient	Problem	Goal term	Goal description
Patient A	Reduced physical exercise tolerance	Short	Walk with stick to front door three times daily
		Long	Walk with stick to library
	Does not know how to use inhalers	Short	Say when and in which order to use
		Long	Demonstrate correct use
	Feels grief and guilt about husband's death	Short and long	Be able to share feelings about husband's death
Patient B	Does not know how to recognize deterioration in	Short	State significance of PEF[a] changes, etc.
	asthma	Long	Act on changes in PEF
	Reduced exercise tolerance;	Short	Pretreat with inhaler
	exercise-induced asthma	Long	Play football regularly

[a]Peak expiratory flow.

never discussed this with anyone. He lived alone; his only child was living abroad. He found it increasingly difficult to get in and out of his second floor apartment, relying upon a neighbor to bring him in shopping and collect his medicines from the pharmacist.

Most of this history was not obtained from Mr. P. on admission. He was bought into hospital after being found semiconscious by his neighbor, who reported that Mr. P. had complained of worsening breathlessness for a week and was awaiting an appointment to see his GP. Mr. P. was in respiratory failure on admission, with signs of a chest infection. The junior doctor on duty prescribed a respiratory stimulant on the basis of the poor blood gases that did not respond to conventional treatment with antibiotics, bronchodilators, and controlled oxygen. Mr. P. became very agitated and confused and seemed to be in obvious respiratory distress. He drank little and became dehydrated and developed a sacral pressure sore. He required intravenous fluids for some days. He was found to be a "difficult and demanding" patient on the ward. After 2 weeks he was discharged home, partly because his bed was urgently needed for an emergency admission. His blood gases had improved by then, but his mobility was poor and he had only once visited the toilet unaided. He was given medicines to take home with him; these were different from those he had been prescribed before. He was told about his medicines before he was discharged by a busy junior doctor who did not have time to check whether he had understood. He did not discuss with anyone his fear of lung cancer and still suspected that this was what was wrong with him. The neighbor was informed of his discharge, and a letter was sent to the GP to ask him to arrange for home help.

Mr. P. returned home to a situation much as before, except that now he was even more limited in his mobility. He had a poor appetite and did not want to bother his neighbor too much about shopping. He became increasingly reclusive and never left his flat. He had two further hospital admissions over the next 2 years, similar but not as severe as the first. On one of these admissions he was prescribed an antidepressant because he was thought to be clinically depressed and to have breathlessness out of proportion to his lung function deficit. He still told no one of his underlying fear of lung cancer. One Monday morning his neighbor became concerned because she could not get him to answer his door and she had not seen him since the Friday morning. The police were called and he was found dead in his apartment, with evidence that he had been trying to use an inhaler.

Examples of Good Management

Miss J.

Miss J. was a 76-year-old woman with severe breathlessness secondary to emphysema, who lived with her sister. She did not require oxygen for hypoxia but was prescribed it because it helped to relieve her breathlessness. She was admitted to the hospital with a chest infection, but she hated being in the hospital and asked to go home. Before her discharge, arrangements were made for an oxygen concentrator to be installed in her home, to avoid the need to change oxygen cylinders. It became clear at home that she was not going to survive, and she found her extreme breathlessness intolerable. She was being visited by a respiratory nurse attached to the hospital. In liaison with the GP, she was started on small doses of morphine to reduce her breathlessness. Her sister had a telephone contact number for the respiratory health worker she could use at any time of day or night, if she was concerned about Miss J. Because of a good response to morphine, Miss J. was started on a morphine infusion, which helped to relieve her severe breathlessness. She was regularly visited by the district nurse to help her sister with her physical care. She died at home after 3 days on the morphine infusion.

Mr. K.

Mr. K. is a 63-year old man with chronic obstructive airways and frequent infective exacerbations. He lives alone in a first floor apartment and is usually able to walk to the local shops. He is an intelligent man and has a good knowledge of his condition and medications. He attends a clinic at the hospital every few months and is admitted to the hospital if an exacerbation fails to respond to treatment that he initiates himself as necessary. He is an anxious man, and it is clear that he has a number of unresolved conflicts and regrets about his life. Following a particularly severe exacerbation of his condition, his mobility was severely reduced, so that he had difficulty getting in and out of his home. He was therefore started on a program of rehabilitation on discharge from the hospital. The coordinator was the respiratory health nurse from the hospital, and there was input from many sources:

> The respiratory health nurse formulated an exercise plan with him and also advised him about nutrition and suitable appliances for his oxygen therapy during exercise.
>
> The occupational therapist provided him with mobility aids in his flat, including wheels on his chair to allow him to move around the room for his hobbies.
>
> He was visited regularly by a community psychiatric nurse, who helped him with his emotional difficulties.
>
> The hospital doctor was informed of the exercise rehabilitation plan and undertook tests of the cardiovascular system because of a previous history of cardiac problems.
>
> The GP was kept fully informed of the program and prescribed appropriate medication.

Mr. K. has made good progress with his rehabilitation. He is now able to get to and from the local shops again, he undertakes his hobbies at home, and he has found benefit from talking about his emotional difficulties.

References

Agle, D.P., Baum, G.L., Chester, E.H., et al. (1973). Multidisciplinary treatment of chronic pulmonary insufficiency. I. Psychological aspects of rehabilitation. J. Psychosom. Med. 35:41–49.

Armitage, S. (1985). Hospital to home: discharge referrals, who's responsible? Nursing Times 81:26–28.

Bagnall, P., and Heslop, A. (1987). Chronic respiratory disease: educating patients at home. Professional Nurse June:293–296.

Bagnall, P., and Sigsworth, J. (1988). Living with lung problems. Professional Nurse September:514–517.

Barstow, R.E. (1974). Coping with emphysema. Nurs. Clin. North Am. 9:137–145.

Beaumont, A., Cockcroft, A., and Guz, A. (1985). A self-paced treadmill walking test for breathless patients. Thorax 40:459–464.

Cockcroft, A. (1985). Exercise for patients with respiratory disease. Update 30:255–262.

Cockcroft, A. (1993). Dyspnoea. In: French's Index of Differential Diagnosis, 13th ed. Edited by H. Ellis, P.R. Fleming, and I. Bouchier. Butterworths, Guildford (in press).

Cockcroft, A., Saunders, M.J., and Berry, G. (1981). Randomized controlled trial of rehabilitation in chronic respiratory disability. Thorax 36:200–203.

Cockcroft, A., Berry, G., Brown, E.B., and Exall, C. (1982). Psychological changes during a controlled trial of rehabilitation in chronic respiratory disability. Thorax 37: 413–416.

Cockcroft, A., Beaumont, A., and Guz, A. (1985). Effects of exercise training on walking distance, exercise ventilation and breathlessness in patients with COAD. Clin. Sci. 69:7p.

Cockcroft, A., Bagnall, P., Heslop, A., Andersson, N., Heaton, R., Batstone, J., Allen, J., Spencer, P., and Guz, A. (1987). Controlled trial of a respiratory health worker visiting patients with chronic respiratory disability. Br. Med. J. 294:225–228.

Cockcroft, A., Adams, L., and Guz, A. (1989). Assessment of breathlessness. Q. J. Med. 268:669–676.

Cohen, S., Evans, G.W., Stokols, D., and Krantz, D.S. (1986). Behaviour, Health and Environmental Stress. Plenum, New York.

Donner, C.F., and Howard, P. (1992). Pulmonary rehabilitation in chronic obstructive pulmonary disease (COPD) with recommendations for its use. Eur. Respir. J. 5: 266–275.

Dudley, D.L., and Pattison, E.M. (1969). Group psychotherapy in patients with severe diffuse obstructive pulmonary syndrome. Am. Rev. Respir. Dis. 100:575.

Elliott, M.W., Adams, L., Cockcroft, A., Macrae, K.D., Murphy, K., and Guz, A. (1991). The language of breathlessness: use of verbal descriptors by patients with cardiopulmonary disease. Am. Rev. Respir. Dis. 144:826–832.

Evans, T.W., Waterhouse, J., and Howard, P. (1983). Clinical experience with the oxygen concentrator. Br. Med. J. 287:459–461.

Fagerhaugh, S.Y. (1975). Getting around with emphysema. In: Chronic Illness and the Quality of Life. Edited by A.L. Strauss. Mosby, St. Louis.

Heller, K., Swindle, R.W. (1983). Social networks, perceived social support and coping with stress. In: Preventive Psychology: Theory, Research and Practice in Community Intervention. Edited by R.D. Felner, L.A. Jason, J. Moritsugu, and S.S. Farber. Pergamon Press, New York, pp.

Hinton, J.M. (1963). The physical and mental distress of the dying. Q. J. Med. 32:1–21.

Jones, I.H. (1984). Cause for complaint: 2. Lack of communication. Nursing Times 80: 51–52.

Jones, P.W. (1992). Breathlessness perception in airways obstruction. Eur. Respir. J. 5:1035–1036.

Knowles, M.S. (1973). The Adult Learner: A Neglected Species. Gulf, Houston.

Littlejohn, P., Baveystock, C.M., Parnell, H., and Jones, P.W. (1991). Randomised controlled trial of the effectiveness of a respiratory health worker in reducing impairment, disability, and handicap due to chronic airflow limitation. Thorax 46:559–564.

Mayou, R., Costa, A., and Williamson, B. (1978). Psychological adjustment in patients one year after myocardial infarction. J. Psychometric Res. 22:447–453.

McGavin, C.R., Gupta, S.P., and McHardy, G.J.R. (1976). Twelve minute walking test for assessing disability in chronic bronchitics. Br. Med. J. 1:822–823.

McGavin, C.R., Gupta, S.P., Lloyd, E.L., and McHardy, G.J.R. (1977). Physical rehabilitation for the chronic bronchitic: results of a controlled trial of exercises in the home. Thorax 32:307–311.

Medical Research Council (1986). Respiratory Symptoms Questionnaire. Medical Research Council, London.

Medical Research Council Working Party. (1981). Long term oxygen therapy in chronic hypoxic cor pulmonale complicating chronic bronchitis and emphysema. Lancet 2: 681–685.

Nocturnal Oxygen Therapy Trial Group. (1980). Continuous or nocturnal oxygen therapy in hypoxaemic chronic obstructive airways disease. Ann. Intern. Med. 93:391–398.

Pritchard, A.P., and David, J.A. (1988). Discharge planning. In: Royal Marsden Manual of Clinical Nursing Procedures. Harper and Row, London, pp. 118–122.

Rosser, R., Denford, J., Heslop, A., Kinston, W., Macklin, D., Minty, K., Moynihan, C., Muir, B., Rein, L., and Guz, A. (1983). Breathlessness and psychiatric morbidity in chronic bronchitis and emphysema: a study of psychotherapeutic management. Psychol. Med. 13:93–110.

Sarason, I.G., Sarason, B.R., and Pierce, G.R. (1988). Social support, personality and health. In: Topics in Health Psychology. Edited by S. Maes, C.D. Spielberger, P.B. Defares, and I.G. Sarason. Wiley, London, pp. 245–256.

Sergysels, R., DeCoster, A., Degre, S., and Denohn, H. (1979). Functional evaluation of a physical rehabilitation program including breathing exercises and bicycle training in chronic obstructive lung disease. Respiration 38:105–111.

Sigsworth, J. (1988). The Denford meeting: airing staff concerns. Professional Nurse December:127–129.

Simon, P.M., Schwartzstein, R.M., Weiss, J.W., Lahive, K., Fencl, V., Teghtsoonian, M., and Weinberger, S.E. (1989). Distinguishable sensations in breathlessness induced in normal volunteers. Am. Rev. Respir. Dis. 140:1021–1027.

Skeet, M. (1971). Home from Hospital. Dan Mason Nursing Research Committee. Macmillan, London.

Strauss, A.L. (1984). Chronic Illness and the Quality of Life, 2nd ed. Mosby, St. Louis.

Viney, L.L., and Westbrook, M.T. (1982). Psychological reactions to chronic illness-related disability as a function of its severity and type. J. Psychosom. Med. 35:513–523.

Waterlow, J. (1985). A risk assessment card. Nursing Times 81:49–55.

Williams, S.J. (1989). Chronic respiratory illness and disability: a critical review of the psychosocial literature. Soc. Sci. Med. 28:791–803.

Williams, S.J., and Bury, M.R. (1989). Impairment, disability, and handicap in chronic respiratory illness. Soc. Sci. Med. 29:609–616.

Wilson, R.C., and Jones, P.W. (1990). Influence of prior ventilatory experience on the estimation of breathlessness during exercise. Clin. Sci. 78:149–153.

Wood, Y.R. (1984). Social support and social networks: nature and measurement. In: Advances in Psychological Assessment, Vol. 6. Edited by P. McReynolds and G.J. Chelune. Jossey-Bass, San Francisco, pp. 312–353.

16

Respiratory Sensations

Some Clinical Perspectives

ABRAHAM GUZ

Charing Cross and Westminster Medical School
University of London
London, England

It was originally intended that this chapter should be an introductory clinical perspective on respiratory sensation. However, other contributors—particularly Schwartzstein and Christiano (Chapter 5); Banzett and Lansing (Chapter 6); Mahler (Chapter 10); Poole-Wilson and Clark (Chapter 11); Laszlo and Higgs (Chapter 12); Jones and Wilson (Chapter 13); Stark, Stark, and Russell (Chapter 14); and Cockcroft and Heslop (Chapter 15)—have been collectively so thorough in their coverage that a general introduction would not contribute in any meaningful way. Instead , this chapter will deal with the following gaps in coverage:

1. Presence or absence of dyspnea and the medulla
2. Individual differences in breathlessness
3. Palliation of breathlessness

This author uses the terms *dyspnea* and *breathlessness* interchangeably; *dyspnea* means breathlessness in Greek.

I. Presence or Absence of Dyspnea and the Medulla

Disease of the medulla affecting the respiratory oscillator may result in partial or complete failure of automatic breathing. Voluntary or behavioral breathing usually remains intact, but this depends on the precise extent of the lesion and whether corticospinal fibers are involved in the pathological process. This typical syndrome, with normal corticospinal control of breathing, is seen in a congenital abnormality as a partial or complete failure to breathe when drowsy or asleep; no anatomical cause has yet been consistently found, and the syndrome (congenital central hypoventilation syndrome) is therefore presumed to be due to some unspecified dysfunction of the automatic respiratory controller. There is usually an absence of response of ventilation to hypercapnia and also an absence of the typical associated air hunger sensation. Voluntary breath holding can continue for an inordinate length of time without any apparent urge to breathe (Shea et al., 1993).

Although poorly documented in the clinical literature, other diseases affecting the brainstem: (particularly the medulla), such as bulbar encephalitis, gliomas, infarcts (Heywood et al., 1993), and motoneuron disease may be responsible for an acquired syndrome that resembles the congenital syndrome with lack of ventilatory responsiveness to hypercapnia and hypoxia and an absence of the expected sensations. This author has had the opportunity to study one such patient with motoneuron disease (predominantly affecting the brainstem) with a near normal vital capacity. Elevation of the end-tidal P_{CO_2} to as high as 85 mmHg was accompanied neither by a ventilatory response nor an urge to breathe. Studying sensation in adults with this syndrome is likely to be more rewarding due to the problem of getting children (aged 6–15 years) to express what they feel when ventilation is stimulated.

This clinical evidence all suggests the need for an intact automatic controller of breathing within the medulla that can respond to stimulation with CO_2 before the typical air hunger is experienced. This view is reinforced by the results of two key studies. First, ventilator-dependent quadriplegics, with the lesion as high as C1–C2, could sense the typical urge to breath, or air hunger, when end-tidal P_{CO_2} was raised by increasing the CO_2 concentration of inspired air via the ventilator (Banzett et al., 1989). The medullary automatic controller is presumably intact, but its activity cannot descend via the bulbospinal fibers to the anterior horn cells of the respiratory musculature. Second, a study in a patient with the "locked-in syndrome" associated with a ventral midbrain/pontine infarct has been made. All voluntary control of breathing (and of other muscles innervated by anterior horn cells below the level of the lesion) was abolished, while sensory pathways remained intact (Munschauer et al., 1991). The medulla was also intact and regular automatic breathing continued with ventilatory sensitivity to CO_2 inhalation well within the normal range, together with the associated air hunger. The results of this study have been confirmed in another patient with the same syndrome by the author.

How might we sense the activation of an intact automatic respiratory controller in the medulla? Recent work in the cat has shown that respiratory-associated firing of both midbrain and thalamic neurons are related to respiratory drive (see Chapter 2) and depend on intact connection with the medulla. A positron emission tomographic (PET) study in an awake man (Corfield et al., 1994, 1995) has now identified increases in relative regional blood flow in supra-brainstem structures during the ventilatory response to inhaled CO_2; such sites, whose anatomical location is further delineated by magnetic resonance imaging, probably indicate neuronal activation. They extend from the upper brainstem, up through the midbrain, hypothalamus, and thalamus. These sites correspond broadly with those found by Eldridge and Chen (see above). Of greatest interest is the further finding by the PET scan study of activation within the limbic system. Areas activated include the cingulate gyrus, the parahippocampus and hippocampus, the fusiform gyrus, and the insula. Such activation of the limbic cortex may explain the unpleasant, uncomfortable effect of the air hunger sensation associated with CO_2 inhalation.

II. Individual Differences in Breathlessness

The intensity of the sensation of breathlessness was found to vary greatly and consistently in different normal subjects given a standard chemical or exercise ventilatory stimulus (Adams et al., 1986). This study was performed before a clear picture had emerged of (1) the semantics of breathlessness (see Chapter 5), (2) the multidimensional nature of breathlessness when the perception of the intensity of the sensation and the distress caused may be confused by the subject who is scaling, and (3) the role of experience, learning, and adaptation in scaling. (For (2) and (3), see Chapter 13). These problems have major clinical importance in the recognition—or nonrecognition—of the severity of an asthma episode, where both chest tightness and urge to breathe are present (see Chapter 12).

Many patients with severe respiratory impairment due to chronic obstructive pulmonary disease (COPD) have psychiatric symptoms of anxiety and/or depression; this has been documented with instruments well-validated in the presence of organic disease (Rutter, 1977; Rosser and Guz, 1981). It is a common clinical experience that a patient's breathlessness may be greater than expected in relation to the functional impairment. In one study (Burns and Howell, 1969) a group of patients with COPD who had what appeared to be "disproportionate" breathlessness were compared with a group of patients with COPD whose breathlessness was considered "proportionate." The disproportionate group had less obstruction, a shorter history of breathlessness, a history of more stressful events in the recent past, more recent bereavements, greater social isolation, a higher incidence of psychiatric illness, and evidence of present psychiatric symptoms. The group's breathlessness had a weak relationship to exercise, varied in relation to social situation, was relieved with alcohol and/or tranquilizers, and was characterized by difficulty in getting air into rather than out of the chest. In addition, anxiety about dying with breathlessness was much more frequent in these patients. They received psychiatric treatment in addition to medical treatment, and, in those who improved psychiatrically, considerable improvements in breathlessness as experienced in daily life were reported. The results of this challenging study have been subjected to much debate; it clearly needs repeating in a more rigorous manner with particular attention to the problem of how to ensure as much therapist contact with the patients in a control proportionate breathlessness group, without giving any form of psychiatric treatment.

III. Palliation of Breathlessness

The treatment of the symptom of breathlessness is best done by treating the underlying condition effectively. A great deal of cardiorespiratory disease is untreatable. This section is therefore concerned only with methods that might palliate the symptom when nothing can be done to alleviate the underlying condition. It must be stressed, however, that new approaches are now available to alleviate, albeit temporarily, dyspnea due to incurable disease within the chest. Optimum treatment of heart failure, including attention to after-load reduction and minimizing excess lung water with effective use of diuretics, can often eliminate breathlessness, at least while at rest. Malignant disease of the bronchi requires meticulous attention to secondary pleural effusions, which may require either medical or surgical ablation of the pleural space, regular aspiration, or the insertion of valves that will ensure the drainage of the pleural fluid into the venous system or the peritoneal cavity. Neoplasms in the larger bronchi that occlude the lumen may need intraluminal surgery or radiotherapy to re-establish a lumen and allow collapsed lobes to expand. Stents may be required to keep the trachea and its bifurcation open. These measures often have a major temporary beneficial effect on the breathlessness experienced during daily life.

Aside from the above interventions, the symptomatic treatment of dyspnea is regarded by most physicians as not very effective, but some have persisted and produced worthwhile results. Unfortunately, enthusiasm by some therapists has gone beyond any definite evidence of benefit with many procedures.

The following approaches may improve dyspnea.

1. Effective management of the patient (see Chapter 15) is of the greatest importance. Patient education, including the development of coping strategies, may remove much of the fear of breathlessness. Where anxiety remains prominent, the careful use of sedatives, including phenothiazines, benzodiazepines,

alcohol, and even opiates may be indicated. But the deliberate induction of drowsiness—an effective therapeutic action—cannot be recommended for the dyspnea of the respiratory cripple because it will shorten life.

2. Reducing respiratory drive may be effective. Hypoxia can be minimized or even eliminated by the continuous administration of oxygen by nasal cannulae or the transtracheal route. This is particularly likely to be effective where the administration of oxygen will minimize increasing desaturation on exercise (Dean et al., 1992). Many patients, however, will not benefit and in some, elimination of hypoxia may promote ventilatory failure with rises in arterial P_{CO_2}. Hypoxic drive may be eliminated, without alleviating the hypoxia, by bilateral carotid body resection. This drastic procedure may be effective therapy for breathlessness, but is unlikely to prolong life given the effects of the serious hypoxia that remains, particularly during sleep (Vermeire et al., 1987; Severinghaus, 1989).

Air administered via nasal cannulae may improve breathlessness in patients with COPD (Liss and Grant, 1988). This remarkable result has no obvious explanation. A similar benefit of administering air via nasal cannulae has been recently found in a single-blind controlled trial in a hospice in patients with advanced cancer within the chest; air was as effective as oxygen in reducing breathlessness at rest in such patients (Booth et al., 1995).

Powerful drives to breathe may arise from the pathological lung, particularly when the lung is infiltrated or "water-logged," or when parts of the lung are collapsed. Such drives to breathe are transmitted to the medullary respiratory controller via vagal afferent fibers. Experience in sectioning a vagus nerve within the chest—particularly on the right side, where this operation can be done below the origin of the right recurrent laryngeal nerve by an approach from the right supraclavicular fossa—has resulted in occasional spectacular results for dyspnea reduction (Guz et al., 1970; Davies et al., 1987).

3. Reducing the sense of effort and improving respiratory muscle function is a sensible approach, but there is no agreement about benefit other than with the following measures:

1. Reducing obesity may be remarkably effective. Weight reduction improves mechanical efficiency and also removes an impedance to descent of the diaphragm with inspiration.
2. Breathing techniques, particularly pursed-lip breathing, slows expiratory flow rates and may improve arterial oxygen saturation and reduce breathlessness.
3. Counteracting the malnutrition that is so often present in the breathless patient with COAD may diminish breathlessness possibly by improving muscle strength (Efthimiou et al., 1988).

4. The role of exercise training in relieving dyspnea is controversial and little hard evidence of benefit for the breathlessness resulting from the ordinary activities of daily living is available. This subject remains one that badly needs carefully designed research protocols with good controls.

The reader will note the tone of skepticism in this author's presentation on palliation of breathlessness. There is a major need for further research in this area.

References

Adams, L., Chronos, N., Lane, R., and Guz, A. (1986). The measurement of breathlesness induced in normal subjects: individual differences. Clin. Sci. 7:131–140.

Banzett, R.B., Lansing, R.W., Reid, M.B., Adams, L., and Brown, R. (1989). Air hunger arising from increased PCO_2 in mechanically ventilated quadriplegics. Respir. Physiol. 76:53–67.

Booth, S., Kelly, M.J., Cox, N.P., Adams, L., and Guz, A. (1995). The treatment of dyspnoea in cancer patients—does oxygen help? Am. J. Respir. Crit. Care Med. (in press).

Burns, B.H., and Howell, J.B.L. (1969). Disproportionately severe breathlessness in chronic bronchitis. Quart. J. Med. 38:277–294.

Corfield, D.R., Fink, G.R., Ramsay, S.C., Murphy, K., Watson, J.D.G., Adams, L., Frackowiak, R.S.J., and Guz, A. (1994). Cortical and sub-cortical activations during CO_2-stimulated breathing in conscious man. J. Physiol. 476:80P.

Corfield, D.R., Fink, G.R., Ramsay, S.C., Murphy, K., Harty, H.R., Watson, J.D.G., Adams, L., Frackowiak, R.S.J., and Guz, A. (1995). Evidence for limbic system activation during CO_2-stimulated breathing in man. J. Physiol. (in press).

Davies, S.F., McQuaid, K.R., Iber, C., McArthur, C.D., Path, M.J., Beebe, D.S., and Helseth, H.K. (1987). Extreme dyspnoea from unilateral pulmonary venous obstruction. Demonstration of a vagal mechanism and relief by right vagotomy. Am. Rev. Respir. Dis. 136:184–188.

Dean, B., Brown, J., Himelman, R.B., Doherty, J., Gold, W.H., and Stulburg, M.S. (1992). Oxygen may improve dyspnoea and exercise performance in chronic obstructive pulmonary disease patients with only mild hypoxemia. Am. Rev. Respir. Dis. 146:941–945.

Efthimiou, J., Fleming, J., Gomes, C., and Spiro, G. (1988). The effect of supplementary oral nutrition in poorly nourished patients with chronic obstructive pulmonary disease. Am. Rev. Respir. Dis. 137:1075–1082.

Guz, A., Noble, M.I.M., Eisele, J.H., and Trenchard, D. (1970). Experimental results of vagal block in cardiopulmonary disease. In: Breathing: Hering-Breuer Centenary Symposium. Edited by J.A. Churchill, CIBA Foundation, London, pp. 315–336.

Heywood, P., Morrell, M.J., Moosavi, S., Stevens, J., and Guz, A. (1993). Ventilatory control awake, asleep and during exercise in man with unilateral rostral ventrolateral medullary lesions. Abstr. XXXII Cong. Intern. Union Physiol. Sci., Glasgow, p. 191.

Liss, H.P., and Grant, B.J. (1988). The effect of nasal flow on breathlesness in patients with chronic obstructive pulmonary disease. Am. Rev. Respir. Dis. 137:1285–1288.

Munschauer, F.E., Mador, J., Ahuja, A., and Jacobs, L. (1991). Selective paralysis of voluntary but not limbically influenced automatic respiration. Arch. Neurol. 48: 1190–1192.

Rosser, R., and Guz, A. (1981). Psychological approaches to breathlessness and its treatment. J. Psychosom. Res. 25:439–447.

Rutter, B.M. (1977). Some psychological concomitants of chronic bronchitis. Psychol. Med. 7:459–464.

Severinghaus, J. (1989). Carotid body resection for COPD? Chest 95:1128–1129.

Shea, S.A., Andres, L.P., Shannon, D.C., Guz, A., and Banzett, R.B. (1993). Respiratory sensations in subjects who lack a ventilatory response to CO_2. Respir. Physiol. 93:203–219.

Vermeire, P., Backer, W.D., Made, R.V., and Bal., J. (1987). Carotid body resection in patients with severe chronic airflow limitation. Clin. Respir. Physiol. 123:1655–1665.

AUTHOR INDEX

Italic numbers give the page on which the complete reference is listed.

A

D

E

H

K

L

M

S

SUBJECT INDEX

B

C

Q

S